Kidney Disease and Transplantation: Principles and Practice

Kidney Disease and Transplantation: Principles and Practice

Editor: Reagen Hu

AMERICAN
MEDICAL PUBLISHERS
www.americanmedicalpublishers.com

AMERICAN
MEDICAL PUBLISHERS
www.americanmedicalpublishers.com

Cataloging-in-Publication Data

Kidney disease and transplantation : principles and practice / edited by Reagen Hu.
p. cm.
Includes bibliographical references and index.
ISBN 978-1-63927-709-4
1. Kidneys--Disease. 2. Kidneys--Transplantation. 3. Kidneys--Disease--Diagnosis.
4. Kidneys--Diseases--Treatment. 5. Nephrology. I. Hu, Reagen.
RC902 .K53 2023
616.61--dc23

American Medical Publishers,
41 Flatbush Avenue,
1st Floor, New York,
NY 11217, USA

ISBN 978-1-63927-709-4 (Hardback)

Contents

Preface

Over the recent decade, advancements and applications have progressed exponentially. This has led to the increased interest in this field and projects are being conducted to enhance knowledge. The main objective of this book is to present some of the critical challenges and provide insights into possible solutions. This book will answer the varied questions that arise in the field and also provide an increased scope for furthering studies.

The disease of the kidney wherein the ability to filter blood and control the blood pressure is affected is known as kidney disease. It can be classified into chronic kidney disease and acute kidney disease. The medical condition in which the kidneys stop working suddenly is known as acute kidney disease. Chronic disease is the medical condition where the kidneys are unable to function properly for more than three months. Diabetes, chronic or uncontrolled high blood pressure, polycystic kidney syndrome and chronic glomerulonephritis are some common causes of kidney disease. Kidney transplantation is a type of surgery performed to replace a diseased kidney with a healthy kidney from a donor. This book aims to shed light on some of the unexplored aspects of kidney disease and transplantation and the recent researches on them. Researchers and students in this field will be greatly assisted by it.

I hope that this book, with its visionary approach, will be a valuable addition and will promote interest among readers. Each of the authors has provided their extraordinary competence in their specific fields by providing different perspectives as they come from diverse nations and regions. I thank them for their contributions.

Editor

1

Eosinophilia and Kidney Disease: More than Just an Incidental Finding?

Philipp Gauckler [1,*], Jae Il Shin [2,3,4,5], Gert Mayer [1] and Andreas Kronbichler [1]

1 Department of Internal Medicine IV (Nephrology and Hypertension), Medical University Innsbruck, 6020 Innsbruck, Austria; gert.mayer@i-med.ac.at (G.M.); andreas.kronbichler@i-med.ac.at (A.K.)
2 Department of Pediatrics, Yonsei University College of Medicine, Seoul 03722, Korea; shinji@yuhs.ac
3 Department of Pediatric Nephrology, Severance Children's Hospital, Seoul 03722, Korea
4 Institute of Kidney Disease Research, Yonsei University College of Medicine, Seoul 03722, Korea
5 Division of Cardiology, Emory University School of Medicine, Atlanta, GA 30322, USA
* Correspondence: philipp.gauckler@i-med.ac.at

Abstract: Peripheral blood eosinophilia (PBE), defined as 500 eosinophils or above per microliter (μL) blood, is a condition that is not uncommon but often neglected in the management of patients with chronic kidney disease (CKD), acute kidney injury (AKI), or patients on renal replacement therapy (RRT). The nature of PBE in the context of kidney diseases is predominantly secondary or reactive and has to be distinguished from primary eosinophilic disorders. Nonetheless, the finding of persistent PBE can be a useful clue for the differential diagnosis of underdiagnosed entities and overlapping syndromes, such as eosinophilic granulomatosis with polyangiitis (EGPA), IgG4-related disease (IgG4-RD), acute interstitial nephritis (AIN), or the hypereosinophilic syndrome (HES). For patients on RRT, PBE may be an indicator for bio-incompatibility of the dialysis material, acute allograft rejection, or *Strongyloides* hyperinfection. In a subset of patients with EGPA, eosinophils might even be the driving force in disease pathogenesis. This improved understanding is already being used to facilitate novel therapeutic options. Mepolizumab has been licensed for the management of EGPA and is applied with the aim to abrogate the underlying immunologic process by blocking interleukin-5. The current article provides an overview of different renal pathologies that are associated with PBE. Further scientific effort is required to understand the exact role and function of eosinophils in these disorders which may pave the way to improved interdisciplinary management of such patients.

Keywords: eosinophilia; CKD; kidney disease; AKI; autoimmune disease; EGPA; interstitial nephritis; IgG4-related disease; vasculitis

---

1. Introduction

The evidence of peripheral blood eosinophilia (PBE), defined as 500 eosinophils or above per microliter (μL) blood, is a condition occasionally seen and often disregarded in the management of patients with chronic kidney disease (CKD), acute kidney injury (AKI), or patients on renal replacement therapy (RRT), either in the context of renal disease or as a consequence of co-morbidities. Diagnostic efforts to determine the etiology of moderately or markedly elevated eosinophil counts are rarely made. This might be explained by the lack of therapeutic consequences, lack of knowledge of eosinophil function and the uncertain diagnostic value of PBE. Classical diseases associated with eosinophilia are atopic conditions such as allergic asthma, autoimmune processes, parasitic infections, and neoplastic disorders.

Although many questions remain regarding the biology of eosinophils, a clearance function in parasitic infections has been postulated [1]. In addition, eosinophils may expand and play a role in a broad range of local and systemic inflammatory diseases [1]. However, only little is known about the functional and prognostic impact of eosinophils in the etiology and progression of these disorders. In the past few years, considerable progress was made in the molecular understanding of different, 'immunologic-driven', systemic disorders that are associated with both, kidney damage and eosinophilia. In fact, various systemic disorders affecting the kidney function may be accompanied by eosinophilia. The discovery of molecular mechanisms that are responsible for specific disease processes has led to a better understanding of eosinophil biology and paved the way for better diagnostics and the development of novel, more specific drug therapies.

In this article, we provide an overview of different renal pathologies that are associated with PBE. A particular focus is set on the meaning of PBE for the diagnosis of underdiagnosed entities, in order to improve the interdisciplinary management of such patients.

2. Eosinophilia, Hypereosinophilia and the Hypereosinophilic Syndrome (HES)

For an in-depth understanding of terminology, it seems to be important to emphasize that definitions and classifications in the field of eosinophilic disorders have changed over the years. Recent recommendations are based primarily on proposals delivered by the World Health Organization (WHO) and the International Cooperative Working Group on Eosinophil Disorders (ICOG-EO) [2,3]. The focus of our work is set on renal pathologies that are associated with PBE. Several classical eosinophilic disorders, including primary hematologic disorders such as eosinophil leukemia, may sometimes also affect the kidney but do not regularly induce persistent kidney damage. For the sake of simplicity, an overview of these eosinophilic disorders is given in Figure 1 and the current definition of HE and HES, as proposed by the ICOG-EO, is highlighted in Table 1.

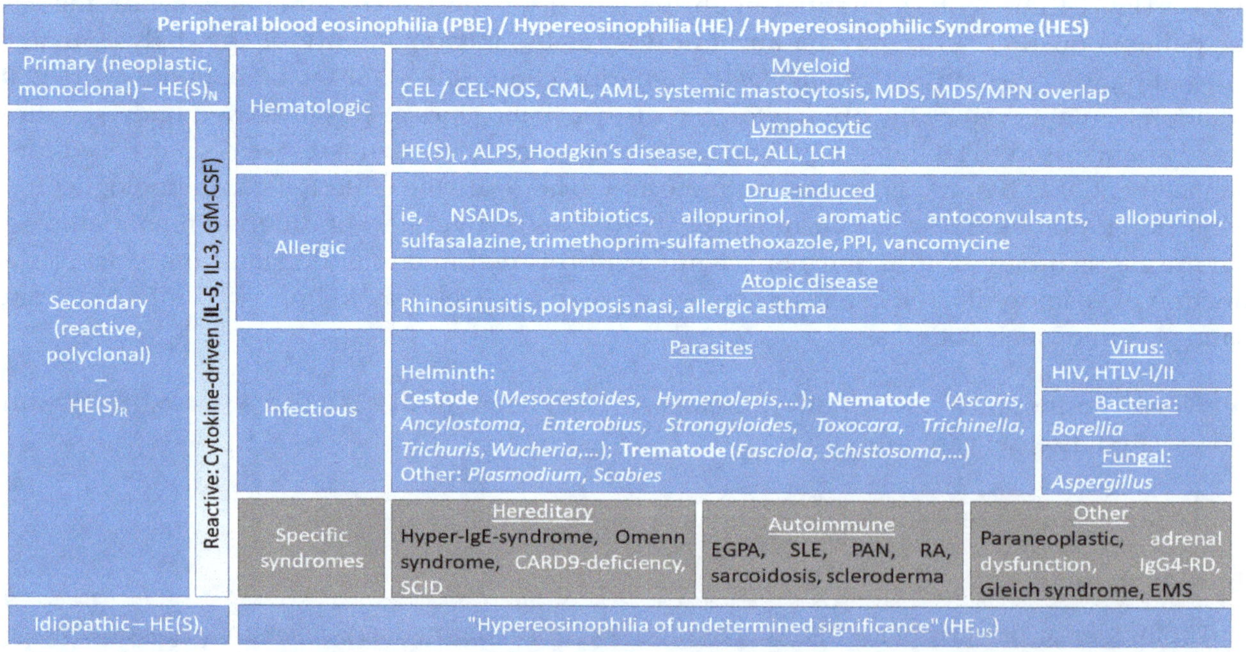

Figure 1. Proposed overview and classification of eosinophilic disorders. Certain specific syndromes (grey boxes) in which the role of eosinophils in the disease mechanism are unclear should be differentiated from 'real' HES, according to the International Cooperative Working Group on Eosinophil Disorders (ICOG-EO) proposal (diseases in black letters are explicitly declared as such [2]). Different diseases leading to increased eosinophilic counts are sub-divided into hematologic, allergic, and infectious disorders, while idiopathic hypereosinophilic syndrome is separated from primary and

secondary forms. IL, interleukin; GM-CSF, granulocyte-macrophage colony-stimulating factor; $HE(S)_M$, myeloid HE(S); $HE(S)_L$, lymphocyte-variant HE(S); CEL, chronic eosinophilic leukemia; NOS, not otherwise specified; CML, chronic myeloid leukemia; AML, acute myeloid leukemia; MDS, myelodysplastic syndromes; MPN, myeloproliferative neoplasms; ALPS, autoimmune-lymphoproliferative syndrome; CTCL, cutaneous T-cell lymphoma; ALL, acute lymphocytic leukemia; LCH, Langerhans cell histiocytosis; NSAID, nonsteroidal anti-inflammatory drugs; PPI, proton-pump inhibitor; HIV, human immunodeficiency virus; HTLV, human T-lymphotropic virus; IgE, immunoglobulin E; CARD9, caspase recruitment domain-containing protein 9; SCID, severe combined immunodeficiency; EGPA, eosinophilic granulomatosis with polyangiitis; SLE, systemic lupus erythematosus; PAN, panarteritis nodosa; RA, rheumatoid arthritis; IgG4-RD, IgG4-related disease; EMS, eosinophilia myalgia syndrome.

Table 1. Definition of hypereosinophilia (HE) and the hypereosinophilic syndrome (HES) proposed by the International Cooperative Working Group on Eosinophil Disorders (ICOG-EO).

Term	Definition and Criteria
Peripheral blood eosinophilia (PBE)	$>0.5 \times 10^9$/L blood
HE	$>1.5 \times 10^9$/L blood on two examinations (interval ≥4 weeks *) and/or tissue HE defined by the following: 1. Percentage of eosinophils in bone marrow section exceeds 20% of all nucleated cells and/or 2. Pathologist is of the opinion that tissue infiltration by eosinophils is extensive and/or 3. Marked deposition of eosinophil granule protein is found (in the absence or presence of major tissue infiltration by eosinophils).
HES	1. Criteria for peripheral blood HE fulfilled * 2. Organ damage and/or dysfunction attributable to tissue HE and 3. Exclusion of other disorders or conditions as major reason for organ damage
Eosinophil-associated single-organ diseases	1. Criteria of HE fulfilled and 2. Single-organ disease

* In the case of evolving life-threatening end-organ damage, the diagnosis can be made immediately to avoid therapeutic delay. Adapted from [2].

2.1. *Biology of Eosinophil Granulocytes*

Eosinophils can enter extravascular tissues and participate in various immunologic reactions relevant to innate immunity. Eosinophil precursors differentiate in the bone marrow in response to different cytokines, such as interleukin (IL)-3, granulocyte-macrophage colony stimulating factor (GM-CSF) and, most importantly, IL-5 before they transit through the blood into various organs, including the thymus, spleen, lymph nodes, uterus, and the gastrointestinal tract. Eosinophils produce and store different bioactive molecules, like eosinophil peroxidase (EP), eosinophil cationic proteins (ECP), and major basic protein (MBP) in their granules. Various conditions facilitate a type 2 helper T (Th2) cell and cytokine-induced activation of eosinophils leading to a release of these molecules with consecutive effects in the affected tissues [4,5]. MBP exerts cytotoxicity to various tissue-adjacent cells. ECP are ribonucleases with antiviral activity and EP is involved in the production of reactive oxygen species (ROS) to digest extracellular pathogens [6]. Other released bioactive molecules like leukotriene C4, platelet activating factor and prostaglandins mediate effects on the tonus of smooth muscle cells, vascular permeability, platelet aggregation and chemotaxis resulting in enhancement, regulation, and repair of inflammation [6,7]. Eosinophils also produce and secrete DNA traps which may be involved in the defense against various pathogens [1]. For a detailed review of the biology and physiology of eosinophils we refer to recent review articles [1,2,4–6].

2.2. *Definitions and Classification of Eosinophil Disorders*

Conditions with an eosinophil count (EC) >500/µL blood are generally referred to as PBE, whereas marked and persistent (examined in two occasions with a minimum of four weeks interval) elevations >1500/µL are categorized as hypereosinophilia (HE). Tissue eosinophilia meeting criteria depicted in Table 1 is also regarded a feature of HE [2]. A percentage greater than 5% of all leukocytes in peripheral blood is commonly regarded as pathological, but relative eosinophil counts are usually not used for diagnostic purposes because the number varies with the total white blood count (WBC). An arbitrary sub-classification, regarded as mild (>350–500/μL), modest (>1500/μL), and severe (>5000/μL) eosinophilia has been proposed [3,7–9].

Different circumstances can lead to an increased proliferation of eosinophils (Figure 1): primary hematologic disorders due to proliferation of neoplastic eosinophils and their progenitor cells have to be distinguished from secondary or reactive eosinophil expansion, induced by a Th2-mediated immunologic cascade of different cytokines (mainly IL-5, but sometimes also IL-3 and GM-CSF) resulting in an accumulation of polyclonal eosinophils [10]. After exclusion of primary and secondary causes, the condition is termed idiopathic (hyper-) eosinophilia. If, in such case, the criteria of HE are fulfilled but no clinical symptoms or organ dysfunction are seen, the term HE of undetermined significance (HE_{us}) is appropriate [2].

In 1975, Chusid et al. introduced the term hypereosinophilic syndrome (HES) for cases with end-organ manifestations that are attributable to HE [11]. Chusid's criteria were used for the definition of HES for nearly four decades and build the groundwork for the current definition, proposed by the WHO and ICOG-EO (see Table 1) [2,3]. Whereas there is consensus about the definition (criteria) of HES, a few open questions remain regarding the classification of rare eosinophilic disorders [9,12].

3. Eosinophilia in Kidney Disease

3.1. Kidney Involvement in the Hypereosinophilic Syndrome

There is a paucity of data linking idiopathic HES to conditions involving the kidney [13]. No case of renal involvement was reported in 50 patients with HES_I [14]. A classical complication of HES is Loeffler's endocarditis which is characterized by progressive heart failure with endomyocardial fibrosis due to eosinophilic infiltration and secondary organ damage provoked by thromboembolic occlusion of larger and smaller vessels [15]. In general, all organ systems can be affected by HES. In a more recent retrospective analysis of HES cases, including primary and secondary (hematologic) forms of HES, skin involvement (69%) was most common, followed by pulmonary (44%), gastrointestinal (38%) and heart (20%) manifestations [16]. Former articles on idiopathic HES describe renal involvement in 0% [14] to 36% [11]. Renal affection seems to occur mostly late in the course of HES, predominantly due to vascular events as a result of thromboembolism or atheroembolism [11,17]. In this regard, it is worth noting that thromboembolism is regarded a major organ manifestation (clinical feature) of HES. A review of cases with HES_I and renal involvement identified certain primary renal parenchymal diseases in association with HES_I. Eosinophilic interstitial nephritis, described as the most common pathologic pattern, followed by infrequent reports of membranous nephropathy (MN) and different other forms of glomerulonephritis, thrombotic microangiopathies (TMA), electrolyte disturbances and the presence of Charcot–Leyden crystals, are further kidney-defined disorders associated with HES_I [18].

3.2. Kidney Diseases Associated with Eosinophilia/Hypereosinophilia

An overview of chronic or acute kidney diseases and special conditions that are associated with eosinophilia is given in Table 2 and a review of these pathologies is provided in the following sections.

Table 2. Overview of conditions associated with renal disease and eosinophilia. Cautious interpretation is necessary, since glucocorticoid treatment can mask eosinophilia.

Category	Kidney Disease	% with Renal Involvement	% with PBE	Exclude
a. Hypersensitivity reactions	AIN	100%	App. 22% [19,20]	ATN
	DRESS	11–57% [21,22]	52–95% [23]	
b. Autoimmune disease	EGPA	App. 26%; Higher prevalence (up to 51.4%) with ANCA-positivity [24,25]	100%; Typically, >1500/µL abs. and >10% rel.; Eosinophilic activity may occasionally be organ-limited without blood eosinophilia [26]	MPA, GPA, HES_I, aspirin-exacerbated respiratory disease, eosinophilic pneumonia, allergic bronchopulmonary aspergillosis, parasitic diseases, allergic conditions, Gleich syndrome, IgG4-RD, diffuse fasciitis with eosinophilia, eosinophilia-myalgia syndrome, eosinophilic myositis, cryoglobulinemic vasculitis, IgA vasculitis
	SLE	app. 50% [27]	<5% [28]	
c. Vascular disease	TMA	App. 77% overall (depending on subtype) [29]	Very rare (number not known)	
	CES	app. 92% [30]	14–71% [31,32]	
d. Other	Kimura's disease	12–18% [33]	100% [34]	ALHE
	TINU syndrome	100%	app. 17% [35]	Sarcoidosis, Sjögren syndrome, SLE, TB
	IgG4-RD	10–15% [36]	app. 30% [36–38]	HES, AAV, malignancies, autoimmune disorders, DI-AIN, MN
e. CKD & RRT	CKD		number not known	
Dialysis	HD-associated eosinophilia		app. 5% (2012) [39], up to 39% in the 1970s [40]	
	PD-associated eosinophilia		<10% (2007) [41], up to 60% in the 1980s [42]	
Kidney transplant	Acute allograft rejection		20–36% (≥4% eosinophils) [43]	(DI-)AIN, *Strongyloides* hyperinfection
	Strongyloides superinfection		app. 34% [44]; 67% of pretransplant patients with chronic *Strongyloides* infection [45]	
f. Renal cell carcinoma			Very rare (number not known)	IgG4-RKD

PBE, peripheral blood eosinophilia; AIN, acute interstitial nephritis; ATN, acute tubular necrosis; DRESS, drug reaction with eosinophilia and systemic symptoms; EGPA, eosinophilic granulomatosis with polyangiitis; ANCA, anti-neutrophil cytoplasmic antibody; MPA, microscopic polyangiitis; GPA, granulomatosis with polyangiitis; HES_I, idiopathic hypereosinophilic syndrome; IgG4-RD, immunoglobulin G4-related disease; CES, cholesterol embolization syndrome; ALHE, angiolymphoid hyperplasia with eosinophilia; TINU, tubulointerstitial nephritis and uveitis; SLE, systemic lupus erythematosus; TMA, thrombotic microangiopathy; TB, tuberculosis; AAV, ANCA-associated vasculitis; DI-AIN, drug-induced-AIN; MN, membranous nephropathy; HD, hemodialysis; PD, peritoneal dialysis; CKD, chronic kidney disease; RRT, renal replacement therapy.

3.2.1. Hypersensitivity Reactions

Eosinophilia is a common feature of hypersensitivity reactions, driven by antigen-activated Th2 cells and a consecutive release of critical cytokines. In all these reactions, IL-5 is considered the most relevant trigger of eosinophil proliferation, accumulation, and function. Basically, any exogenous antigen can provoke a hypersensitivity reaction with possible affection of the kidney function.

Tubulointerstitial nephritis (TIN) is the histologic pattern found in acute interstitial nephritis (AIN) and other immune-mediated kidney diseases. AIN is found in about 5–18% of kidney biopsies performed in the setting of AKI and an increasing tendency in prevalence is seen in the last years [46]. Drug-induced AIN accounts for about three-quarters of the cases and basically any drug can trigger the disease. Antibiotics, non-steroidal anti-inflammatory drugs (NSAIDs) and proton-pump-inhibitors (PPIs) are the most frequent agents leading to AIN. Other possible causes of AIN are infections and autoimmune diseases like sarcoidosis, Sjögren syndrome, IgG4-related disease (IgG4-RD), or the tubuloinsterstitial nephritis and uveitis (TINU)-syndrome. Blood eosinophilia is seen in about 20% of the cases [19]. Urinalysis may reveal unspecific results like mid-range proteinuria, hematuria, pyuria, or abnormalities in the tubular function including Fanconi syndrome or renal tubular acidosis (RTA). Urinary eosinophils appear to be a poor diagnostic predictor with a rather low positive-predictive value, irrespective of using the traditional cut-off of >1% or a higher cut-off of >5% [19,47]. The classical clinical hypersensitivity-triad of fever, skin rash, and eosinophilia is rarely found and considering the subtle clinical signs and the multitude of possible triggers, it is not surprising that only in about half of the cases AIN was the suspected diagnosis before biopsy [19,48]. Potential triggers, especially drugs, should be withdrawn if possible. In the case of uncertainty or in absence of clinical improvement after drug withdrawal, an early kidney biopsy should be performed to verify the diagnosis. The role of corticosteroids in the therapy of AIN is controversially discussed [19,49–51]. Until now, no clear recommendation can be made, but two recent large retrospective studies suggest a benefit of steroid treatment. Prendecki et al. showed an improvement of GFR and a lower prevalence of ESRD after 6 and 25 months [52]. Fernandez-Juarez et al. showed a greater recovery of kidney function at six months when steroid treatment is started early [53]. General outcome and prognosis of AIN depends on the delay until the causative trigger is identified and removed as well as the degree of tubular atrophy and interstitial fibrosis on biopsy. Approximately half of the patients show full recovery, while the other half develops CKD or, in a small number, remains on RRT [19,20]. Relapses may occur after terminating an initially successful corticosteroid therapy. In some of these patients, an underlying systemic disease may be diagnosed. Drug-induced AIN can evolve into corticosteroid-dependent AIN even when the causative agent has been stopped [46].

A specific condition is the drug reaction with eosinophilia and systemic symptoms (DRESS) syndrome, which is a potentially life-threatening hypersensitivity reaction to a medication or its reactive metabolites. The precise pathogenesis is not fully understood and different theories like an underlying versus a secondarily-induced reactivation of different herpes viruses was proposed [54,55]. Among the known causative drugs, aromatic anticonvulsants (e.g., carbamazepine and phenytoine), allopurinol, sulfasalazine, trimethoprim-sulfamethoxazole, PPI, vancomycin, and minocycline are most frequently reported [56,57]. Clinical features, beside the typical cutaneous eruptions, are systemic symptoms including fever, eosinophilia, and different organ manifestations. PBE is present in the majority of the cases, whereas marked eosinophilia is described in approximately 30% [23,58,59]. The prevalence of renal involvement is ranging between 10% and 57% with highest rates described in association with allopurinol [21–23]. The histological pattern and the clinical findings are similar to those seen in AIN. Identification and withdrawal of the causative drug is the principal therapeutic challenge in DRESS. Systemic corticosteroids (suggested starting dose 1 mg/kg/day of prednisone or equivalent with slow tapering over 6–8 weeks) and a supportive therapy to control hemodynamics, fever and cutaneous symptoms are indicated, while prophylactic antibiotic therapy should be avoided [59]. Some patients show no response or have contraindications towards corticosteroid treatment. In this setting, alternative immunosuppressive or immunomodulatory therapeutic measures such as intravenous immunoglobulins (IVIG), plasma exchange, cyclophosphamide, cyclosporine, mycophenolate mofetil, and rituximab (RTX) have shown efficacy in selected cases [60–62].

Among 824 patients receiving outpatient parenteral antibiotics, 25% developed eosinophilia in a prospective cohort study. Most patients did not develop hypersensitivity reactions, while DRESS occurred in 0.8%. Eosinophilia increased the risk of developing renal injury (HR = 2.13, $p = 0.0009$) [63]. Drug-induced kidney injury seems to be an underestimated entity and eosinophilia might be a helpful diagnostic tool in these patients.

3.2.2. Autoimmune Reactions and Related Diseases

The main vasculitic glomerulopathy associated with eosinophilia is eosinophilic granulomatosis with polyangiitis (EGPA, Churg-Strauss syndrome). EGPA differs from other anti-neutrophil cytoplasmic antibody (ANCA)-associated vasculitides (AAV), since patients have severe asthma as well as blood and tissue eosinophilia [26]. The American College of Rheumatology diagnostic criteria are asthma, eosinophilia, mono-polyneuropathy, pulmonary infiltrates, non-fixed paranasal sinus abnormalities, and extravascular eosinophils with at least four of six criteria to be fulfilled for diagnosis [64]. Patients with EGPA show a low frequency of ANCA-positivity (30–40%) with myeloperoxidase (MPO)-ANCA predominance [24,65–67]. ANCA-positivity is associated with a higher prevalence of renal disease [24,25], involvement of the upper airways and peripheral neuropathy. ANCA-negative EGPA, in contrast, shows more cardiac manifestations (including pericarditis and cardiomyopathy) and pleural effusions which are both usually associated with eosinophil-mediated disorders [24,25,65]. The linkage between ANCA-positivity and glomerulonephritis has been implemented in the revised Chapel Hill consensus conference nomenclature of vasculitides in 2012 [68]. More recently, two different disease phenotypes of EGPA have been discussed and different underlying pathophysiological processes suggested, but until now there is not enough evidence to split EGPA into different disease entities (see Figure 2). In fact, EGPA should be regarded as one syndrome with different phenotypes [69]. AAV have a clear genetic background and two genome-wide association studies (GWASs) showed distinct human leukocyte antigen (HLA) gene-variants for the three AAV-subtypes [70]. Vaglio et al. found the HLA-DRB4 gene and HLA-DRB1*07 allele as genetic risk factors for EGPA, correlating with a vasculitic phenotype and ANCA-positivity [71]. Moreover, IL-10.2 haplotype is associated with ANCA-negative EGPA and an increased IL-10 production [72]. A GWAS in the specific context of EGPA is ongoing and promises new insights into the pathophysiological understanding of this Janus-like disease.

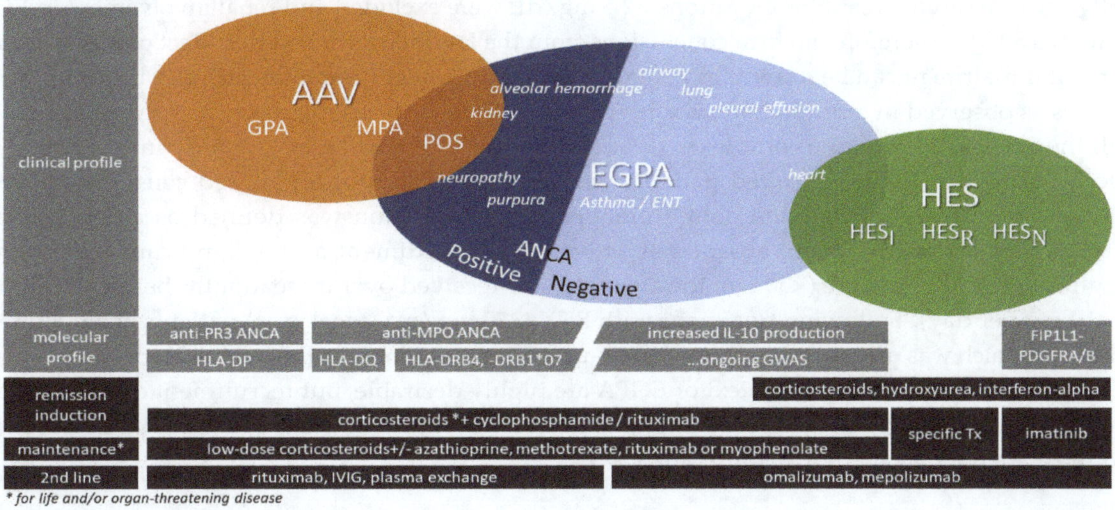

Figure 2. Eosinophil granulomatosis with polyangiitis (EPGA) and overlapping syndromes. The clinical profile of EGPA has distinct but also overlapping symptoms. In the clinical assessment, specific investigations are often needed, since ANCA is negative in most patients. There is a clear overlap between EGPA with a predominant heart involvement and idiopathic hypereosinophilic syndrome (HES_I). On the other hand, polyangiitis overlap syndrome (POS) has been described for cases that fulfill diagnostic criteria for granulomatosis with polyangiitis (GPA) and EGPA and there is a particular overlap between microscopic polyangiitis (MPA) and EGPA in those with a positive ANCA test presenting with peripheral neuropathy and in some cases kidney and pulmonary disease. A clear distinction is not always possible but should be the aim of the initial investigation. Treatment approaches overlap in some situations. ANCA, anti-neutrophil cytoplasmic antibody; AAV, ANCA-associated vasculitis; GPA, granulomatosis with polyangiitis; MPA, microscopic polyangiitis; POS, polyangiitis overlap syndrome; EGPA, eosinophilic granulomatosis with polyangiitis; ENT, ear,

nose, and throat; HES, hypereosinophilic syndrome (I = idiopathic, R = reactive, N = neoplastic); PR3, proteinase 3; MPO, myeloperoxidase; IL-5, interleukin-5; FIP1L1-PDGFRA/B, gene fusion of fibroblast growth factor receptor 1 and platelet-derived growth factor receptor α/β; HLA, human leukocyte antigen; IVIG, intravenous immunoglobulins. According to the EGPA Consensus Task Force, glucocorticoids are the principal therapy to achieve EGPA remission, defined as absence of a clinical systemic manifestation (excluding asthma and/or ear, nose and throat manifestation). In life- and/or organ-threatening disease, remission-induction should include additional immunosuppression (e.g., cyclophosphamide). These patients usually need a maintenance therapy with azathioprine or methotrexate [26]. ANCA-positivity reflects activation of B-cells which could explain the good response seen in studies investigating the effect of RTX [73]. Given the retrospective analyses of RTX efficacy in EGPA, a lower grade of recommendation for the treatment has been issued compared to GPA/MPA according to the EULAR/ERA-EDTA recommendations [74–76]. In the largest trial of RTX in EGPA patients (41 cases) until now, Mohammad et al. showed good response rates after one year. Prednisolone could be reduced during follow-up. Interestingly, ANCA-positivity was found to be associated with a higher remission-rate at 12 months compared to ANCA-negative patients (80% vs. 36%) [77]. Other agents employed to reduce corticosteroid doses and maintain remission of EGPA include drugs targeting relevant pro-inflammatory components of the involved immune system. For example, omalizumab (anti-IgE antibody) and mepolizumab (anti-IL-5 antibody) are currently being investigated in several eosinophil disorders like asthma and HES [73]. One randomized controlled trial assigned patients either to mepolizumab or placebo and showed significant higher efficacy rates in the mepolizumab arm, which was achieved in approximately half of the mepolizumab-treated patients [78]—An observation that again adds fuel to the fire in the discussion about different disease phenotypes. Reslizumab and benralizumab are other antibodies targeting IL-5 and its receptor, being tested in phase II trials in patients with eosinophil-driven diseases, including EGPA (ClinicalTrials.gov identifier: NCT02947945; NCT03010436) [79]. In the so-far published clinical trials investigating anti-IL-5 targeted-therapy in EGPA patients, only one patient with glomerulonephritis was enrolled, partly because serum-creatinine elevations >2.5 mg/dL were excluded and renal involvement in EGPA is rare [78,80,81]. Therefore, no firm conclusions from the landmark trial on the effect of mepolizumab on renal impairment can be drawn. In general, renal involvement resembles similar histopathologic features as observed in granulomatosis with polyangiitis (GPA) and microscopic polyangiitis (MPA) with the absence of immune complexes ('pauci-immune') in most cases. A study investigating the efficacy of RTX in EGPA recruited patients with either >25% dysmorphic red cells, red cell casts, or biopsy-proven pauci-immune glomerulonephritis. Remission was defined as a composite of stabilization of renal function, absence of active urinary sediment and a significant reduction of the glucocorticoid exposure (<50% of the average dose received over three months before enrollment or <10 mg per day). Following treatment with RTX (375 mg/m^2/week $\times$ 4) patients achieved renal remission which was prolonged during a follow-up period of 12 months [82]. Clinical trials particularly looking at renal disease in the context of EGPA are highly desirable, but recruitment of such patients remains difficult, partly because only one-quarter of EGPA patients present with renal involvement and most are not managed by nephrologists.

Nasal involvement in GPA is characterized by epistaxis, crusting, rhinorrhoe, and classical signs of sinusitis [83], while extensive nasal polyposis or rhinitis (either allergic or non-allergic) are the hallmarks of nasal involvement in EGPA [84]. However, polyangiitis overlap syndrome (POS) of GPA and EGPA was suggested in a few cases that fulfilled diagnostic criteria (e.g., ACR criteria) for both, GPA and EGPA [85–88]. In respect thereof, patients with typical vasculitis lesions, marked eosinophilia and PR3-ANCA positivity may be classified as POS in the absence of asthma. The optimal therapy for POS is not known but it seems important to identify these patients. Long term high dose steroid exposure to control disease activity is necessary in many patients with EGPA [77], which is different to patients with GPA.

On the other hand, ANCA-negative EGPA might be difficult to separate from HES_I because of overlapping clinical presentation and biomarker profiles [89]. Findings like the recent publication of a FIP1L1-PDGFRA-positive case of EGPA support the idea of overlapping syndromes that should be characterized by clinical appearance together with their biomarker profiles rather than finding an explicit diagnosis-label [90]. Given the fact that EGPA is a heterogeneous entity with potentially overlapping diseases carrying different biomarker profiles, patients could benefit from different treatment options like RTX for ANCA-positive EGPA, omalizumab or mepolizumab for ANCA-negative EGPA and imatinib for EGPA patients with mutations in TK fusion genes [91]. Testing for FIP1L1-PDGFRA mutation should therefore be performed routinely in all cases with HE, regardless of clinical presentation, suspected EGPA or ANCA-status. [92].

In systemic lupus erythematosus (SLE), kidney involvement in form of lupus nephritis occurs in about half of the patients [27]. PBE is a rare finding in subjects with SLE. Moreover, differential blood count has not been measured in most studies [28]. Harvey et al. reported PBE of 3% or more in 15 of 46 patients with SLE but only two patients had absolute eosinophil counts over 400/μL [93]. Reports of marked eosinophilia in association with SLE are restricted to single-case reports of SLE with concomitant Loeffler endocarditis [94,95], Wells' syndrome [96], eosinophilic pleuritis [97], or EGPA and HES [98].

Kargili et al. explored the prevalence of eosinophilia in other rheumatologic diseases in a retrospective analysis of 1000 cases between 2001 and 2002. Eosinophilia was seen in 26 of 293 patients with fibromyalgia (8.9%), 3 of 182 patients with rheumatoid arthritis (1.65%), and none of 12 patients with scleroderma, but the low prevalence might be explained by the frequent use of corticosteroids among these patients [99]. A recent study analyzed the eosinophil count to lymphocyte ratio (proportion of eosinophils to lymphocytes within the leukocyte count) in 344 patients with SLE and observed lower eosinophil counts in subjects with SLE compared to other autoimmune disorders. In line, the eosinophil-lymphocyte ratio in cases with SLE was lower compared to the diseased and healthy controls [100].

3.2.3. Vascular Diseases

Thrombotic microangiopathy (TMA) is characterized by a clinical presentation with microangiopathic hemolytic anemia, thrombocytopenia, and frequent renal and neurological involvement. TMA may occur in many disease processes but is typically associated with hemolytic uremic syndrome (HUS) and thrombotic thrombocytopenic purpura (TTP) [101]. Renal involvement is typical in HUS and rather uncommon in TTP. The overall prevalence and the outcome of AKI in TMA is therefore determined by the TMA subtype [29]. Low evidence exists for an association of PBE and thrombotic microangiopathies (TMA). Eight reported cases of TMA with PBE were diagnosed as HES [17,102–106]. Recently, one case of atypical HUS with AIN and PBE was reported and the first two case reports of concomitant atypical HUS and EGPA were published [107,108]. Activated eosinophils are known to favor thrombosis by various mechanisms. Endothelial cell damage is supposed to be mediated by degranulation of bioactive molecules, like EP, ECP, and MBP. Additionally, these molecules showed direct effects on coagulation, e.g., by inactivation of endothelial cell-expressed thrombomodulin and induction of tissue factor activity in endothelial cells [109,110]. Nonetheless, this observation appears interesting because thrombosis is a major link between HE and eosinophil-mediated organ damage observed in HES [109]. Whereas arterial thrombosis shows a higher incidence in HES, EGPA appears to have a predominance of venous thrombosis [109]. Vascular thrombosis is the main clinical feature of HES and also seen in EGPA, whilst TMA is less frequently reported in these patients. Nonetheless, the co-existence of HE with TMA or with any other thrombotic event should be sufficient to diagnose HES.

A primary non-renal disease that is worth noting because of its frequent impact on kidney function and association with eosinophilia is the cholesterol embolization syndrome (CES). It is a systemic disease with distal showering of cholesterol crystals out of atheromatous plaques from the aorta or other major arteries. CES has a male preponderance, present at an older age (>50% over 70 years), and shares the same risk factors with atherosclerosis. CES can occur spontaneously but is mainly induced iatrogenic, e.g., after aortic surgery or arterial invasive procedures such as angiography or left heart catheterization. Moreover, the use of anticoagulation (both, heparin and oral anticoagulants) have been linked with CES [111,112]. Beside skin lesions (commonly livedo reticularis limited to the lower limbs and trunk), the kidney is the most common site of involvement, followed by the spleen, pancreas, gastrointestinal tract, and adrenal glands [111,113]. Atheroembolic renal disease (AERD) is seen either in the form of AKI by acute rupture of unstable plaques or in a chronic but progressive way due to slow release of eroded atherosclerotic lesions [112]. In a prospective study, Fukumoto et al. found CES in 1.4% of 1786 patients who underwent left-heart catheterization. 64% of the reported CES-cases had renal damage. Blood eosinophil count was significantly higher than in patients without CES but did not reach the threshold for HE. Interestingly, CES with renal involvement showed a greater increase of eosinophil counts (from 220/μL to 535/μL) compared to CES without renal dysfunction (from 302/μL to 339/μL) [114]. In general, the presence of eosinophilia in CES is ranging from 14% to 71% [31,32]. The overall incidence of renal involvement in CES was 92.2% in a review of 22 studies [30]. CES is possibly an underdiagnosed entity because biopsy is rarely performed and clinical signs of CES are often subtle, especially when the disease progress is slow. An autopsy study showed a higher prevalence (25–30%) of CES after angiography [115]. Recent estimations by Mayo and Swartz revealed that 5–10% of all AKIs could be due to atheroembolism [116]. Among cardiac patients, the stage of CKD seems to correlate positively with the peripheral eosinophil count, so subclinical cholesterol embolization might play a role in this subset of patients [117]. Light microscopy of renal biopsy shows atheroemboli in interlobular and arcuate arteries, but also in arterioles and glomeruli with typical appearance as lance-shaped clefts, due to dissolution of cholesterol crystals during formalin fixation [113]. Given the high frequency of skin involvement, biopsy of skin lesions is suggested for diagnostic purposes [111]. The overall prognosis is poor with mortality rates ranging from 58% to 90% and RRT is necessary in about half of the patients [30,112]. A specific therapy for CES is not established. Withdrawal of anticoagulants, if possible, is proposed by some authors, while the role of steroids remains controversial [111,118]. Lipid-lowering therapies with statins or low-density lipoprotein (LDL)-apheresis are being used in case reports but until now there are no randomized trials that support this strategy [119,120]. Considering the lack of therapeutic options for CES, prevention of further episodes is crucial. This includes the limitation of anticoagulation and the restriction of vascular-invasive procedures for patients at risk as far as possible [111].

3.2.4. Other Diseases Presenting with Eosinophilia

Kimura's disease (KD) is a rare benign chronic inflammatory disorder mainly affecting young Asian men and commonly presenting with recurrent subcutaneous masses (of head and neck), lymphadenopathy, marked eosinophilia, and elevated IgE levels. Since the first reported case in 1937 in China, about 400 cases have been described in the literature, however, some cases of non-Asians with KD have been reported in the last years [121–127]. The main differential diagnosis is angiolymphoid hyperplasia with eosinophilia (ALHE). Both share significant overlap in clinical symptoms (soft tissue masses in the head and neck region) but can be distinguished by both clinical and histologic features. Systemic manifestations are rarely found in ALHE and therefore kidney involvement is more suggestive for KD [128]. Coexisting renal disease is common in KD and described in about 12–18% of the patients with about two-thirds of them developing nephrotic syndrome [33]. On kidney biopsy, various pathologies including minimal change disease (MCD), mesangial proliferative glomerulonephritis (MsPGN), focal segmental glomerulosclerosis (FSGS), IgM nephropathy, IgA nephropathy, and MN are described [33,129]. MsPGN, MN, and MCD are the most common histological lesions associated with KD [130–132]. The etiopathogenesis of KD is still not understood. Considering the regularly present eosinophilia and elevated IL-5 and IgE-levels, an abnormal T-cell stimulation to a hypersensitivity type reaction is suggested [33,133].

Chim et al. showed clonality in T-cell receptor studies in a case of KD. They propose that an initial immunologic response to an unidentified pathogen or stimuli may lead to prolonged lymphoid stimulation and eventually clonal proliferation in some cases, which has been suggested to be a pathogenetic factor of MCD as well [134,135]. First line treatment of KD includes surgical excision and radiation therapy. Oral corticosteroids are used in coexisting renal disease with good response but recurrence of proteinuria after termination of steroid therapy is frequent [33,129,136].

Another rare disease combining eosinophilia and kidney injury is tubulointerstitial nephritis and uveitis (TINU) syndrome. It has been described in 1975 by Dobrin et al., while meanwhile about 200 cases have been reported [137,138]. The incidence is highest in children, but all ages may be affected. Patients may initially present with azotemia as first finding and may later develop uveitis, but most cases are diagnosed by an ophthalmologist and abnormal kidney function is found during investigation of the underlying cause, although nephritis typically precedes uveitis in TINU syndrome [139]. Given the high number of cases with 'idiopathic' uveitis and the often subtle clinical signs of TIN, it is not surprising that TINU is regarded as a considerably underdiagnosed entity [35]. Mandeville et al. reviewed 133 cases of TINU syndrome and found blood eosinophilia in 17% of patients [35]. This number correlates roughly with the incidence of eosinophilia described in the setting of AIN without uveitis and in both diseases the role of eosinophils in the pathogenesis is unclear. TINU syndrome is thought to arise from a coincidence of certain host susceptibility factors and environmental triggers, leading to an autoimmune-mediated process [138]. Potential HLA risk alleles (depending on geographic background) for TINU, compared to TIN without uveitis or uveitis without TIN, are DRB1*01, DQA1*01, and DQB1*05 [140–143]. Modified C-reactive protein (CRP) might play a role as a target autoantigen in TINU syndrome [144]. Interestingly, TINU syndrome can recur after kidney transplantation [145]. In general, the degree of AKI in TINU is not severe and renal function often recovers spontaneously. In the large retrospective review by Mandeville et al., 80% of the patients received systemic corticosteroids and 9% further immunosuppressive therapy because of recurrent disease. About half of the patients had recurrence of uveitis, but ophthalmologic prognosis was good. Only 11% of the patients had persistent renal dysfunction, 5 out of 133 patients required dialysis and two of them underwent chronic dialysis [35].

IgG4-Related Disease (IgG4-RD) is a recently recognized fibroinflammatory disorder, characterized by IgG4-positive lymphoplasmacytic tissue infiltration, storiform fibrosis, and commonly elevated serum IgG4-levels [146]. Elevated serum IgG4-levels had been associated with autoimmune pancreatitis (AIP) before, but in 2003 a new disease entity was born when systemic manifestations in eight patients with autoimmune pancreatitis were identified and associated with tissue infiltration of IgG4-positive plasma cells [147,148]. IgG4-RD can virtually affect any organ and like AIP, several diseases formerly believed to be organ-limited—like Mikulicz's syndrome of salivary and lacrimal glands, Ormond's disease with retroperitoneal fibrosis, or Riedel thyroiditis—now fall within the spectrum of IgG4-RD [146]. The pathogenesis is not fully understood. Although not yet proven, autoimmunity seems to be the initial immunologic stimulus for a Th2 cell mediated immune response [146]. Recently the intracellular protein annexin A11 was identified as an IgG4-recognizing autoantigen. This finding led to the hypothesis that occupational antigens (especially industrial dust, gases, oils, and solvents [149]) or food and animal antigens [150] may cause tissue injuries in target organs with consecutive release of intracellular antigens like annexin A11 that trigger autoimmune response in genetically susceptible individuals (HLA DRB1*04:05-DQB1*04:01) [151–153]. The role of the IgG4 antibody in IgG4-RD is complex and some unique characteristics distinguish IgG4 from other antibody subclasses. Because of unstable disulfide bonds between the heavy chains of the IgG4 molecule, an exchange reaction with other antibodies called 'Fab-arm exchange' is continuously performed. The resulting asymmetric, bispecific IgG4 molecules are unable to cross-link antigens and to form immune complexes [146,154]. An animal model showed that both IgG1 and IgG4 can induce specific lesions of IgG4-RD, while IgG4 simultaneously appears to have an inhibitory effect on the pathogenic activity of IgG1 [155]. It remains unclear, whether IgG4 itself is the driving force or a compensatory reaction to reduce tissue injury. Regulation of IgG4 production is dependent on Th2 cells and therefore linked to IgE response and eosinophilia. The latter is seen in about 30% of patients with IgG4-RD [37,38,156]. In the setting of allergic reactions, high IgG4 levels reflect an enhanced production of IL-10 and other anti-inflammatory cytokines and therefore are associated with a decrease of allergic symptoms [154]. Two cohort studies examined the prevalence of atopy, eosinophilia and IgE in patients with IgG4-RD. Atopy was present in 31% (22 of 70) in a retrospective US-cohort study and in 43% (22 of 51) patients of a Japanese-cohort which roughly corresponds to the prevalence of allergic-symptoms in the respective population. Interestingly, both studies showed no significant differences in the frequency of eosinophilia, serum levels of IgG4 and IgE or mean concentrations of IgE and IgG4, and peripheral blood cell counts between the allergy groups and the non-allergy groups. These observations support the suggestion that eosinophilia and IgE elevations are inherent characteristics of IgG4-RD immune response and not caused by an underlying allergic condition [37,38].

The kidney itself has been proven to be 'special' among the organs affected by IgG4-RD. IgG4-related TIN is the leading renal involvement and less frequently IgG4-related MN can be diagnosed. Thus, two different histopathologic types of lesions are common within one organ. Other glomerular lesions associated with IgG4-RD are IgA nephropathy and mild mesangial immune complex glomerulonephritis not otherwise specified [157]. These types of kidney manifestations need to be distinguished from secondary kidney affection in the course of IgG4-RD due to other organ manifestations, like retroperitoneal fibrosis with consecutive postrenal function impairment. The kidney is involved in about 10–15% of the patients with IgG4-RD [36]. Most data about IgG4-related kidney disease (IgG4-RKD) is obtained by a Japanese cohort study of 23 patients and an American (Mayo Clinic) cohort of 35 patients with biopsy-proven IgG4-related TIN [158,159]. Deduced by the collected data, both studies separately proposed diagnostic criteria for IgG4-related TIN, sharing the typical histologic pattern as the only obligatory criterion plus one (Mayo Clinic criteria), respectively two (Japanese Society of Nephrology criteria) other features, including radiologic abnormalities, total IgG and IgG4 serum-levels, and extra-renal organ involvement [159,160]. In both studies, patients were predominantly male with an average age of approximately 65 years. At the time of diagnosis, nearly all patients had extrarenal manifestations. Beside renal dysfunction, typical laboratory findings were elevated total IgG and/or IgG4 levels, hypocomplemententemia, PBE, and a positive ANA test [158,159]. Radiographic abnormalities consisted of multiple, bilateral lesions, or masses (69.6% and 78.3%) seen in MRI or CT [158,159]. A recent study showed improved diagnostic sensitivity of these lesions on MRI including diffusion-weighted imaging (DWI) [161].

It is important to recognize IgG4-related inflammatory pseudotumor and distinguish it from renal malignant tumor to avoid unnecessary nephrectomy [162]. Another mimicker of IgG4-RKD is AAV, which can be present with elevated serum IgG4 levels and similar organ manifestations compared to IgG4-RD [163]. Moreover, AAV can be associated with both peripheral and tissue eosinophilia, and biopsy specimens may even show IgG4-positive lymphoplasmacytic infiltrations with storiform fibrosis [164]. Constitutional symptoms such as fever, ANCA-positivity and elevated CRP may be helpful to establish the diagnosis of AAV, on the other hand ANCA-positivity does not exclude IgG4-RD [151,165]. ANCA in AAV are most often IgG1 and IgG4 and its speculated that IgG4-RD might trigger AAV in patients with a vulnerable genetic background [165]. RTX might be preferentially used in overlapping syndromes of IgG4-RD and AAV to treat both diseases. On the other side of the clinical spectrum of IgG4-RD, there is a significant overlap with HES. In a comparative case series, Carruthers et al. evaluated cases of IgG4-RD and lymphocyte-variant HES and found elevated serum IgG4-levels (90% and 42%), PBE (26% and 100%), increased serum IgE (60% and 62%) and clonal T-cell receptor gene rearrangement by PCR (52% and 77%) in a significant number of cases in both diseases [166].

In HES, kidney involvement is rare, patients often present with cardiac, pulmonary, or cutaneous manifestations and the disease rarely affects more than three organs, whereas IgG4-RD typically shows multiple organ manifestations [166]. A final diagnosis of IgG4-RD is made after exclusion of

IgG4-mimicking diseases, principally through pathological evaluation of biopsy specimens [165,167]. Histopathological features on light microscopy are dense lymphoplasmacytic infiltrates of mainly IgG4-positive plasma cells (>10 IgG4-positive plasma cells per high power field, and/or >40% IgG4/IgG-positive plasma cells in the most affected areas), usually accompanied by interstitial fibrosis with a 'storiform' pattern. Immunofluorescence microscopy reveals granular tubular basement membrane immune deposits with a positive staining for IgG4, IgG1, IgG3, and C3 complement. In contrast, IgG4-related MN (about 7–10% of cases) does not exhibit the typical fibroinflammatory pattern of IgG4-RD. Instead, granular glomerular capillary wall deposits of IgG (usually with IgG4-dominance) and negative staining for phospholipase A2 receptor (PLA_2R) are usually seen in IgG4-related MN [168]. Screening for serum antibodies against M-type PLA_2R, in contrast to most primary MN cases, is negative in its IgG4-related form [169]. Interestingly, primary or idiopathic MN also characteristically shows IgG4 predominance in the glomerular immune complex deposits [168]. Patients with known IgG4-related TIN or IgG4-RD with other organ manifestations who develop proteinuria have a suspected diagnosis of MN, but in absence of already diagnosed IgG4-RD, differential diagnosis of IgG4-related MN can be challenging and effort must be made to rule out primary MN and secondary causes of MN, such as autoimmune disorders (SLE, rheumatoid arthritis, and Sjögren syndrome), infections, neoplasms, or causative drugs [169].

The optimal treatment for IgG4-RD is not known due to the lack of RCT evaluating different therapeutic options. In an international symposium among experts, an initial therapy with steroids was proposed for all symptomatic patients. Asymptomatic patients with involvement of important organs like the kidneys, should also receive early steroid therapy to prevent irreversible organ damage. For some subsets of patients, like asymptomatic IgG4-RD with lymphadenopathy or mild submandibular gland enlargement, "watchful waiting" may be appropriate [167]. The typical initial regimen for both IgG4-RD and IgG4-RKD, is an administration of prednisone (e.g., 30–40 mg/day for two to four weeks) with a stepwise tapering depending on the clinical response [167,170,171]. Although the initial response to glucocorticoids is often good, relapse rates after steroid tapering are high and long-term steroid therapy exposes to major adverse side effects [170,172]. Azathioprine, mycophenolate mofetil, and methotrexate are therefore being used frequently as steroid-sparing agents for induction and maintenance therapy but evidence of clinical trials is still lacking [146]. B-cell depleting agents, such as RTX, appear to be an attractive alternative (even without concomitant glucocorticoid therapy) for both induction and maintenance therapy in IgG4-RD and clinical trials are ongoing (ClinicalTrials.gov identifier: NCT01584388) [173–175]. For the use of RTX in IgG4-RKD there is even less evidence, but especially in patients with aggressive IgG-RD and renal involvement, treatment with RTX might have beneficial effects in terms of long-term preservation of renal function [171]. Patients with AAV-overlapping disease are possibly a subgroup that is suited for RTX to treat both diseases [163]. The optimal strategy for RTX as maintenance therapy (e.g., need for retreatment or application intervals) is unclear but baseline elevations of IgG4, IgE, and PBE before treatment with RTX predict disease-relapses independently and could be helpful for therapy monitoring [175].

Several other renal pathologies have been associated with PBE in selected cases. In diabetic nephropathy, PBE is rarely present and might be related to a drug-induced hypersensitivity reaction [176,177] or a consequence of an accompanying interstitial nephritis [178,179]. Interestingly, the predictive value of PBE for diagnosing a *Strongyloides* infection in an endemic community appears to be particularly high in patients with type 2 diabetes mellitus [180].

Various forms of renal pathologies may be caused by the human immunodeficiency virus (HIV), either by the infection itself, its treatment or as a complication of the acquired immunodeficiency syndrome (AIDS) [181]. In general, the association of PBE and HIV-infection is complex. PBE is not an infrequent finding among HIV-infected patients but no association with concomitant kidney disease attributable to HIV has been proposed so far. Al Mohajer et al. found PBE in 9.7% (65/671) among antiretroviral therapy (ART)-naive HIV-patients in a single-center cohort [182]. Patients with eosinophilia were more likely to present with skin rash, while treatment to suppress the HIV viral load did not result in the resolution of eosinophilia. A potential parasite-endemic risk should be assessed to rule out *Strongyloides* or *Schistosoma* infection and in the case of suspected infection empirical therapy with ivermectin or praziquantel may be considered [183,184]. Reported cases of HIV-infected patients with PBE and impaired kidney function are usually a consequence of the side effects, toxicity, or hypersensitivity reactions of antiretroviral treatment [185–187]. Thomas et al. propose an association of HLA-B*53:01, a prevalent allele among African individuals, with the risk of raltegravir-induced DRESS syndrome [188]. A systematic review of DRESS-cases in HIV-patients found five different antiretrovirals in 35 reported cases [187]. Eosinophilia was seen in 51.4% (18/35) of the cases, while 28.6% (10/35) of the cases presented with kidney affection. Of note, efavirenz (6/35 cases) was associated with the most severe renal failure. These observations need to be confirmed in larger, prospective studies.

For primary glomerulopathies such as MN [131,189,190], IgA nephropathy [191–194], or FSGS [195–197], an association with PBE was mainly found when described in the context of primary eosinophilia-associated diseases like Kimura's disease, EGPA, IgG4-RKD, or HES.

3.2.5. Chronic Kidney Disease, Dialysis, and Kidney Transplantation

Slightly elevated peripheral blood eosinophil levels without meeting the criteria for PBE were seen in a prospective cohort study comparing leukocyte counts among US veterans with versus without CKD [198]. Among patients with type 2 diabetes, eosinophilia was associated with albuminuria [199]. Solak et al. investigated pruritus among patients with CKD and showed a mean prevalence of eosinophilia in 18.9% of the patients, interestingly without significant differences between CKD Stages 2 to 5. Patients who suffered pruritus had significantly elevated numbers of peripheral blood eosinophils ($p = 0.005$, OR 3.209) [200]. Studies of uremic patients showed bone marrow eosinophilia without elevated PBE, but high circulating levels of ECP. These findings of an abnormal eosinophil homeostasis suggest an accelerated turnover of peripheral eosinophils due to uremia [201,202].

Hemodialysis-associated eosinophilia (HAE) is not uncommon among patients on hemodialysis and is mostly induced by allergy to components of the dialysis circuit [39]. Dialyzer reactions were quite frequent in the 1970s with a reported prevalence of PBE in up to 39% of all patients on maintenance dialysis [40]. Ethylene oxide, the commonly used sterilizing agent of that time, was associated with allergic reactions and HAE [203–205]. Traditional cellulosic membranes of cellophane (Kolff dialyzer) or cuprophane (Kiil dialyzer) are derived from cotton and showed limited biocompatibility because of activation of the complement cascade [206]. Using steam and gamma irradiation as modern sterilization techniques instead of ethylene oxide and replacing traditional cellophane and cuprophane membranes by ester modified cellulose or synthetic polymer based membranes, the prevalence of hemodialysis-associated reactions decreased [39]. Modified cellulose membranes primarily provide low-flux dialysis, whereas synthetic membranes are preferred for high-flux dialysis [39]. Even though less frequent, hypersensitivity reactions are also described with modern dialyzer membranes and it was realized that the dialyzer bio-incompatibility depends on the membrane composition [207]. Anaphylactoid reactions within the first minutes of hemodialysis were reported with high-flux polyacrylonitrile AN69® capillary dialyzers [208]. The reported cases were linked to a concomitant ACE inhibitor treatment that might aggravate increased bradykinin concentrations which are reported in patients using polyacrylonitrile membranes [208,209]. Simon et al. showed a higher incidence of anaphylactoid reactions (AR) in patients dialyzed with synthetic membranes than in patients dialyzed with cellulose membranes [210]. More recently, Hildebrand et al. investigated eosinophilia in three hemodialysis facilities among current hemodialysis patients and showed an increase in the prevalence of HAE (defined as greater than 1000 eosinophils/μL) from 1.5% in 2007 (historical cohort of patients dialyzing at the same facilities) to 4.7% in 2012 [39]. ACE inhibitor treatment again correlated with the presence of eosinophilia (41.7% vs. 12.5%, $p = 0.049$). In the follow up period, no difference was seen in the mean number of hospital admission days (12 months follow-up) or in mortality rates (29 months follow-up) between patients on dialysis with or without HAE. Eosinophilia was absent at dialysis initiation in all patients but one, suggesting that eosinophilia can occur in dialysis as a subclinical effect of the dialysis process. The reason for the reported increasing prevalence of HAE remains unclear, but the overall prognosis for asymptomatic eosinophilia among dialysis patients appears to be good [39]. For patients with peri-dialytic symptoms, eosinophilia and also complement C3a and C5a may be indicative parameters for membrane bio-incompatibility. In these cases, changing the hemodialysis membrane might be beneficial [207,211].

PBE in patients undergoing peritoneal dialysis tends to be mild, episodic, and is often associated with peritoneal fluid eosinophilia (PFE) [42]. The latter was mainly reported in the context of eosinophilic peritonitis (EP), a condition defined as an absolute EC in the peritoneal effluent greater than 100/μL, or a relative EC greater than 10% of the total WBC count when the absolute number of eosinophils in the peritoneal effluent is greater than 40/μL [212,213]. In analogue to HAE, the prevalence of eosinophilia associated with peritoneal dialysis decreased within the last decades. Chan et al. studied PFE in a prospective cohort among 23 patients on continuous ambulatory peritoneal dialysis (CAPD) in the 1980s and found PFE in 60.8% of all patients with 57% of those showing PBE [214]. Identified risk factors associated with EP are exposure to vancomycin, infections (fungal or viral) after a recent catheter replacement or treatment with icodextrin, a polymer used to increase ultrafiltration in order to treat volume overload in ESRD [215,216]. More recent data from a prospective study of 48 patients undergoing CAPD suggested a smaller prevalence of PFE of less than 10% and shows no significant correlation between PBE and PFE [41]. PBE is typically detected in asymptomatic patients following catheter replacement and usually resolves spontaneously within a few days [41,213], although the course can be chronic or recurring with permanent changes in membrane function [217]. Considering the favorable prognosis, a steroid treatment in general is not recommended [214]. In severe cases with abdominal symptoms who require further peritoneal dialysis, corticosteroid therapy showed good effects in case reports for both intraperitoneal and systemic application forms [218–220]. Montelukast, a leukotriene receptor antagonist, might be a therapeutic option but until now is only reported in one single case [221].

In kidney transplant recipients (KTR), both PBE and tissue eosinophilia are primarily associated with acute allograft rejection (AAR) [43,222–226]. In this context, tissue eosinophilia in the kidney allograft appears to be a specific and sensitive indicator of irreversible and severe acute (vascular) rejection and should be considered as a predictor of poor transplant outcome [223,225,226]. In a retrospective analysis of 71 patients with AAR, Hongwei et al. found a higher mean level of peripheral blood eosinophils in all grades of AAR (1.5–3.0%) than in controls (0.0–0.9%) and PBE was defined as a relative count of $\geq$4%, which was present in 20–36% of the patients [43]. Weir et al. found a correlation between the percentage of PBE and the severity and outcome of AAR. Patients with peripheral blood eosinophil percentages $\geq$4% had a higher irreversible rejection rate (37.9% versus 22.4% compared to those with peripheral blood eosinophil percentages <4%, $p < 0.01$). The absolute EC, however, showed no significant correlation [227]. A current single-center renal allograft biopsy study with 1217 KTR confirmed the correlation between the presence of tissue eosinophils and an impaired allograft outcome but detected no PBE in their study cohort [226]. The latter might be explained by a relatively high maintenance dose of 10 mg prednisone per day among all included patients. With respect to the data provided by Hongwei et al. and Weir et al., peripheral blood eosinophil levels appear to be only slightly elevated in AAR and concomitant immunosuppressive therapy with corticosteroids presumably hinders diagnosis.

Two other conditions should be considered as differential diagnosis of eosinophilia in KTR. Firstly, delayed graft function with PBE is suggestive for AIN. Trimethoprim-sulfamethoxazole is one agent frequently prescribed after kidney transplantation that is associated with drug-induced AIN [228,229]. In contrast to AAR, increasing the steroid doses is less effective and the most striking treatment is withdrawal of the offending agent. Drug-induced TIN is a reversible injury that should be considered in the differential diagnosis of renal allograft dysfunction accompanied by eosinophilia.

A quite uncommon differential diagnosis, but one with a potentially fatal outcome is *Strongyloides* hyperinefction. *Strongyloides stercoralis* is an intestinal nematode prevalent in tropical and subtropical regions, currently believed to infect an estimated 370 million people worldwide [230–232]. Due to autoinfection, larvae may persist undetected for years in immunocompetent hosts or cause only slight clinical symptoms. Immunocompromised patients are at risk of a hyperinfection syndrome due to an uncontrolled multiplication of parasites with potentially life-threatening dissemination to all internal organs [231]. A retrospective multicenter study and review of the literature analyzed clinical features of *Strongyloides* hyperinfection in 133 patients and found fever (80.8%), respiratory (88.6%), and gastrointestinal (71.1%) symptoms as the most common clinical manifestations. PBE was observed in only 34.3% of the cases, probably due to underlying immunosuppressive therapy [44]. Immunosuppressive therapy in general and treatment with glucocorticoids in particular, especially when used as high-dose therapy in transplant rejection, is associated with an augmented risk for *Strongyloides* hyperinfection [233]. *Strongyloides* infection in KTR is well documented in endemic regions, but a quantity of reported cases in non-endemic areas is suspected to be donor-derived [45,234–240]. The American Transplant Society recommends pretransplant *Strongyloides stercoralis* IgG-antibody testing and stool screening for recipients and donors from endemic areas, with gastrointestinal symptoms or with PBE [241]. A survey of physicians found that only 9% of US physicians-in-training could recognize a person in need of screening for strongyloidiasis and treatment errors occurred often among providers unfamiliar with immigrant health (e.g., prescription of empiric corticosteroids) [242]. A retrospective analysis of the Centers for Disease Control and Prevention (CDC) illustrates the deficient screening of high-risk donors and data provided by the New York Organ Donor Network (NYODN) confirms the effectiveness of a targeted donor screening prior to transplantation [238,240]. A recent survey of US Organ Procurement Organizations showed again widespread uncertainty related to donor screening for *Strongyloides stercoralis* and continuing education and advocacy on the importance of targeted donor screening is emphasized by the US Center for Global Health [243]. Nonetheless, eosinophilia, fever, and gastrointestinal and/or respiratory symptoms in a KTR should prompt further diagnostic steps. The current demographic changes due to increased global migratory movements (case reports in Europe are to date restricted to Spain and Italy) demand a certain awareness for screening and therapy approaches [244–246]. Sensitivity rates of serology testing are quite high (about 90%), but false-negative results can occur especially in immunocompromised patients. Once hyperinfection is considered, larvae are usually found in stool specimens but invasive methods to obtain tissue specimens by skin biopsy or gastroscopy might be necessary for definite diagnosis [45]. Therapy differs from almost all other causes of eosinophilia hence that intensified immunosuppressive therapy can have fatal consequences. Mortality rates in KTR with *Strongyloides* hyperinfection are up to 50% [247,248]. Antihelmintic therapy with oral ivermectin is the first-line therapy in hyperinfection syndrome and decreasing the steroid dose might be beneficial [45,233].

3.2.6. Renal Cell Carcinoma

Renal cell carcinoma (RCC) is in general managed by urologists but nevertheless, suspected masses might be diagnosed by either radiologists or doctors of internal medicine by performing ultrasound or initially detected by the presence of urinary red cells. RCC can induce various paraneoplastic syndromes, such as hypercalcemia, arterial hypertension, or production of erythropoietin [249–251]. Paraneoplastic PBE is rarely described in RCC and restricted to case reports of patients with different RCC-subtypes, such as clear cell RCC and chromophobe RCC but mostly appears to reflect an advanced disease phase with widespread metastasis [252–256].

Beside RCC, paraneoplastic PBE is described in a variety of other malignancies, such as gastrointestinal tumors, sarcoma, lung cancer, prostate cancer, cervix cancer, and sarcoma [256–259]. Release of eosinophilopoietic cytokines by the tumor appears to be an underlying mechanism for reactive eosinophil proliferation in these patients [260]. Other authors linked the presence of PBE to necrosis of the tumor or its metastasis [255,256]. In paraneoplastic eosinophilia, tumor-associated tissue eosinophilia (TATE) is distinguished from tumor-associated blood eosinophilia (TABE). Both may occur simultaneously or separately and their association remains unclear [253]. It is noteworthy that tumors with TATE alone are associated with a better prognosis whilst TABE is associated with a poor prognosis and advanced tumor stadium [255].

3.2.7. Eosinophilia on Nephrology Consultation Service

The largest study up to date was published by Diskin et al. in 2011 in form of a prospective cross-sectional study evaluating the prevalence of eosinophilia on a nephrology consultation service [261]. In 2009, 1339 patients on nephrology consultation service of Auburn University (Auburn, AL, USA) had an assessment of the EC. Reasons for consultation were CKD or ESRD in over 50% of cases and no diagnosed case of parasitic infection was seen. The strongest correlation with an increased EC was seen in unspecific conditions like the presence of vascular disease, pleural effusions, and cirrhosis, while a negative correlation was found for total WBC count and beta-blocker use [261]. No correlation between an increased EC and the aforementioned kidney diseases associated with eosinophilia like vasculitis, TIN, or patients on RRT was observed, mainly impacted by the low number of patients in these subgroups.

4. Proposed Approach for the Management of Unexplained Eosinophilia and Acute Kidney Injury

4.1. First Step Approach for the Patient with Unexplained Peripheral Blood Eosinophilia

As shown in Figure 3, every patient should undergo a basic assessment. This includes a clinical status with focus on signs of organ involvement and a thorough past medical history assessment that addresses symptoms of organ involvement, exposures, and prior eosinophil counts. The history of exposures should include a travel history, past and current medications including over-the-counter medications, foods, and occupational or recreational exposures.

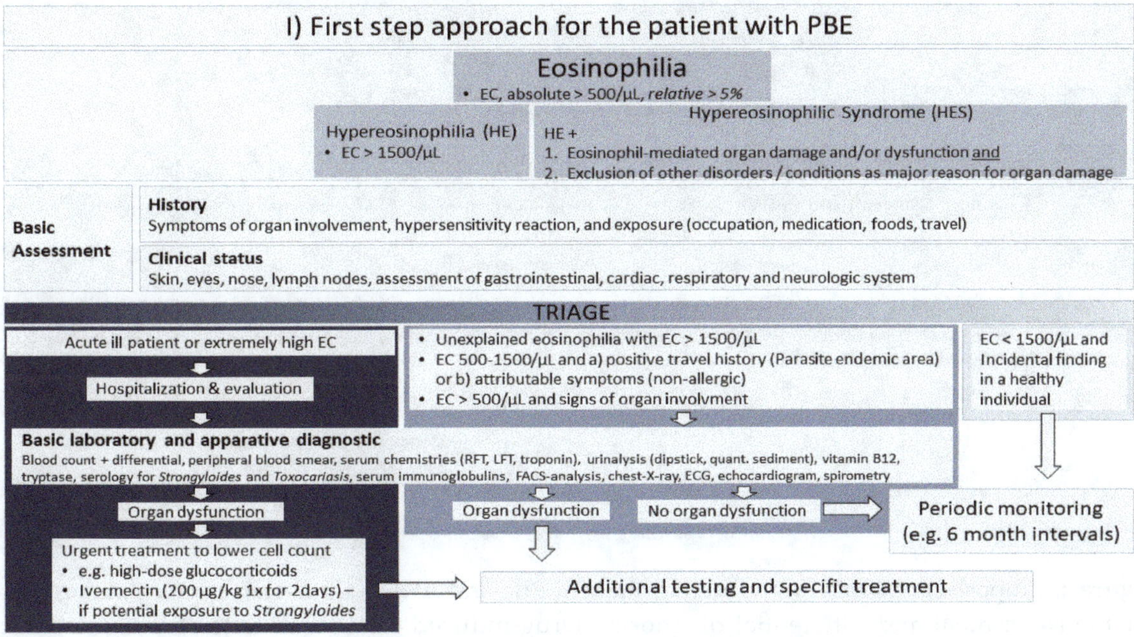

Figure 3. Proposed approach for the initial management of unexplained eosinophilia. When PBE is detected, a systematic management should include a basic assessment, an evaluation of urgency, and the screening for organ dysfunctions. EC, eosinophil count; HE, hypereosinophilia; HES, hypereosinophilic syndrome; RFT, renal function tests; LFT, liver function tests; FACS, fluorescence-activated cell scanning; ECG, electrocardiogram.

Patients with mild or modest PBE (EC < 1500/µL) and no signs of organ involvement should not undergo further evaluation or treatment and can be monitored in intervals of six months. Patients that appear acutely ill with extremely high EC need hospitalization and prompt evaluation.

In life-threatening conditions, urgent treatment with high-dose glucocorticoids to lower EC is indicated. To prevent potentially fatal *Strongyloides* hyperinfection syndrome, accompanying empirical prophylaxis with ivermectin 200 μg/kg is recommended in those with potential exposure. Patients with marked HE (EC > 1500/μL) or patients with modest eosinophilia (EC from 500 to 1500/μL) and signs of organ involvement or positive history of exposures should be screened for organ dysfunction. If organ dysfunction is excluded, periodic monitoring should be performed.

In the case of organ dysfunction, an efficient diagnostic algorithm to exclude serious underlying diseases that require specific treatment is indicated. The WHO suggests the exclusion of secondary (reactive) causes of eosinophilia as the first step [3], including exclusion of allergy/atopy, hypersensitivity conditions, drug reactions, autoimmune diseases, pulmonary eosinophilic diseases, allergic gastroenteritis, and metabolic conditions such as adrenal insufficiency. To exclude an underlying infection, serology for *Strongyloides* species should be performed in all patients. Additional tests, such as repeated ova and parasite testing, stool culture and antibody testing for specific parasites and other infections may be indicated depending on the exposure history. We recommend that additional tests should depend on individual patient characteristics and the results of the initial assessment. Selected patients should be screened for primary or secondary causes of eosinophilia, starting with those investigations that appear more likely to be informative.

4.2. Approach for the Patient with PBE and AKI

When PBE and AKI is present, a three-step approach as shown in Figure 4 should be considered. We emphasize that evidence for such recommendations is lacking and to our knowledge, no such proposal has been made to this point.

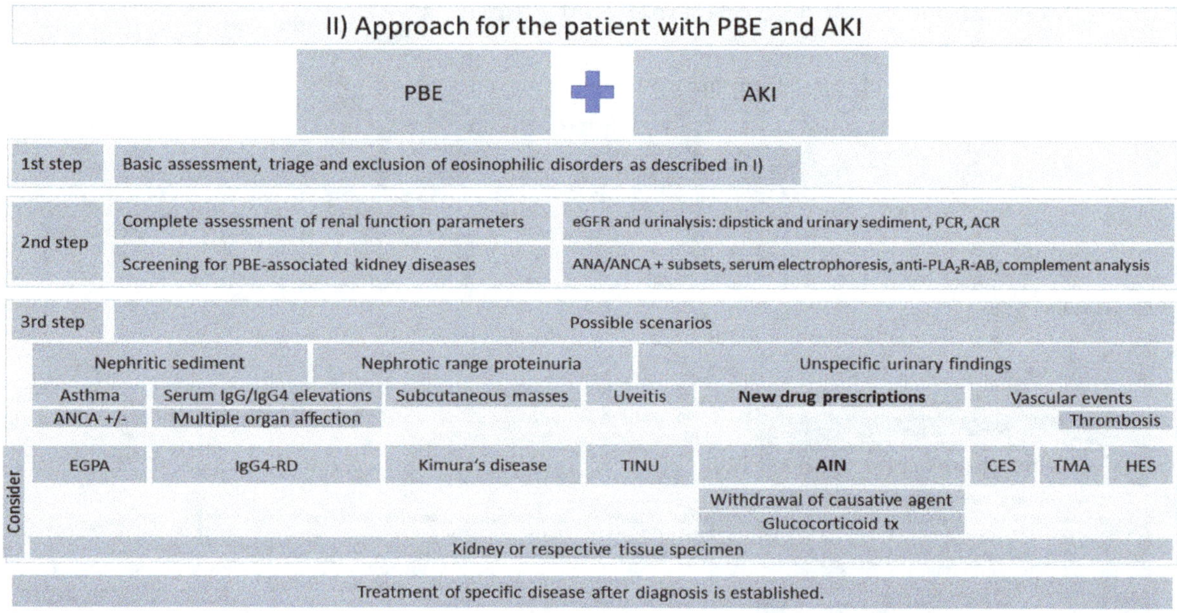

Figure 4. Proposed approach for the management of PBE and AKI. A three-step approach is suggested for the assessment and differential diagnosis. Drug-induced AIN (bold letters) is a comparably frequent finding and prompt identification of the culprit drug is decisive for prognosis. PBE, peripheral blood eosinophilia; AKI, acute kidney injury; HE, hypereosinophilia; EC, eosinophil count; eGFR, estimated glomerular filtration rate; PCR, protein-creatinine ratio; ACR albumin-creatinine ratio; ANA, antinuclear antibody; ANCA, anti-neutrophil cytoplasmic antibody; anti-PLA2R-AB, anti-phospholipase-A2-receptor antibody; IgG, immunoglobulin G; EGPA, eosinophilic granulomatosis with polyangiitis; IgG4-RD, IgG4-related disease; TINU, tubulointerstitial nephritis and uveitis; AIN, acute interstitial nephritis; CES, cholesterol embolization syndrome; TMA, thrombotic microangiopathy; HES, hypereosinophilic syndrome.

As a first step, we recommend a basic assessment to rule out classical eosinophilic disorders, including hematologic neoplasia, parasitic infection, and allergies (see Figure 1).

After exclusion of classical eosinophilic disorders, a thorough assessment of renal function parameters and screening for PBE-associated kidney diseases is recommended. Distinguishing nephritic and nephrotic syndrome might be helpful to narrow down possible underlying kidney diseases. In the case of unspecific urinary findings, PBE can be a useful diagnostic marker for AIN which is the most frequent entity associated with PBE. We recommend screening for recent changes in the patient's medication list with a focus set on PPIs, NSAIDs, and antibiotics, but generally any drug can cause AIN. Prompt withdrawal of any potential causative agents is pivotal. In the absence of kidney function recovery within three to five days following discontinuation of potential causative agents, kidney biopsy is recommended and early steroid treatment and more specific immunosuppressive measures should be considered.

5. Conclusions

In classical eosinophilic disorders such as HES, in which eosinophils are the driving force of pathogenesis and organ damage, renal involvement is rare and possibly occurs late in the course of disease, e.g., as a consequence of thromboembolism. Nevertheless, a variety of different diseases that typically affect kidney function are associated with PBE. Here, the presence of PBE may be a helpful diagnostic marker for rare or underdiagnosed entities with only subtle clinical signs such as AIN or CES or in overlapping syndromes like EGPA/HES/GPA or IgG4-RD.

When marked PBE is present, classical eosinophilic disorders such as an underlying hematologic neoplasm, parasitic infections, or allergic conditions need to be excluded first. Patients with AKI and PBE should be investigated for culprit drugs of AIN (frequent). A history of recent vascular interventions should be assessed to evaluate CES (rare). It is noteworthy that both entities may also appear in a slowly progressive form.

In patients undergoing hemodialysis or peritoneal dialysis, eosinophilia might be an indicator for bio-incompatibility of the dialysis material. In KTR, eosinophilia is associated with AAR and portends a poor transplant outcome. Before initiation of high-dose steroid treatment, an infection with *Strongyloides stercoralis* should be excluded to avoid a potentially fatal *Strongyloides* hyperinfection syndrome. The role of eosinophils in immune-mediated diseases like EGPA and IgG4-RD is incompletely understood. Novel insights into EGPA establish the concept of a disease with two different phenotypes. ANCA-positive patients show a vasculitis phenotype with typical renal involvement, whereas the ANCA-negative phenotype shares clinical overlap with HES. Until now, it is unclear if different EGPA-phenotypes should receive tailored therapy, for instance anti-IL-5 therapy with mepolizumab for ANCA-negative EGPA. From our current knowledge, no concrete statement of this treatment approach on renal outcome can be made. Therefore, clinical trials particularly looking at renal disease in the context of EGPA are highly desirable.

6. Future Perspectives

Eosinophilia is a frequent finding in patients seen in a general nephrology practice. Taking this into count, there is a clear need to recommend routine differential blood count assessment, at least in the context of a first visit. In our opinion, large, multi-national cohorts should be assessed to describe the frequency of eosinophilia in specific renal diseases. In patients from endemic regions, *Strongyloides* must be ruled out before kidney transplantation and awareness to detect a potential infection following transplantation needs to be increased. With this review, our aim was to summarize eosinophilia in kidney diseases to strengthen further research efforts in this field. Studies are needed to add missing pieces to the puzzles, i.e., if an EC above the normal level before initiation of drugs potentially leading to AIN increases the risk to develop interstitial nephritis. We will particularly focus on diseases leading to nephrotic syndrome and if eosinophilia in this context is predictive of future flares. In diseases with a known association with eosinophilia, further efforts need to be undertaken to define the different phenotypes. As an example, approaches to propose specific biomarkers related to eosinophil-biology have failed to show promising results in EGPA, such as eotaxin-3 or TARC/CCL17 [262]. Phenotyping of these patients is essential to rule out such shortcomings and to draw firm conclusions.

Author Contributions: P.G. and A.K. designed the study. P.G. wrote the first draft of the manuscript, J.I.S., G.M. and A.K. critically revised the manuscript. All authors read and approved the final manuscript.

Acknowledgments: We are grateful to Peter Valent who critically revised our manuscript.

References

1. Radonjic-Hoesli, S.; Valent, P.; Klion, A.D.; Wechsler, M.E.; Simon, H.U. Novel targeted therapies for eosinophil-associated diseases and allergy. *Annu. Rev. Pharmacol. Toxicol.* **2015**, *55*, 633–656. [CrossRef] [PubMed]
2. Valent, P.; Klion, A.D.; Horny, H.P.; Roufosse, F.; Gotlib, J.; Weller, P.F.; Hellmann, A.; Metzgeroth, G.; Leiferman, K.M.; Arock, M.; et al. Contemporary consensus proposal on criteria and classification of eosinophilic disorders and related syndromes. *J. Allergy Clin. Immunol.* **2012**, *130*, 607–612.e9. [CrossRef] [PubMed]
3. Gotlib, J. World Health Organization-defined eosinophilic disorders: 2017 update on diagnosis, risk stratification, and management. *Am. J. Hematol.* **2017**, *92*, 1243–1259. [CrossRef] [PubMed]
4. Hogan, S.P.; Rosenberg, H.F.; Moqbel, R.; Phipps, S.; Foster, P.S.; Lacy, P.; Kay, A.B.; Rothenberg, M.E. Eosinophils: Biological properties and role in health and disease. *Clin. Exp. Allergy* **2008**, *38*, 709–750. [CrossRef] [PubMed]
5. Gleich, G.J. Mechanisms of eosinophil-associated inflammation. *J. Allergy Clin. Immunol.* **2000**, *105*, 651–663. [CrossRef] [PubMed]
6. Ramirez, G.A.; Yacoub, M.R.; Ripa, M.; Mannina, D.; Cariddi, A.; Saporiti, N.; Ciceri, F.; Castagna, A.; Colombo, G.; Dagna, L. Eosinophils from Physiology to Disease: A Comprehensive Review. *Biomed. Res. Int.* **2018**, *2018*, 9095275. [CrossRef] [PubMed]
7. Roufosse, F.; Weller, P.F. Practical approach to the patient with hypereosinophilia. *J. Allergy Clin. Immunol.* **2010**, *126*, 39–44. [CrossRef]
8. Rothenberg, M.E. Eosinophilia. *N. Engl. J. Med.* **1998**, *338*, 1592–1600. [CrossRef]
9. Kahn, J.E.; Groh, M.; Lefevre, G. (A Critical Appraisal of) Classification of Hypereosinophilic Disorders. *Front. Med.* **2017**, *4*, 216. [CrossRef]
10. Sanderson, C.J. Interleukin-5, eosinophils, and disease. *Blood* **1992**, *79*, 3101–3109.
11. Chusid, M.J.; Dale, D.C.; West, B.C.; Wolff, S.M. The hypereosinophilic syndrome: Analysis of fourteen cases with review of the literature. *Medicine* **1975**, *54*, 1–27. [CrossRef] [PubMed]
12. Valent, P.; Horny, H.P.; Bochner, B.S.; Haferlach, T.; Reiter, A. Controversies and open questions in the definitions and classification of the hypereosinophilic syndromes and eosinophilic leukemias. *Semin. Hematol.* **2012**, *49*, 171–181. [CrossRef] [PubMed]
13. Spry, C.J. The hypereosinophilic syndrome: Clinical features, laboratory findings and treatment. *Allergy* **1982**, *37*, 539–551. [CrossRef] [PubMed]
14. Fauci, A.S.; Harley, J.B.; Roberts, W.C.; Ferrans, V.J.; Gralnick, H.R.; Bjornson, B.H. NIH conference. The idiopathic hypereosinophilic syndrome. Clinical, pathophysiologic, and therapeutic considerations. *Ann. Intern. Med.* **1982**, *97*, 78–92. [CrossRef] [PubMed]
15. Spry, C.J.; Davies, J.; Tai, P.C.; Olsen, E.G.; Oakley, C.M.; Goodwin, J.F. Clinical features of fifteen patients with the hypereosinophilic syndrome. *Q. J. Med.* **1983**, *52*, 1–22. [PubMed]
16. Ogbogu, P.U.; Bochner, B.S.; Butterfield, J.H.; Gleich, G.J.; Huss-Marp, J.; Kahn, J.E.; Leiferman, K.M.; Nutman, T.B.; Pfab, F.; Ring, J.; et al. Hypereosinophilic syndrome: A multicenter, retrospective analysis of clinical characteristics and response to therapy. *J. Allergy Clin. Immunol.* **2009**, *124*, 1319.e3–1325.e3. [CrossRef] [PubMed]

17. Liapis, H.; Ho, A.K.; Brown, D.; Mindel, G.; Gleich, G. Thrombotic microangiopathy associated with the hypereosinophilic syndrome. *Kidney Int.* **2005**, *67*, 1806–1811. [CrossRef]
18. Shehwaro, N.; Langlois, A.L.; Gueutin, V.; Izzedine, H. Renal involvement in idiopathic hypereosinophic syndrome. *Clin. Kidney J.* **2013**, *6*, 272–276. [CrossRef]
19. Muriithi, A.K.; Leung, N.; Valeri, A.M.; Cornell, L.D.; Sethi, S.; Fidler, M.E.; Nasr, S.H. Biopsy-proven acute interstitial nephritis, 1993–2011: A case series. *Am. J. Kidney Dis.* **2014**, *64*, 558–566. [CrossRef]
20. Baker, R.J.; Pusey, C.D. The changing profile of acute tubulointerstitial nephritis. *Nephrol. Dial. Transplant.* **2004**, *19*, 8–11. [CrossRef]
21. Kano, Y.; Ishida, T.; Hirahara, K.; Shiohara, T. Visceral involvements and long-term sequelae in drug-induced hypersensitivity syndrome. *Med. Clin. N. Am.* **2010**, *94*, 743–759. [CrossRef] [PubMed]
22. Wei, C.H.; Chung-Yee Hui, R.; Chang, C.J.; Ho, H.C.; Yang, C.H.; Lin, Y.J.; Chung, W.H. Identifying prognostic factors for drug rash with eosinophilia and systemic symptoms (DRESS). *Eur. J. Dermatol.* **2011**, *21*, 930–937.
23. Watanabe, H. Recent Advances in Drug-Induced Hypersensitivity Syndrome/Drug Reaction with Eosinophilia and Systemic Symptoms. *J. Immunol. Res.* **2018**, *2018*, 5163129. [CrossRef]
24. Sinico, R.A.; Di Toma, L.; Maggiore, U.; Bottero, P.; Radice, A.; Tosoni, C.; Grasselli, C.; Pavone, L.; Gregorini, G.; Monti, S.; et al. Prevalence and clinical significance of antineutrophil cytoplasmic antibodies in Churg-Strauss syndrome. *Arthritis Rheum.* **2005**, *52*, 2926–2935. [CrossRef] [PubMed]
25. Durel, C.A.; Berthiller, J.; Caboni, S.; Jayne, D.; Ninet, J.; Hot, A. Long-Term Followup of a Multicenter Cohort of 101 Patients with Eosinophilic Granulomatosis with Polyangiitis (Churg-Strauss). *Arthritis Care Res.* **2016**, *68*, 374–387. [CrossRef] [PubMed]
26. Groh, M.; Pagnoux, C.; Baldini, C.; Bel, E.; Bottero, P.; Cottin, V.; Dalhoff, K.; Dunogue, B.; Gross, W.; Holle, J.; et al. Eosinophilic granulomatosis with polyangiitis (Churg-Strauss) (EGPA) Consensus Task Force recommendations for evaluation and management. *Eur. J. Intern. Med.* **2015**, *26*, 545–553. [CrossRef] [PubMed]
27. Bertsias, G.K.; Tektonidou, M.; Amoura, Z.; Aringer, M.; Bajema, I.; Berden, J.H.; Boletis, J.; Cervera, R.; Dorner, T.; Doria, A.; et al. Joint European League Against Rheumatism and European Renal Association-European Dialysis and Transplant Association (EULAR/ERA-EDTA) recommendations for the management of adult and paediatric lupus nephritis. *Ann. Rheum. Dis.* **2012**, *71*, 1771–1782. [CrossRef] [PubMed]
28. Anzai, M.; Maezawai, R.; Ohara, T.; Kodama, K.; Fukuda, T.; Kurasawa, K. Systemic lupus erythematosus associated with facial edema, overproduction of interleukin-5, and eosinophilia. *J. Clin. Rheumatol.* **2008**, *14*, 361–362. [CrossRef]
29. Kang, E.; Yoo, S.H.; Oh, D.; Joo, K.W.; Kim, Y.S.; Yoon, S.S.; Kim, I.; Park, S.; Lee, H.; Koh, Y. Clinical dissection of thrombotic microangiopathy. *Ann. Hematol.* **2017**, *96*, 1715–1726. [CrossRef] [PubMed]
30. Agrawal, A.; Ziccardi, M.R.; Witzke, C.; Palacios, I.; Rangaswami, J. Cholesterol embolization syndrome: An under-recognized entity in cardiovascular interventions. *J. Interv. Cardiol.* **2018**, *31*, 407–415. [CrossRef]
31. Thadhani, R.I.; Camargo, C.A., Jr.; Xavier, R.J.; Fang, L.S.; Bazari, H. Atheroembolic renal failure after invasive procedures. Natural history based on 52 histologically proven cases. *Medicine* **1995**, *74*, 350–358. [CrossRef] [PubMed]
32. Lye, W.C.; Cheah, J.S.; Sinniah, R. Renal cholesterol embolic disease. Case report and review of the literature. *Am. J. Nephrol.* **1993**, *13*, 489–493. [CrossRef] [PubMed]
33. Rajpoot, D.K.; Pahl, M.; Clark, J. Nephrotic syndrome associated with Kimura disease. *Pediatr. Nephrol.* **2000**, *14*, 486–488. [CrossRef] [PubMed]
34. Matsuo, T.; Tanaka, T.; Kinomura, M. Nephrotic syndrome during the tapering of oral steroids after pathological diagnosis of Kimura disease from a lacrimal gland mass: Case report and review of 10 Japanese patients. *J. Clin. Exp. Hematop.* **2017**, *57*, 147–152. [CrossRef] [PubMed]
35. Mandeville, J.T.; Levinson, R.D.; Holland, G.N. The tubulointerstitial nephritis and uveitis syndrome. *Surv. Ophthalmol.* **2001**, *46*, 195–208. [CrossRef]
36. Brito-Zeron, P.; Ramos-Casals, M.; Bosch, X.; Stone, J.H. The clinical spectrum of IgG4-related disease. *Autoimmun. Rev.* **2014**, *13*, 1203–1210. [CrossRef] [PubMed]
37. Della Torre, E.; Mattoo, H.; Mahajan, V.S.; Carruthers, M.; Pillai, S.; Stone, J.H. Prevalence of atopy, eosinophilia, and IgE elevation in IgG4-related disease. *Allergy* **2014**, *69*, 269–272. [CrossRef]

38. Saeki, T.; Kobayashi, D.; Ito, T.; Tamura, M.; Yoshikawa, S.; Yamazaki, H. Comparison of clinical and laboratory features of patients with and without allergic conditions in IgG4-related disease: A single-center experience in Japan. *Mod. Rheumatol.* **2018**, *28*, 845–848. [CrossRef]
39. Hildebrand, S.; Corbett, R.; Duncan, N.; Ashby, D. Increased prevalence of eosinophilia in a hemodialysis population: Longitudinal and case control studies. *Hemodial. Int.* **2016**, *20*, 414–420. [CrossRef]
40. Hoy, W.E.; Cestero, R.V. Eosinophilia in maintenance hemodialysis patients. *J. Dial* **1979**, *3*, 73–87. [CrossRef]
41. Jo, Y.I.; Song, J.O.; Park, J.H.; Lee, J.H.; Shin, S.K. Idiopathic eosinophilic peritonitis in continuous ambulatory peritoneal dialysis: Experience with percutaneous catheter placement. *Nephrology* **2007**, *12*, 437–440. [CrossRef] [PubMed]
42. Chandran, P.K.; Humayun, H.M.; Daugirdas, J.T.; Nawab, Z.M.; Gandhi, V.C.; Ing, T.S. Blood eosinophilia in patients undergoing maintenance peritoneal dialysis. *Arch. Intern. Med.* **1985**, *145*, 114–116. [CrossRef]
43. Hongwei, W.; Nanra, R.S.; Stein, A.; Avis, L.; Price, A.; Hibberd, A.D. Eosinophils in acute renal allograft rejection. *Transpl. Immunol.* **1994**, *2*, 41–46. [CrossRef]
44. Geri, G.; Rabbat, A.; Mayaux, J.; Zafrani, L.; Chalumeau-Lemoine, L.; Guidet, B.; Azoulay, E.; Pene, F. Strongyloides stercoralis hyperinfection syndrome: A case series and a review of the literature. *Infection* **2015**, *43*, 691–698. [CrossRef]
45. Roxby, A.C.; Gottlieb, G.S.; Limaye, A.P. Strongyloidiasis in transplant patients. *Clin. Infect. Dis.* **2009**, *49*, 1411–1423. [CrossRef]
46. Praga, M.; Sevillano, A.; Aunon, P.; Gonzalez, E. Changes in the aetiology, clinical presentation and management of acute interstitial nephritis, an increasingly common cause of acute kidney injury. *Nephrol. Dial. Transplant.* **2015**, *30*, 1472–1479. [CrossRef] [PubMed]
47. Muriithi, A.K.; Nasr, S.H.; Leung, N. Utility of urine eosinophils in the diagnosis of acute interstitial nephritis. *Clin. J. Am. Soc. Nephrol.* **2013**, *8*, 1857–1862. [CrossRef] [PubMed]
48. Praga, M.; Gonzalez, E. Acute interstitial nephritis. *Kidney Int.* **2010**, *77*, 956–961. [CrossRef]
49. Clarkson, M.R.; Giblin, L.; O'Connell, F.P.; O'Kelly, P.; Walshe, J.J.; Conlon, P.; O'Meara, Y.; Dormon, A.; Campbell, E.; Donohoe, J. Acute interstitial nephritis: Clinical features and response to corticosteroid therapy. *Nephrol. Dial. Transplant.* **2004**, *19*, 2778–2783. [CrossRef]
50. Gonzalez, E.; Gutierrez, E.; Galeano, C.; Chevia, C.; de Sequera, P.; Bernis, C.; Parra, E.G.; Delgado, R.; Sanz, M.; Ortiz, M.; et al. Early steroid treatment improves the recovery of renal function in patients with drug-induced acute interstitial nephritis. *Kidney Int.* **2008**, *73*, 940–946. [CrossRef]
51. Moledina, D.G.; Perazella, M.A. Treatment of Drug-Induced Acute Tubulointerstitial Nephritis: The Search for Better Evidence. *Clin. J. Am. Soc. Nephrol.* **2018**. [CrossRef] [PubMed]
52. Prendecki, M.; Tanna, A.; Salama, A.D.; Tam, F.W.; Cairns, T.; Taube, D.; Cook, H.T.; Ashby, D.; Duncan, N.D.; Pusey, C.D. Long-term outcome in biopsy-proven acute interstitial nephritis treated with steroids. *Clin. Kidney J.* **2017**, *10*, 233–239. [CrossRef] [PubMed]
53. Fernandez-Juarez, G.; Perez, J.V.; Caravaca-Fontan, F.; Quintana, L.; Shabaka, A.; Rodriguez, E.; Gadola, L.; de Lorenzo, A.; Cobo, M.A.; Oliet, A.; et al. Duration of Treatment with Corticosteroids and Recovery of Kidney Function in Acute Interstitial Nephritis. *Clin. J. Am. Soc. Nephrol.* **2018**. [CrossRef] [PubMed]
54. Kano, Y.; Hiraharas, K.; Sakuma, K.; Shiohara, T. Several herpesviruses can reactivate in a severe drug-induced multiorgan reaction in the same sequential order as in graft-versus-host disease. *Br. J. Dermatol.* **2006**, *155*, 301–306. [CrossRef] [PubMed]
55. Roujeau, J.C.; Dupin, N. Virus Reactivation in Drug Reaction with Eosinophilia and Systemic Symptoms (Dress) Results from a Strong Drug-Specific Immune Response. *J. Allergy Clin. Immunol. Pract.* **2017**, *5*, 811–812. [CrossRef] [PubMed]
56. Descamps, V.; Ranger-Rogez, S. DRESS syndrome. *Joint Bone Spine* **2014**, *81*, 15–21. [CrossRef] [PubMed]
57. Cacoub, P.; Musette, P.; Descamps, V.; Meyer, O.; Speirs, C.; Finzi, L.; Roujeau, J.C. The DRESS syndrome: A literature review. *Am. J. Med.* **2011**, *124*, 588–597. [CrossRef]
58. Roujeau, J.C.; Stern, R.S. Severe adverse cutaneous reactions to drugs. *N. Engl. J. Med.* **1994**, *331*, 1272–1285. [CrossRef]
59. De, A.; Rajagopalan, M.; Sarda, A.; Das, S.; Biswas, P. Drug Reaction with Eosinophilia and Systemic Symptoms: An Update and Review of Recent Literature. *Indian J. Dermatol.* **2018**, *63*, 30–40. [CrossRef]
60. Kito, Y.; Ito, T.; Tokura, Y.; Hashizume, H. High-dose intravenous immunoglobulin monotherapy for drug-induced hypersensitivity syndrome. *Acta Derm. Venereol.* **2012**, *92*, 100–101. [CrossRef]

61. Joly, P.; Janela, B.; Tetart, F.; Rogez, S.; Picard, D.; D'Incan, M.; Descamps, V.; Collet, E.; Roujeau, J.C.; Musette, P. Poor benefit/risk balance of intravenous immunoglobulins in DRESS. *Arch. Dermatol.* **2012**, *148*, 543–544. [CrossRef] [PubMed]
62. Husain, Z.; Reddy, B.Y.; Schwartz, R.A. DRESS syndrome: Part II. Management and therapeutics. *J. Am. Acad. Dermatol.* **2013**, *68*, 709.e1-9. [CrossRef] [PubMed]
63. Blumenthal, K.G.; Youngster, I.; Rabideau, D.J.; Parker, R.A.; Manning, K.S.; Walensky, R.P.; Nelson, S.B. Peripheral blood eosinophilia and hypersensitivity reactions among patients receiving outpatient parenteral antibiotics. *J. Allergy Clin. Immunol.* **2015**, *136*, 1288.e1–1294.e1. [CrossRef] [PubMed]
64. Masi, A.T.; Hunder, G.G.; Lie, J.T.; Michel, B.A.; Bloch, D.A.; Arend, W.P.; Calabrese, L.H.; Edworthy, S.M.; Fauci, A.S.; Leavitt, R.Y. The American College of Rheumatology 1990 criteria for the classification of Churg-Strauss syndrome (allergic granulomatosis and angiitis). *Arthritis Rheum.* **1990**, *33*, 1094–1100. [CrossRef] [PubMed]
65. Comarmond, C.; Pagnoux, C.; Khellaf, M.; Cordier, J.F.; Hamidou, M.; Viallard, J.F.; Maurier, F.; Jouneau, S.; Bienvenu, B.; Puechal, X.; et al. Eosinophilic granulomatosis with polyangiitis (Churg-Strauss): Clinical characteristics and long-term followup of the 383 patients enrolled in the French Vasculitis Study Group cohort. *Arthritis Rheum.* **2013**, *65*, 270–281. [CrossRef]
66. Sable-Fourtassou, R.; Cohen, P.; Mahr, A.; Pagnoux, C.; Mouthon, L.; Jayne, D.; Blockmans, D.; Cordier, J.F.; Delaval, P.; Puechal, X.; et al. Antineutrophil cytoplasmic antibodies and the Churg-Strauss syndrome. *Ann. Intern. Med.* **2005**, *143*, 632–638. [CrossRef] [PubMed]
67. Healy, B.; Bibby, S.; Steele, R.; Weatherall, M.; Nelson, H.; Beasley, R. Antineutrophil cytoplasmic autoantibodies and myeloperoxidase autoantibodies in clinical expression of Churg-Strauss syndrome. *J. Allergy Clin. Immunol.* **2013**, 131. [CrossRef]
68. Jennette, J.C.; Falk, R.J.; Bacon, P.A.; Basu, N.; Cid, M.C.; Ferrario, F.; Flores-Suarez, L.F.; Gross, W.L.; Guillevin, L.; Hagen, E.C.; et al. 2012 revised International Chapel Hill Consensus Conference Nomenclature of Vasculitides. *Arthritis Rheum.* **2013**, *65*, 1–11. [CrossRef]
69. Chaigne, B.; Terrier, B.; Thieblemont, N.; Witko-Sarsat, V.; Mouthon, L. Dividing the Janus vasculitis? Pathophysiology of eosinophilic granulomatosis with polyangitis. *Autoimmun. Rev.* **2016**, *15*, 139–145. [CrossRef]
70. Alberici, F.; Martorana, D.; Vaglio, A. Genetic aspects of anti-neutrophil cytoplasmic antibody-associated vasculitis. *Nephrol. Dial. Transplant.* **2015**, *30* (Suppl. 1), i37–i45. [CrossRef]
71. Vaglio, A.; Martorana, D.; Maggiore, U.; Grasselli, C.; Zanetti, A.; Pesci, A.; Garini, G.; Manganelli, P.; Bottero, P.; Tumiati, B.; et al. HLA-DRB4 as a genetic risk factor for Churg-Strauss syndrome. *Arthritis Rheum.* **2007**, *56*, 3159–3166. [CrossRef] [PubMed]
72. Wieczorek, S.; Hellmich, B.; Arning, L.; Moosig, F.; Lamprecht, P.; Gross, W.L.; Epplen, J.T. Functionally relevant variations of the interleukin-10 gene associated with antineutrophil cytoplasmic antibody-negative Churg-Strauss syndrome, but not with Wegener's granulomatosis. *Arthritis Rheum.* **2008**, *58*, 1839–1848. [CrossRef] [PubMed]
73. Navarro-Mendoza, E.P.; Tobon, G.J. Eosinophilic Granulomatosis with Polyangiitis: Newer Therapies. *Curr. Rheumatol. Rep.* **2018**, *20*, 23. [CrossRef] [PubMed]
74. Yates, M.; Watts, R.; Bajema, I.; Cid, M.; Crestani, B.; Hauser, T.; Hellmich, B.; Holle, J.; Laudien, M.; Little, M.A.; et al. Validation of the EULAR/ERA-EDTA recommendations for the management of ANCA-associated vasculitis by disease content experts. *RMD Open* **2017**, *3*, e000449. [CrossRef] [PubMed]
75. Stone, J.H.; Merkel, P.A.; Spiera, R.; Seo, P.; Langford, C.A.; Hoffman, G.S.; Kallenberg, C.G.; St Clair, E.W.; Turkiewicz, A.; Tchao, N.K.; et al. Rituximab versus cyclophosphamide for ANCA-associated vasculitis. *N. Engl. J. Med.* **2010**, *363*, 221–232. [CrossRef]
76. Jones, R.B.; Tervaert, J.W.; Hauser, T.; Luqmani, R.; Morgan, M.D.; Peh, C.A.; Savage, C.O.; Segelmark, M.; Tesar, V.; van Paassen, P.; et al. Rituximab versus cyclophosphamide in ANCA-associated renal vasculitis. *N. Engl. J. Med.* **2010**, *363*, 211–220. [CrossRef]
77. Mohammad, A.J.; Hot, A.; Arndt, F.; Moosig, F.; Guerry, M.J.; Amudala, N.; Smith, R.; Sivasothy, P.; Guillevin, L.; Merkel, P.A.; Jayne, D.R. Rituximab for the treatment of eosinophilic granulomatosis with polyangiitis (Churg-Strauss). *Ann. Rheum. Dis.* **2016**, *75*, 396–401. [CrossRef]
78. Wechsler, M.E.; Akuthota, P.; Jayne, D.; Khoury, P.; Klion, A.; Langford, C.A.; Merkel, P.A.; Moosig, F.; Specks, U.; Cid, M.C.; et al. Mepolizumab or Placebo for Eosinophilic Granulomatosis with Polyangiitis. *N. Engl. J. Med.* **2017**, *376*, 1921–1932. [CrossRef]

79. Raffray, L.; Guillevin, L. Treatment of Eosinophilic Granulomatosis with Polyangiitis: A Review. *Drugs* **2018**. [CrossRef]
80. Kim, S.; Marigowda, G.; Oren, E.; Israel, E.; Wechsler, M.E. Mepolizumab as a steroid-sparing treatment option in patients with Churg-Strauss syndrome. *J. Allergy Clin. Immunol.* **2010**, *125*, 1336–1343. [CrossRef]
81. Moosig, F.; Gross, W.L.; Herrmann, K.; Bremer, J.P.; Hellmich, B. Targeting interleukin-5 in refractory and relapsing Churg-Strauss syndrome. *Ann. Intern. Med.* **2011**, *155*, 341–343. [CrossRef] [PubMed]
82. Cartin-Ceba, R.; Keogh, K.A.; Specks, U.; Sethi, S.; Fervenza, F.C. Rituximab for the treatment of Churg-Strauss syndrome with renal involvement. *Nephrol. Dial. Transplant.* **2011**, *26*, 2865–2871. [CrossRef] [PubMed]
83. Kuhn, D.; Hospowsky, C.; Both, M.; Hey, M.; Laudien, M. Manifestation of granulomatosis with polyangiitis in head and neck. *Clin. Exp. Rheumatol.* **2018**, *36* (Suppl. 111), 78–84. [PubMed]
84. Seccia, V.; Baldini, C.; Latorre, M.; Gelardi, M.; Dallan, I.; Cristofani-Mencacci, L.; Sellari-Franceschini, S.; Bartoli, M.L.; Bacci, E.; Paggiaro, P. Focus on the Involvement of the Nose and Paranasal Sinuses in Eosinophilic Granulomatosis with Polyangiitis (Churg-Strauss Syndrome): Nasal Cytology Reveals Infiltration of Eosinophils as a Very Common Feature. *Int. Arch. Allergy Immunol.* **2018**, *175*, 61–69. [CrossRef] [PubMed]
85. Potter, M.B.; Fincher, R.K.; Finger, D.R. Eosinophilia in Wegener's granulomatosis. *Chest* **1999**, *116*, 1480–1483. [CrossRef] [PubMed]
86. Shoda, H.; Kanda, H.; Tanaka, R.; Komagata, Y.; Misaki, Y.; Yamamoto, K. Wegener's granulomatosis with eosinophilia. *Intern. Med.* **2005**, *44*, 750–753. [CrossRef] [PubMed]
87. Uematsu, H.; Takata, S.; Sueishi, K.; Inoue, H. Polyangiitis overlap syndrome of granulomatosis with polyangiitis (Wegener's granulomatosis) and eosinophilic granulomatosis with polyangiitis (Churg-Strauss syndrome). *BMJ Case Rep.* **2014**, *2014*. [CrossRef]
88. Kroegel, C.; Foerster, M.; Quickert, S.; Slevogt, H.; Neumann, T. Vasculitides and eosinophilic pulmonary diseases. *Internist* **2018**, *59*, 898–910. [CrossRef]
89. Khoury, P.; Zagallo, P.; Talar-Williams, C.; Santos, C.S.; Dinerman, E.; Holland, N.C.; Klion, A.D. Serum biomarkers are similar in Churg-Strauss syndrome and hypereosinophilic syndrome. *Allergy* **2012**, *67*, 1149–1156. [CrossRef]
90. Emmi, G.; Silvestri, E.; Marconi, R.; Carrai, V.; Fanelli, T.; Zucchini, P.; Marasca, R.; Vannucchi, A.M.; Emmi, L.; Prisco, D.; et al. First report of FIP1L1-PDGFRalpha-positive eosinophilic granulomatosis with polyangiitis. *Rheumatology* **2015**, *54*, 1751–1753. [CrossRef]
91. Beketova, T.V.; Volkov, M.Y.; Naryshkin, E.A.; Novoselova, T.M.; Nasonov, E.L. Imatinib mesylate use in refractory eosinophilic granulomatosis with polyangiitis: A literature review and a case report. *Clin. Rheumatol.* **2018**, *37*, 1729–1735. [CrossRef] [PubMed]
92. Groh, M.; Kahn, J.E.; Puechal, X.; Guillevin, L. Comment on: First report of FIP1L1-PDGFRalpha-positive eosinophilic granulomatosis with polyangiitis. *Rheumatology* **2016**, *55*, 384–385. [CrossRef] [PubMed]
93. Harvey, A.M.; Shulman, L.E.; Tumulty, P.A.; Conley, C.L.; Schoenrich, E.H. Systemic lupus erythematosus: Review of the literature and clinical analysis of 138 cases. *Medicine* **1954**, *33*, 291–437. [CrossRef] [PubMed]
94. Thomeer, M.; Moerman, P.; Westhovens, R.; Van den Eeckhout, A.; Dequeker, J.; Demedts, M. Systemic lupus erythematosus, eosinophilia and Loffler's endocarditis. An unusual association. *Eur. Respir. J.* **1999**, *13*, 930–933. [CrossRef] [PubMed]
95. Aydogdu, S.; Ucar, O.; Cetin, M. A case of systemic lupus erythematosus presenting with hypereosinophilia and Loeffler endocarditis. *Acta Cardiol.* **2010**, *65*, 571–573. [CrossRef] [PubMed]
96. Yin, G.; Xie, Q. Systemic lupus erythematosus associated with Wells' syndrome. *Rheumatol. Int.* **2012**, *32*, 1087–1089. [CrossRef] [PubMed]
97. Kojima, T.; Umeno, M.; Takaki, K.; Tanaka, M.; Takeda, T.; Nagasawa, K. A case of SLE with the onset of pleuritis showing eosinophilia and elevation of serum IgE. *Fukuoka Igaku Zasshi* **1996**, *87*, 97–101.
98. Fukui, S.; Iwamoto, N.; Tsuji, S.; Umeda, M.; Nishino, A.; Nakashima, Y.; Suzuki, T.; Horai, Y.; Koga, T.; Kawashiri, S.Y.; et al. Eosinophilic Granulomatosis with Polyangiitis With Thrombotic Microangiopathy: Is Simultaneous Systemic Lupus Erythematosus Associated with Clinical Manifestations? A Case Report and Review of the Literature. *Medicine* **2015**, *94*, e1943. [CrossRef]
99. Kargili, A.; Bavbek, N.; Kaya, A.; Kosar, A.; Karaaslan, Y. Eosinophilia in rheumatologic diseases: A prospective study of 1000 cases. *Rheumatol. Int.* **2004**, *24*, 321–324. [CrossRef] [PubMed]

100. Yang, Z.; Zhang, Z.; Lin, F.; Ren, Y.; Liu, D.; Zhong, R.; Liang, Y. Comparisons of neutrophil-, monocyte-, eosinophil-, and basophil-lymphocyte ratios among various systemic autoimmune rheumatic diseases. *APMIS* **2017**, *125*, 863–871. [CrossRef] [PubMed]
101. Brocklebank, V.; Wood, K.M.; Kavanagh, D. Thrombotic Microangiopathy and the Kidney. *Clin. J. Am. Soc. Nephrol.* **2018**, *13*, 300–317. [CrossRef] [PubMed]
102. Ohguchi, H.; Sugawara, T.; Harigae, H. Thrombotic thrombocytopenic purpura complicated with hypereosinophilic syndrome. *Intern. Med.* **2009**, *48*, 1687–1690. [CrossRef] [PubMed]
103. Yuste, C.; Quiroga, B.; Verde, E.; Barraca, D.; Reque, J.E.; Perez de Jose, A.; Luno, J. The non-casual relation between eosinophilia and thrombotic microangiopathy. *Transfus. Apher. Sci.* **2012**, *47*, 365–367. [CrossRef] [PubMed]
104. Langlois, A.L.; Shehwaro, N.; Rondet, C.; Benbrik, Y.; Maloum, K.; Gueutin, V.; Rouvier, P.; Izzedine, H. Renal thrombotic microangiopathy and FIP1L1/PDGFRalpha-associated myeloproliferative variant of hypereosinophilic syndrome. *Clin. Kidney J.* **2013**, *6*, 418–420. [CrossRef] [PubMed]
105. Chaudhary, L.N.; Bailey, N.G.; Vos, J.A.; Stotler, C.J. Unique association of myeloid neoplasm with eosinophilia and abnormalities of PDGFRA with TTP. *W. V. Med. J.* **2013**, *109*, 6–9. [PubMed]
106. Mulvey, J.J.; Magro, C.; Chadburn, A. Resolution of a steroid-resistant, hypereosinophilic immune diathesis with mepolizumab and concomitant amelioration of a mixed thrombotic microangiopathy. *Blood Cells Mol. Dis.* **2018**, *69*, 38–42. [CrossRef] [PubMed]
107. Basak, R.; Wang, X.; Keane, C.; Woroniecki, R. Atypical presentation of atypical haemolytic uraemic syndrome. *BMJ Case Rep.* **2018**, *2018*. [CrossRef] [PubMed]
108. Cao, M.; Ferreiro, T.; Leite, B.N.; Pita, F.; Bolanos, L.; Valdes, F.; Alonso, A.; Vazquez, E.; Mosquera, J.; Trigas, M.; et al. Two cases of atypical hemolytic uremic syndrome (aHUS) and eosinophilic granulomatosis with polyangiitis (EGPA): A possible relationship. *CEN Case Rep.* **2017**, *6*, 91–97. [CrossRef]
109. Maino, A.; Rossio, R.; Cugno, M.; Marzano, A.V.; Tedeschi, A. Hypereosinophilic syndrome, Churg-Strauss syndrome and parasitic diseases: Possible links between eosinophilia and thrombosis. *Curr. Vasc. Pharmacol.* **2012**, *10*, 670–675. [CrossRef]
110. Roufosse, F. L4. Eosinophils: How they contribute to endothelial damage and dysfunction. *Presse Med.* **2013**, *42*, 503–507. [CrossRef]
111. Li, X.; Bayliss, G.; Zhuang, S. Cholesterol Crystal Embolism and Chronic Kidney Disease. *Int. J. Mol. Sci.* **2017**, *18*, 1120. [CrossRef]
112. Scolari, F.; Ravani, P.; Gaggi, R.; Santostefano, M.; Rollino, C.; Stabellini, N.; Colla, L.; Viola, B.F.; Maiorca, P.; Venturelli, C.; et al. The challenge of diagnosing atheroembolic renal disease: Clinical features and prognostic factors. *Circulation* **2007**, *116*, 298–304. [CrossRef]
113. Lusco, M.A.; Najafian, B.; Alpers, C.E.; Fogo, A.B. AJKD Atlas of Renal Pathology: Cholesterol Emboli. *Am. J. Kidney Dis.* **2016**, *67*, e23–e24. [CrossRef]
114. Fukumoto, Y.; Tsutsui, H.; Tsuchihashi, M.; Masumoto, A.; Takeshita, A.; Cholesterol Embolism Study (CHEST). Investigators The incidence and risk factors of cholesterol embolization syndrome, a complication of cardiac catheterization: A prospective study. *J. Am. Coll. Cardiol.* **2003**, *42*, 211–216. [CrossRef]
115. Ramirez, G.; O'Neill, W.M., Jr.; Lambert, R.; Bloomer, H. Cholesterol embolization: A complication of angiography. *Arch. Intern. Med.* **1978**, *138*, 1430–1432. [CrossRef] [PubMed]
116. Mayo, R.R.; Swartz, R.D. Redefining the incidence of clinically detectable atheroembolism. *Am. J. Med.* **1996**, *100*, 524–529. [CrossRef]
117. Ishii, R.; Fujita, S.; Kizawa, S.; Sakane, K.; Morita, H.; Ozeki, M.; Sohmiya, K.; Hoshiga, M.; Ishizaka, N. Association between absolute blood eosinophil count and CKD stages among cardiac patients. *Heart Vessels* **2016**, *31*, 198–205. [CrossRef] [PubMed]
118. Igarashi, Y.; Akimoto, T.; Kobayashi, T.; Iwazu, Y.; Miki, T.; Otani-Takei, N.; Imai, T.; Sugase, T.; Masuda, T.; Takeda, S.I.; et al. Performing Anticoagulation: A Puzzling Case of Cholesterol Embolization Syndrome. *Clin. Med. Insights Case Rep.* **2017**, 10. [CrossRef]
119. Ishiyama, K.; Sato, T.; Taguma, Y. Low-Density Lipoprotein Apheresis Ameliorates Renal Prognosis of Cholesterol Crystal Embolism. *Ther. Apher. Dial.* **2015**, *19*, 355–360. [CrossRef]
120. Scolari, F.; Ravani, P.; Pola, A.; Guerini, S.; Zubani, R.; Movilli, E.; Savoldi, S.; Malberti, F.; Maiorca, R. Predictors of renal and patient outcomes in atheroembolic renal disease: A prospective study. *J. Am. Soc. Nephrol.* **2003**, *14*, 1584–1590. [CrossRef]

121. Deng, W.Y.; Ye, S.B.; Luo, R.Z.; Yan, S.M.; Gao, Y.F.; Yang, Y.Z.; Guo, Z.M.; Chen, Y.F. Notch-1 and Ki-67 receptor as predictors for the recurrence and prognosis of Kimura's disease. *Int. J. Clin. Exp. Pathol.* **2014**, *7*, 2402–2410. [PubMed]
122. Glibbery, N.; Muscat, K.; Cascarini, L. Kimura's disease of the parotid gland with cutaneous features in a Caucasian female patient. *J. Surg. Case Rep.* **2018**, *2018*, rjy067. [CrossRef] [PubMed]
123. Drouillard, M.; Steve, M.; Ranoarivony, T.; Souraud, J.B. Kimura's disease in a 50-year-old Tunisian man. *Eur. Ann. Otorhinolaryngol. Head Neck Dis.* **2017**, *134*, 127–129. [CrossRef] [PubMed]
124. Osuch-Wojcikiewicz, E.; Bruzgielewicz, A.; Lachowska, M.; Wasilewska, A.; Niemczyk, K. Kimura's Disease in a Caucasian Female: A Very Rare Cause of Lymphadenopathy. *Case Rep. Otolaryngol.* **2014**, *2014*, 415865. [CrossRef] [PubMed]
125. McKelvie, P.A.; Lyons, B.; Barnett, G.; Allen, P.W. Kimura's disease in two Caucasians, one with multiple recurrences associated with prominent IgG4 production. *Pathology* **2012**, *44*, 275–278. [CrossRef] [PubMed]
126. Noel, N.; Meignin, V.; Rosenstingl, S.; Ronco, P.; Boffa, J.J. Nephrotic syndrome associated with immune thrombocytopenia revealing Kimura's disease in a non-Asian male. *NDT Plus* **2009**, *2*, 452–454. [CrossRef] [PubMed]
127. Muller-Richter, U.D.; Moralis, A.; Reuther, T.; Kochel, M.; Reichert, T.E.; Driemel, O. Kimura's disease in a white man. *Head Neck* **2011**, *33*, 138–140. [CrossRef]
128. De Bastos, J.T.; da Rocha, C.R.M.; Silva, P.M.C.; de Freitas, B.M.P.; Cassia, F.F.; Avelleira, J.C.R. Angiolymphoid hyperplasia with eosinophilia versus Kimura's disease: A case report and a clinical and histopathological comparison. *An. Bras. Dermatol.* **2017**, *92*, 392–394. [CrossRef]
129. Rathore, S.S.; Arora, P.; Usha; Prakash, J. Mesangioproliferative glomerulonephritis in a patient with Kimura's disease presenting as Nephrotic syndrome. *Saudi J. Kidney Dis. Transpl.* **2015**, *26*, 115–118. [CrossRef]
130. Wang, D.Y.; Mao, J.H.; Zhang, Y.; Gu, W.Z.; Zhao, S.A.; Chen, Y.F.; Liu, A.M. Kimura disease: A case report and review of the Chinese literature. *Nephron Clin. Pract.* **2009**, *111*, c55–c61. [CrossRef]
131. Okura, T.; Miyoshi, K.; Irita, J.; Enomoto, D.; Nagao, T.; Kukida, M.; Tanino, A.; Kudo, K.; Higaki, J. Kimura's disease associated with membranous nephropathy with IgG4 and phospholipase A2 receptor-positive staining of the glomerular basement membrane. *Intern. Med.* **2014**, *53*, 1435–1440. [CrossRef] [PubMed]
132. Obata, Y.; Furusu, A.; Nishino, T.; Ichinose, H.; Ohnita, A.; Iwasaki, K.; Taguchi, T.; Kohno, S. Membranous nephropathy and Kimura's disease manifesting a hip mass. A case report with literature review. *Intern. Med.* **2010**, *49*, 1405–1409. [CrossRef] [PubMed]
133. Kar, I.B.; Sethi, A.K. Kimura's Disease: Report of a Case & Review of Literature. *J. Maxillofac. Oral. Surg.* **2013**, *12*, 109–112.
134. Chim, C.S.; Liang, R.; Fung, A.; Kwong, Y.L.; Shek, T.W. Further analysis of clonality in Kimura's disease. *Am. J. Surg. Pathol.* **2003**, *27*, 703–704. [CrossRef]
135. Kim, S.H.; Park, S.J.; Han, K.H.; Kronbichler, A.; Saleem, M.A.; Oh, J.; Lim, B.J.; Shin, J.I. Pathogenesis of minimal change nephrotic syndrome: An immunological concept. *Korean J. Pediatr.* **2016**, *59*, 205–211. [CrossRef] [PubMed]
136. Zhu, S.L.; Wei, P.F.; Chen, J.H.; Zhao, Z.F.; Xu, Q.N.; Ye, L. Diagnosis and treatment of a patient with Kimura's disease associated with nephrotic syndrome and lymphadenopathy of the epitrochlear nodes. *BMC Nephrol.* **2015**, *16*, 10-015-0007-7. [CrossRef] [PubMed]
137. Dobrin, R.S.; Vernier, R.L.; Fish, A.L. Acute eosinophilic interstitial nephritis and renal failure with bone marrow-lymph node granulomas and anterior uveitis. A new syndrome. *Am. J. Med.* **1975**, *59*, 325–333. [CrossRef]
138. Clive, D.M.; Vanguri, V.K. The Syndrome of Tubulointerstitial Nephritis with Uveitis (TINU). *Am. J. Kidney Dis.* **2018**, *72*, 118–128. [CrossRef]
139. Azar, R.; Verove, C.; Boldron, A. Delayed onset of uveitis in TINU syndrome. *J. Nephrol.* **2000**, *13*, 381–383.
140. Reddy, A.K.; Hwang, Y.S.; Mandelcorn, E.D.; Davis, J.L. HLA-DR, DQ class II DNA typing in pediatric panuveitis and tubulointerstitial nephritis and uveitis. *Am. J. Ophthalmol.* **2014**, *157*, 678.e1-2–686.e1-2. [CrossRef]
141. Peräsaari, J.; Saarela, V.; Nikkilä, J.; Ala-Houhala, M.; Arikoski, P.; Kataja, J.; Rönnholm, K.; Merenmies, J.; Nuutinen, M.; Jahnukainen, T. HLA associations with tubulointerstitial nephritis with or without uveitis in Finnish pediatric population: A nation-wide study. *Tissue Antigens* **2013**, *81*, 435–441. [CrossRef] [PubMed]

142. Levinson, R.D.; Park, M.S.; Rikkers, S.M.; Reed, E.F.; Smith, J.R.; Martin, T.M.; Rosenbaum, J.T.; Foster, C.S.; Sherman, M.D.; Holland, G.N. Strong associations between specific HLA-DQ and HLA-DR alleles and the tubulointerstitial nephritis and uveitis syndrome. *Investig. Ophthalmol. Vis. Sci.* **2003**, *44*, 653–657. [CrossRef]
143. Mackensen, F.; David, F.; Schwenger, V.; Smith, L.K.; Rajalingam, R.; Levinson, R.D.; Austin, C.R.; Houghton, D.; Martin, T.M.; Rosenbaum, J.T. HLA-DRB1*0102 is associated with TINU syndrome and bilateral, sudden-onset anterior uveitis but not with interstitial nephritis alone. *Br. J. Ophthalmol.* **2011**, *95*, 971–975. [CrossRef]
144. Tan, Y.; Yu, F.; Qu, Z.; Su, T.; Xing, G.Q.; Wu, L.H.; Wang, F.M.; Liu, G.; Yang, L.; Zhao, M.H. Modified C-reactive protein might be a target autoantigen of TINU syndrome. *Clin. J. Am. Soc. Nephrol.* **2011**, *6*, 93–100. [CrossRef]
145. Onyekpe, I.; Shenoy, M.; Denley, H.; Riad, H.; Webb, N.J. Recurrent tubulointerstitial nephritis and uveitis syndrome in a renal transplant recipient. *Nephrol. Dial. Transplant.* **2011**, *26*, 3060–3062. [CrossRef] [PubMed]
146. Stone, J.H.; Zen, Y.; Deshpande, V. IgG4-related disease. *N. Engl. J. Med.* **2012**, *366*, 539–551. [CrossRef] [PubMed]
147. Hamano, H.; Kawa, S.; Horiuchi, A.; Unno, H.; Furuya, N.; Akamatsu, T.; Fukushima, M.; Nikaido, T.; Nakayama, K.; Usuda, N.; et al. High serum IgG4 concentrations in patients with sclerosing pancreatitis. *N. Engl. J. Med.* **2001**, *344*, 732–738. [CrossRef] [PubMed]
148. Kamisawa, T.; Funata, N.; Hayashi, Y.; Eishi, Y.; Koike, M.; Tsuruta, K.; Okamoto, A.; Egawa, N.; Nakajima, H. A new clinicopathological entity of IgG4-related autoimmune disease. *J. Gastroenterol.* **2003**, *38*, 982–984. [CrossRef] [PubMed]
149. De Buy Wenniger, L.J.; Culver, E.L.; Beuers, U. Exposure to occupational antigens might predispose to IgG4-related disease. *Hepatology* **2014**, *60*, 1453–1454. [CrossRef] [PubMed]
150. Culver, E.L.; Vermeulen, E.; Makuch, M.; van Leeuwen, A.; Sadler, R.; Cargill, T.; Klenerman, P.; Aalberse, R.C.; van Ham, S.M.; Barnes, E.; et al. Increased IgG4 responses to multiple food and animal antigens indicate a polyclonal expansion and differentiation of pre-existing B cells in IgG4-related disease. *Ann. Rheum. Dis.* **2015**, *74*, 944–947. [CrossRef] [PubMed]
151. Akiyama, M.; Takeuchi, T. IgG4-Related Disease: Beyond Glucocorticoids. *Drugs Aging* **2018**, *35*, 275–287. [CrossRef] [PubMed]
152. Hubers, L.M.; Vos, H.; Schuurman, A.R.; Erken, R.; Oude Elferink, R.P.; Burgering, B.; van de Graaf, S.F.J.; Beuers, U. Annexin A11 is targeted by IgG4 and IgG1 autoantibodies in IgG4-related disease. *Gut* **2018**, *67*, 728–735. [CrossRef] [PubMed]
153. Kawa, S.; Ota, M.; Yoshizawa, K.; Horiuchi, A.; Hamano, H.; Ochi, Y.; Nakayama, K.; Tokutake, Y.; Katsuyama, Y.; Saito, S.; et al. HLA DRB10405-DQB10401 haplotype is associated with autoimmune pancreatitis in the Japanese population. *Gastroenterology* **2002**, *122*, 1264–1269. [CrossRef] [PubMed]
154. Aalberse, R.C.; Stapel, S.O.; Schuurman, J.; Rispens, T. Immunoglobulin G4: An odd antibody. *Clin. Exp. Allergy* **2009**, *39*, 469–477. [CrossRef] [PubMed]
155. Shiokawa, M.; Kodama, Y.; Kuriyama, K.; Yoshimura, K.; Tomono, T.; Morita, T.; Kakiuchi, N.; Matsumori, T.; Mima, A.; Nishikawa, Y.; et al. Pathogenicity of IgG in patients with IgG4-related disease. *Gut* **2016**, *65*, 1322–1332. [CrossRef] [PubMed]
156. Stone, J.H.; Brito-Zeron, P.; Bosch, X.; Ramos-Casals, M. Diagnostic Approach to the Complexity of IgG4-Related Disease. *Mayo Clin. Proc.* **2015**, *90*, 927–939. [CrossRef] [PubMed]
157. Zhang, P.; Cornell, L.D. IgG4-Related Tubulointerstitial Nephritis. *Adv. Chronic Kidney Dis.* **2017**, *24*, 94–100. [CrossRef]
158. Saeki, T.; Nishi, S.; Imai, N.; Ito, T.; Yamazaki, H.; Kawano, M.; Yamamoto, M.; Takahashi, H.; Matsui, S.; Nakada, S.; et al. Clinicopathological characteristics of patients with IgG4-related tubulointerstitial nephritis. *Kidney Int.* **2010**, *78*, 1016–1023. [CrossRef]
159. Raissian, Y.; Nasr, S.H.; Larsen, C.P.; Colvin, R.B.; Smyrk, T.C.; Takahashi, N.; Bhalodia, A.; Sohani, A.R.; Zhang, L.; Chari, S.; et al. Diagnosis of IgG4-related tubulointerstitial nephritis. *J. Am. Soc. Nephrol.* **2011**, *22*, 1343–1352. [CrossRef]
160. Kawano, M.; Saeki, T.; Nakashima, H.; Nishi, S.; Yamaguchi, Y.; Hisano, S.; Yamanaka, N.; Inoue, D.; Yamamoto, M.; Takahashi, H.; et al. Proposal for diagnostic criteria for IgG4-related kidney disease. *Clin. Exp. Nephrol.* **2011**, *15*, 615–626. [CrossRef]

161. Kim, B.; Kim, J.H.; Byun, J.H.; Kim, H.J.; Lee, S.S.; Kim, S.Y.; Lee, M.G. IgG4-related kidney disease: MRI findings with emphasis on the usefulness of diffusion-weighted imaging. *Eur. J. Radiol.* **2014**, *83*, 1057–1062. [CrossRef] [PubMed]
162. Cai, Y.I.; Li, H.Z.; Zhang, Y.S. IgG4-related inflammatory pseudotumor of the kidney mimicking renal cell carcinoma: A case report. *Oncol. Lett.* **2016**, *11*, 3438–3440. [CrossRef] [PubMed]
163. Danlos, F.X.; Rossi, G.M.; Blockmans, D.; Emmi, G.; Kronbichler, A.; Durupt, S.; Maynard, C.; Luca, L.; Garrouste, C.; Lioger, B.; et al. Antineutrophil cytoplasmic antibody-associated vasculitides and IgG4-related disease: A new overlap syndrome. *Autoimmun. Rev.* **2017**, *16*, 1036–1043. [CrossRef] [PubMed]
164. Chang, S.Y.; Keogh, K.A.; Lewis, J.E.; Ryu, J.H.; Cornell, L.D.; Garrity, J.A.; Yi, E.S. IgG4-positive plasma cells in granulomatosis with polyangiitis (Wegener's): A clinicopathologic and immunohistochemical study on 43 granulomatosis with polyangiitis and 20 control cases. *Hum. Pathol.* **2013**, *44*, 2432–2437. [CrossRef] [PubMed]
165. Della-Torre, E.; Lanzillotta, M.; Campochiaro, C.; Bozzalla, E.; Bozzolo, E.; Bandiera, A.; Bazzigaluppi, E.; Canevari, C.; Modorati, G.; Stone, J.H.; et al. Antineutrophil cytoplasmic antibody positivity in IgG4-related disease: A case report and review of the literature. *Medicine* **2016**, *95*, e4633. [CrossRef]
166. Carruthers, M.N.; Park, S.; Slack, G.W.; Dalal, B.I.; Skinnider, B.F.; Schaeffer, D.F.; Dutz, J.P.; Law, J.K.; Donnellan, F.; Marquez, V.; et al. IgG4-related disease and lymphocyte-variant hypereosinophilic syndrome: A comparative case series. *Eur. J. Haematol.* **2017**, *98*, 378–387. [CrossRef] [PubMed]
167. Khosroshahi, A.; Wallace, Z.S.; Crowe, J.L.; Akamizu, T.; Azumi, A.; Carruthers, M.N.; Chari, S.T.; Della-Torre, E.; Frulloni, L.; Goto, H.; et al. International Consensus Guidance Statement on the Management and Treatment of IgG4-Related Disease. *Arthritis Rheumatol.* **2015**, *67*, 1688–1699. [CrossRef] [PubMed]
168. Najafian, B.; Fogo, A.B.; Lusco, M.A.; Alpers, C.E. AJKD Atlas of Renal Pathology: IgG4-Related Tubulointerstitial Nephritis. *Am. J. Kidney Dis.* **2017**, *69*, e19–e20. [CrossRef]
169. Alexander, M.P.; Larsen, C.P.; Gibson, I.W.; Nasr, S.H.; Sethi, S.; Fidler, M.E.; Raissian, Y.; Takahashi, N.; Chari, S.; Smyrk, T.C.; et al. Membranous glomerulonephritis is a manifestation of IgG4-related disease. *Kidney Int.* **2013**, *83*, 455–462. [CrossRef]
170. Yamamoto, M.; Takahashi, H.; Shinomura, Y. Mechanisms and assessment of IgG4-related disease: Lessons for the rheumatologist. *Nat. Rev. Rheumatol.* **2014**, *10*, 148–159. [CrossRef]
171. Quattrocchio, G.; Barreca, A.; Demarchi, A.; Solfietti, L.; Beltrame, G.; Fenoglio, R.; Ferro, M.; Mesiano, P.; Murgia, S.; Del Vecchio, G.; et al. IgG4-related kidney disease: The effects of a Rituximab-based immunosuppressive therapy. *Oncotarget* **2018**, *9*, 21337–21347. [CrossRef] [PubMed]
172. Wallace, Z.S.; Deshpande, V.; Mattoo, H.; Mahajan, V.S.; Kulikova, M.; Pillai, S.; Stone, J.H. IgG4-Related Disease: Clinical and Laboratory Features in One Hundred Twenty-Five Patients. *Arthritis Rheumatol.* **2015**, *67*, 2466–2475. [CrossRef] [PubMed]
173. Carruthers, M.N.; Topazian, M.D.; Khosroshahi, A.; Witzig, T.E.; Wallace, Z.S.; Hart, P.A.; Deshpande, V.; Smyrk, T.C.; Chari, S.; Stone, J.H. Rituximab for IgG4-related disease: A prospective, open-label trial. *Ann. Rheum. Dis.* **2015**, *74*, 1171–1177. [CrossRef]
174. Salvadori, M.; Tsalouchos, A. Immunoglobulin G4-related kidney diseases: An updated review. *World J. Nephrol.* **2018**, *7*, 29–40. [CrossRef]
175. Wallace, Z.S.; Mattoo, H.; Mahajan, V.S.; Kulikova, M.; Lu, L.; Deshpande, V.; Choi, H.K.; Pillai, S.; Stone, J.H. Predictors of disease relapse in IgG4-related disease following rituximab. *Rheumatology* **2016**, *55*, 1000–1008. [CrossRef]
176. Shilpa, R.; Sreekrishnan, T.P.; Kumar, K.P.G.; Neethu, C.M. A Case Report on Pregabalin-Induced Eosinophilia. *Consult. Pharm.* **2018**, *33*, 317–320. [CrossRef]
177. Alharbi, M.; Jhinger, R.K.; Wuerz, T.; Walkty, A. Marked peripheral eosinophilia due to prolonged administration of posaconazole. *JMM Case Rep.* **2017**, *4*, e005100. [CrossRef]
178. Fogo, A.B. Quiz page. Diabetic nephropathy with superimposed acute interstitial nephritis. *Am. J. Kidney Dis.* **2003**, *41*, A47, E1–E3.
179. Dai, D.F.; Sasaki, K.; Lin, M.Y.; Smith, K.D.; Nicosia, R.F.; Alpers, C.E.; Najafian, B. Interstitial eosinophilic aggregates in diabetic nephropathy: Allergy or not? *Nephrol. Dial. Transplant.* **2015**, *30*, 1370–1376. [CrossRef]
180. Hays, R.; Thompson, F.; Esterman, A.; McDermott, R. Strongyloides stercoralis, Eosinophilia, and Type 2 Diabetes Mellitus: The Predictive Value of Eosinophilia in the Diagnosis of S stercoralis Infection in an Endemic Community. *Open Forum Infect. Dis.* **2016**, *3*, ofw029. [CrossRef]

181. Cohen, S.D.; Kopp, J.B.; Kimmel, P.L. Kidney Diseases Associated with Human Immunodeficiency Virus Infection. *N. Engl. J. Med.* **2017**, *377*, 2363–2374. [CrossRef] [PubMed]
182. Al Mohajer, M.; Villarreal-Williams, E.; Andrade, R.A.; Giordano, T.P.; Serpa, J.A. Eosinophilia and associated factors in a large cohort of patients infected with human immunodeficiency virus. *South Med. J.* **2014**, *107*, 554–558. [CrossRef] [PubMed]
183. Sivaram, M.; White, A.; Radcliffe, K.W. Eosinophilia: Clinical significance in HIV-infected individuals. *Int. J. STD AIDS* **2012**, *23*, 635–638. [CrossRef] [PubMed]
184. Chou, A.; Serpa, J.A. Eosinophilia in patients infected with human immunodeficiency virus. *Curr. HIV/AIDS Rep.* **2015**, *12*, 313–316. [CrossRef]
185. Knudtson, E.; Para, M.; Boswell, H.; Fan-Havard, P. Drug rash with eosinophilia and systemic symptoms syndrome and renal toxicity with a nevirapine-containing regimen in a pregnant patient with human immunodeficiency virus. *Obstet. Gynecol.* **2003**, *101*, 1094–1097.
186. Angel-Moreno-Maroto, A.; Suarez-Castellano, L.; Hernandez-Cabrera, M.; Perez-Arellano, J.L. Severe efavirenz-induced hypersensitivity syndrome (not-DRESS) with acute renal failure. *J. Infect.* **2006**, *52*, e39–e40. [CrossRef] [PubMed]
187. Brandariz, D.; Smithson, A.; Anton-Vazquez, V. Drug reaction with eosinophilia and systemic symptoms related to antiretroviral treatment in human immunodeficiency virus patients. *Indian J. Sex. Transm. Dis. AIDS* **2017**, *38*, 163–170.
188. Thomas, M.; Hopkins, C.; Duffy, E.; Lee, D.; Loulergue, P.; Ripamonti, D.; Ostrov, D.A.; Phillips, E. Association of the HLA-B*53:01 Allele with Drug Reaction with Eosinophilia and Systemic Symptoms (DRESS) Syndrome During Treatment of HIV Infection with Raltegravir. *Clin. Infect. Dis.* **2017**, *64*, 1198–1203. [CrossRef]
189. Akosa, A.B.; Sherif, A.; Maidment, C.G. Kimura's disease and membranous nephropathy. *Nephron* **1991**, *58*, 472–474. [CrossRef]
190. Frigui, M.; Hmida, M.B.; Jallouli, M.; Kechaou, M.; Frikha, F.; Bahloul, Z. Membranous glomerulopathy associated with idiopathic hypereosinophilic syndrome. *Saudi J. Kidney Dis. Transpl.* **2010**, *21*, 320–322.
191. Yim, H.E.; Yoo, K.H.; Won, N.H.; Hong, Y.S.; Lee, J.W. Churg-Strauss syndrome in a child with IgA nephropathy. *Clin. Nephrol.* **2009**, *71*, 306–309. [CrossRef] [PubMed]
192. Natov, S.N.; Strom, J.A.; Ucci, A. Relapsing nephrotic syndrome in a patient with Kimura's disease and IgA glomerulonephritis. *Nephrol. Dial. Transplant.* **1998**, *13*, 2358–2363. [CrossRef]
193. Kitazawa, A.; Koda, R.; Yoshino, A.; Ueda, Y.; Takeda, T. An IgA1-lambda-type monoclonal immunoglobulin deposition disease associated with membranous features in a patient with IgG4-related kidney disease: A case report. *BMC Nephrol.* **2018**, *19*, 330. [CrossRef] [PubMed]
194. Takeda, S.; Takazakura, E.; Fukui, Y. Tubulointerstitial nephritis in a patient with eosinophilic fasciitis and IgA nephropathy. *Nephron* **1995**, *69*, 314–317. [CrossRef] [PubMed]
195. Patil, S.B.; Vanikar, A.V.; Gumber, M.R.; Kute, V.B.; Shah, P.R.; Patel, H.V.; Trivedi, H.L. Churg-Strauss syndrome presenting with acute kidney injury in a case of primary focal segmental glomerulosclerosis. *Int. Urol. Nephrol.* **2014**, *46*, 211–215. [CrossRef] [PubMed]
196. Romao, J.E.; Saldanha, L.B.; Ianez, L.E.; Sabbaga, E. Recurrence of focal segmental glomerulosclerosis associated with Kimura's disease after kidney transplantation. *Am. J. Kidney Dis.* **1998**, *31*, E3. [CrossRef] [PubMed]
197. Dede, F.; Ayli, D.; Atilgan, K.G.; Yuksel, C.; Duranay, M.; Sener, D.; Turker, F. Focal segmental glomerulosclerosis associating Kimura disease. *Ren. Fail.* **2005**, *27*, 353–355. [CrossRef] [PubMed]
198. Agarwal, R.; Light, R.P. Patterns and prognostic value of total and differential leukocyte count in chronic kidney disease. *Clin. J. Am. Soc. Nephrol.* **2011**, *6*, 1393–1399. [CrossRef]
199. Fukui, M.; Tanaka, M.; Hamaguchi, M.; Senmaru, T.; Sakabe, K.; Shiraishi, E.; Harusato, I.; Yamazaki, M.; Hasegawa, G.; Nakamura, N. Eosinophil count is positively correlated with albumin excretion rate in men with type 2 diabetes. *Clin. J. Am. Soc. Nephrol.* **2009**, *4*, 1761–1765. [CrossRef]
200. Solak, B.; Acikgoz, S.B.; Sipahi, S.; Erdem, T. Epidemiology and determinants of pruritus in pre-dialysis chronic kidney disease patients. *Int. Urol. Nephrol.* **2016**, *48*, 585–591. [CrossRef]
201. Gabizon, D.; Kaufman, S.; Shaked, U.; Evans, S.Y.; Modai, D. Eosinophilia in uremia. *Nephron* **1981**, *29*, 36–39. [CrossRef] [PubMed]
202. Hallgren, R.; Grefberg, N.; Venge, P. Elevated circulating levels of eosinophil cationic protein in uremia as signs of abnormal eosinophil homeostasis. *Nephron* **1984**, *36*, 10–14. [CrossRef] [PubMed]

203. Rockel, A.; Klinke, B.; Hertel, J.; Baur, X.; Thiel, C.; Abdelhamid, S.; Fiegel, P.; Walb, D. Allergy to dialysis materials. *Nephrol. Dial. Transplant.* **1989**, *4*, 646–652. [PubMed]
204. Rumpf, K.W.; Seubert, S.; Seubert, A.; Lowitz, H.D.; Valentin, R.; Rippe, H.; Ippen, H.; Scheler, F. Association of ethylene-oxide-induced IgE antibodies with symptoms in dialysis patients. *Lancet* **1985**, *2*, 1385–1387. [CrossRef]
205. Bommer, J.; Ritz, E. Ethylene oxide (ETO) as a major cause of anaphylactoid reactions in dialysis (a review). *Artif. Organs* **1987**, *11*, 111–117. [CrossRef]
206. Vienken, J.; Diamantoglou, M.; Henne, W.; Nederlof, B. Artificial dialysis membranes: From concept to large scale production. *Am. J. Nephrol.* **1999**, *19*, 355–362. [CrossRef] [PubMed]
207. Zhang, D.L.; Liu, J.; Cui, W.Y.; Ji, D.Y.; Zhang, Y.; Liu, W.H. Differences in bio-incompatibility among four biocompatible dialyzer membranes using in maintenance hemodialysis patients. *Ren. Fail.* **2011**, *33*, 682–691. [CrossRef]
208. Tielemans, C.; Madhoun, P.; Lenaers, M.; Schandene, L.; Goldman, M.; Vanherweghem, J.L. Anaphylactoid reactions during hemodialysis on AN69 membranes in patients receiving ACE inhibitors. *Kidney Int.* **1990**, *38*, 982–984. [CrossRef]
209. Ebo, D.G.; Bosmans, J.L.; Couttenye, M.M.; Stevens, W.J. Haemodialysis-associated anaphylactic and anaphylactoid reactions. *Allergy* **2006**, *61*, 211–220. [CrossRef]
210. Simon, P.; Potier, J.; Thebaud, H.E. Risk factors for acute hypersensitivity reactions in hemodialysis. *Nephrologie* **1996**, *17*, 163–170.
211. Li, Z.; Ma, L.; Zhao, S. Effect of polyflux membranes on the improvement of hemodialysis-associated eosinophilia: A case series. *Ren. Fail.* **2016**, *38*, 65–69. [CrossRef] [PubMed]
212. Lee, S.; Schoen, I. Eosinophilia of peritoneal fluid and peripheral blood associated with chronic peritoneal dialysis. *Am. J. Clin. Pathol.* **1967**, *47*, 638–640. [CrossRef] [PubMed]
213. Oh, S.Y.; Kim, H.; Kang, J.M.; Lim, S.H.; Park, H.D.; Jung, S.S.; Lee, K.B. Eosinophilic peritonitis in a patient with continuous ambulatory peritoneal dialysis (CAPD). *Korean J. Intern. Med.* **2004**, *19*, 121–123. [CrossRef] [PubMed]
214. Chan, M.K.; Chow, L.; Lam, S.S.; Jones, B. Peritoneal eosinophilia in patients on continuous ambulatory peritoneal dialysis: A prospective study. *Am. J. Kidney Dis.* **1988**, *11*, 180–183. [CrossRef]
215. Tzvi-Behr, S.; Frishberg, Y.; Ben-Shalom, E.; Rinat, C.; Becker-Cohen, R. Eosinophilia in a peritoneal dialysis patient: Answers. *Pediatr. Nephrol.* **2018**, *33*, 1507–1508. [CrossRef] [PubMed]
216. MacGinley, R.; Cooney, K.; Alexander, G.; Cohen, S.; Goldsmith, D.J. Relapsing culture-negative peritonitis in peritoneal dialysis patients exposed to icodextrin solution. *Am. J. Kidney Dis.* **2002**, *40*, 1030–1035. [CrossRef] [PubMed]
217. Nakamura, Y.; Okada, H.; Yasui, A.; Koh, T.; Yamane, T. Sclerosing encapsulating peritonitis associated with recurrent eosinophilic peritonitis. *Nephrol. Dial. Transplant.* **1999**, *14*, 768–770. [CrossRef]
218. Asghar, R.; Woodrow, G.; Turney, J.H. A case of eosinophilic peritonitis treated with oral corticosteroids. *Perit. Dial. Int.* **2000**, *20*, 579–580.
219. Thakur, S.S.; Unikowsky, B.; Prichard, S. Eosinophilic peritonitis in CAPD: Treatment with prednisone and diphenhydramine. *Perit. Dial. Int.* **1997**, *17*, 402–403.
220. Leung, A.C.; Orange, G.; Henderson, I.S. Intraperitoneal hydrocortisone in eosinophilic peritonitis associated with continuous ambulatory peritoneal dialysis. *Br. Med. J.* **1983**, *286*, 766. [CrossRef]
221. Forbes, T.A.; Lunn, A.J. Montelukast: A novel therapeutic option in eosinophilic peritonitis. *Pediatr. Nephrol.* **2014**, *29*, 1279–1282. [CrossRef] [PubMed]
222. Shalev, O.; Rubinger, D.; Barlatzky, Y.; Kopolovic, J.; Drukker, A. Eosinophilia associated with acute allograft kidney rejection. *Nephron* **1982**, *31*, 182–183. [CrossRef] [PubMed]
223. Kormendi, F.; Amend, W.J., Jr. The importance of eosinophil cells in kidney allograft rejection. *Transplantation* **1988**, *45*, 537–539. [CrossRef] [PubMed]
224. Almirall, J.; Campistol, J.M.; Sole, M.; Andreu, J.; Revert, L. Blood and graft eosinophilia as a rejection index in kidney transplant. *Nephron* **1993**, *65*, 304–309. [CrossRef] [PubMed]
225. Meleg-Smith, S.; Gauthier, P.M. Abundance of interstitial eosinophils in renal allografts is associated with vascular rejection. *Transplantation* **2005**, *79*, 444–450. [CrossRef] [PubMed]

226. Vanikar, A.V.; Kanodia, K.V.; Patel, R.D.; Suthar, K.S.; Nigam, L.A.; Thakkar, U.G.; Patel, H.V.; Kute, V.B.; Trivedi, H.L. Repercussions of eosinophils in a renal allograft—Predictor of early graft loss! *Saudi J. Kidney Dis. Transpl.* **2017**, *28*, 1034–1040. [CrossRef] [PubMed]
227. Weir, M.R.; Hall-Craggs, M.; Shen, S.Y.; Posner, J.N.; Alongi, S.V.; Dagher, F.J.; Sadler, J.H. The prognostic value of the eosinophil in acute renal allograft rejection. *Transplantation* **1986**, *41*, 709–712. [CrossRef]
228. Acuna, M.; Ramos, A.; Santonja, C.; Barat, A.; Egido, J.; Ortiz, A. Delayed graft function and cotrimoxazole. *Transplant. Proc.* **2011**, *43*, 2502–2504. [CrossRef]
229. Josephson, M.A.; Chiu, M.Y.; Woodle, E.S.; Thistlethwaite, J.R.; Haas, M. Drug-induced acute interstitial nephritis in renal allografts: Histopathologic features and clinical course in six patients. *Am. J. Kidney Dis.* **1999**, *34*, 540–548. [CrossRef]
230. Genta, R.M. Global prevalence of strongyloidiasis: Critical review with epidemiologic insights into the prevention of disseminated disease. *Rev. Infect. Dis.* **1989**, *11*, 755–767. [CrossRef]
231. Olsen, A.; van Lieshout, L.; Marti, H.; Polderman, T.; Polman, K.; Steinmann, P.; Stothard, R.; Thybo, S.; Verweij, J.J.; Magnussen, P. Strongyloidiasis—The most neglected of the neglected tropical diseases? *Trans. R. Soc. Trop. Med. Hyg.* **2009**, *103*, 967–972. [CrossRef] [PubMed]
232. Bisoffi, Z.; Buonfrate, D.; Montresor, A.; Requena-Mendez, A.; Munoz, J.; Krolewiecki, A.J.; Gotuzzo, E.; Mena, M.A.; Chiodini, P.L.; Anselmi, M.; et al. Strongyloides stercoralis: A plea for action. *PLoS Negl. Trop. Dis.* **2013**, *7*, e2214. [CrossRef]
233. Keiser, P.B.; Nutman, T.B. Strongyloides stercoralis in the Immunocompromised Population. *Clin. Microbiol. Rev.* **2004**, *17*, 208–217. [CrossRef] [PubMed]
234. Hamilton, K.W.; Abt, P.L.; Rosenbach, M.A.; Bleicher, M.B.; Levine, M.S.; Mehta, J.; Montgomery, S.P.; Hasz, R.D.; Bono, B.R.; Tetzlaff, M.T.; et al. Donor-derived Strongyloides stercoralis infections in renal transplant recipients. *Transplantation* **2011**, *91*, 1019–1024. [CrossRef] [PubMed]
235. Roseman, D.A.; Kabbani, D.; Kwah, J.; Bird, D.; Ingalls, R.; Gautam, A.; Nuhn, M.; Francis, J.M. Strongyloides stercoralis transmission by kidney transplantation in two recipients from a common donor. *Am. J. Transplant.* **2013**, *13*, 2483–2486. [CrossRef]
236. Le, M.; Ravin, K.; Hasan, A.; Clauss, H.; Muchant, D.G.; Pasko, J.K.; Cipollina, G.; Abanyie, F.; Montgomery, S.P.; Loy, M.; et al. Single donor-derived strongyloidiasis in three solid organ transplant recipients: Case series and review of the literature. *Am. J. Transplant.* **2014**, *14*, 1199–1206. [CrossRef] [PubMed]
237. Abdalhamid, B.A.; Al Abadi, A.N.; Al Saghier, M.I.; Joudeh, A.A.; Shorman, M.A.; Amr, S.S. Strongyloides stercoralis infection in kidney transplant recipients. *Saudi J. Kidney Dis. Transpl.* **2015**, *26*, 98–102. [CrossRef] [PubMed]
238. Abanyie, F.A.; Gray, E.B.; Delli Carpini, K.W.; Yanofsky, A.; McAuliffe, I.; Rana, M.; Chin-Hong, P.V.; Barone, C.N.; Davis, J.L.; Montgomery, S.P.; et al. Donor-derived Strongyloides stercoralis infection in solid organ transplant recipients in the United States, 2009–2013. *Am. J. Transplant.* **2015**, *15*, 1369–1375. [CrossRef]
239. Galiano, A.; Trelis, M.; Moya-Herraiz, A.; Sanchez-Plumed, J.; Merino, J.F. Donor-derived Strongyloides stercoralis hyperinfection syndrome after simultaneous kidney/pancreas transplantation. *Int. J. Infect. Dis.* **2016**, *51*, 19–21. [CrossRef]
240. Kim, J.H.; Kim, D.S.; Yoon, Y.K.; Sohn, J.W.; Kim, M.J. Donor-Derived Strongyloidiasis Infection in Solid Organ Transplant Recipients: A Review and Pooled Analysis. *Transplant. Proc.* **2016**, *48*, 2442–2449. [CrossRef]
241. Fischer, S.A.; Avery, R.K.; AST Infectious Disease Community of Practice. Screening of donor and recipient prior to solid organ transplantation. *Am. J. Transplant.* **2009**, *9* (Suppl. 4), S7–S18. [CrossRef] [PubMed]
242. Boulware, D.R.; Stauffer, W.M.; Hendel-Paterson, B.R.; Rocha, J.L.; Seet, R.C.; Summer, A.P.; Nield, L.S.; Supparatpinyo, K.; Chaiwarith, R.; Walker, P.F. Maltreatment of Strongyloides infection: Case series and worldwide physicians-in-training survey. *Am. J. Med.* **2007**, *120*, 545.e1–545.e8. [CrossRef] [PubMed]
243. Abanyie, F.A.; Valice, E.; Delli Carpini, K.W.; Gray, E.B.; McAuliffe, I.; Chin-Hong, P.V.; Handali, S.; Montgomery, S.P.; Huprikar, S. Organ donor screening practices for Strongyloides stercoralis infection among US organ procurement organizations. *Transpl. Infect. Dis.* **2018**, *20*, e12865. [CrossRef] [PubMed]
244. Mascarello, M.; Gobbi, F.; Angheben, A.; Gobbo, M.; Gaiera, G.; Pegoraro, M.; Lanzafame, M.; Buonfrate, D.; Concia, E.; Bisoffi, Z. Prevalence of Strongyloides stercoralis infection among HIV-positive immigrants attending two Italian hospitals, from 2000 to 2009. *Ann. Trop. Med. Parasitol.* **2011**, *105*, 617–623. [CrossRef] [PubMed]

245. Ramirez-Olivencia, G.; Espinosa, M.A.; Martin, A.B.; Nunez, N.I.; de Las Parras, E.R.; Nunez, M.L.; Puente, S.P. Imported strongyloidiasis in Spain. *Int. J. Infect. Dis.* **2014**, *18*, 32–37. [CrossRef] [PubMed]
246. Martinez-Perez, A.; Roure Diez, S.; Belhassen-Garcia, M.; Torrus-Tendero, D.; Perez-Arellano, J.L.; Cabezas, T.; Soler, C.; Diaz-Menendez, M.; Navarro, M.; Trevino, B.; et al. Management of severe strongyloidiasis attended at reference centers in Spain. *PLoS Negl. Trop. Dis.* **2018**, *12*, e0006272. [CrossRef]
247. DeVault, G.A., Jr.; King, J.W.; Rohr, M.S.; Landreneau, M.D.; Brown, S.T., 3rd; McDonald, J.C. Opportunistic infections with Strongyloides stercoralis in renal transplantation. *Rev. Infect. Dis.* **1990**, *12*, 653–671. [CrossRef]
248. Morgan, J.S.; Schaffner, W.; Stone, W.J. Opportunistic strongyloidiasis in renal transplant recipients. *Transplantation* **1986**, *42*, 518–524. [CrossRef]
249. Bedke, J.; Buse, S.; Kurosch, M.; Haferkamp, A.; Jager, D.; Hohenfellner, M. Paraneoplastic syndrome in renal cell carcinoma. *Urologe A* **2007**, *46*, 45–48. [CrossRef]
250. Da Silva, J.L.; Lacombe, C.; Bruneval, P.; Casadevall, N.; Leporrier, M.; Camilleri, J.P.; Bariety, J.; Tambourin, P.; Varet, B. Tumor cells are the site of erythropoietin synthesis in human renal cancers associated with polycythemia. *Blood* **1990**, *75*, 577–582. [PubMed]
251. Hegemann, M.; Kroeger, N.; Stenzl, A.; Bedke, J. Rare and changeable as a chameleon: Paraneoplastic syndromes in renal cell carcinoma. *World J. Urol.* **2018**, *36*, 849–854. [CrossRef] [PubMed]
252. Zhou, W.W.; Guan, Y.Y.; Liu, X.M. Paraneoplastic Eosinophilia in Clear Cell Renal Cell Carcinoma. *Chin. Med. J.* **2015**, *128*, 2271–2272. [PubMed]
253. Wei, Y.B.; Yan, B.; Yin, Z.; Yang, J.R. Chromophobe renal cell carcinoma associated with eosinophilia: A report of three cases. *Exp. Ther. Med.* **2014**, *8*, 91–94. [CrossRef] [PubMed]
254. Rajpara, A.; Liolios, A.; Fraga, G.; Blackmon, J. Recurrent paraneoplastic wells syndrome in a patient with metastatic renal cell cancer. *Dermatol. Online J.* **2014**, *20*, 13030/qt35w8r1g3. [PubMed]
255. Lowe, D.; Jorizzo, J.; Hutt, M.S. Tumour-associated eosinophilia: A review. *J. Clin. Pathol.* **1981**, *34*, 1343–1348. [CrossRef] [PubMed]
256. Todenhofer, T.; Wirths, S.; von Weyhern, C.H.; Heckl, S.; Horger, M.; Hennenlotter, J.; Stenzl, A.; Kanz, L.; Schwentner, C. Severe paraneoplastic hypereosinophilia in metastatic renal cell carcinoma. *BMC Urol.* **2012**, *12*, 7. [CrossRef] [PubMed]
257. Rojas, G.J.; Castro, D.M.; Vigo-Guevara, G.L.; Ferrua, M.; Barriga-Maldonado, V.; Rotta-Escalante, R. Hypereosinophilic encephalopathy with multiple cerebral infarctions in neighbouring vascular territories associated with prostate cancer. *Rev. Neurol.* **2006**, *43*, 762–764.
258. Santos, R.P.; Carvalho, S.D.; Ferreira, O.; Brito, C. Wells syndrome associated with lung cancer. *BMJ Case Rep.* **2017**, *2017*, bcr-2017-220323. [CrossRef]
259. Balian, A.; Bonte, E.; Naveau, S.; Foussat, A.; Bouchet-Delbos, L.; Berrebi, D.; Vons, C.; Capron, F.; Chaput, J.C.; Emilie, D. Intratumoral production of interleukin-5 leading to paraneoplastic peripheral eosinophilia in hepatocellular carcinoma. *J. Hepatol.* **2001**, *34*, 355–356. [CrossRef]
260. Anagnostopoulos, G.K.; Sakorafas, G.H.; Kostopoulos, P.; Margantinis, G.; Tsiakos, S.; Terpos, E.; Pavlakis, G.; Fortun, P.; Arvanitidis, D. Disseminated colon cancer with severe peripheral blood eosinophilia and elevated serum levels of interleukine-2, interleukine-3, interleukine-5, and GM-CSF. *J. Surg. Oncol.* **2005**, *89*, 273–275. [CrossRef]
261. Diskin, C.J.; Stokes, T.J.; Dansby, L.M.; Radcliff, L.; Carter, T.B. The prevalence and meaning of eosinophilia in renal diseases on a nephrology consultation service. *Nephrol. Dial. Transplant.* **2011**, *26*, 2549–2558. [CrossRef] [PubMed]
262. Dejaco, C.; Oppl, B.; Monach, P.; Cuthbertson, D.; Carette, S.; Hoffman, G.; Khalidi, N.; Koening, C.; Langford, C.; McKinnon-Maksimowicz, K.; et al. Serum biomarkers in patients with relapsing eosinophilic granulomatosis with polyangiitis (Churg-Strauss). *PLoS ONE* **2015**, *10*, e0121737. [CrossRef] [PubMed]

2

Urinary Biomarkers α-GST and π-GST for Evaluation and Monitoring in Living and Deceased Donor Kidney Grafts

Shadi Katou [1,*], Brigitta Globke [2], M. Haluk Morgul [1], Thomas Vogel [1], Benjamin Struecker [1], Natalie Maureen Otto [3], Anja Reutzel-Selke [2], Marion Marksteiner [2], Jens G. Brockmann [1], Andreas Pascher [1] and Volker Schmitz [1]

1 Department of General, Visceral and Transplantation Surgery, Universitätsklinikum Münster, 48189 Münter, Germany; haluk.morguel@ukmuenster.de (M.H.M.); thomas.vogel@ukmuenster.de (T.V.); benjamin.struecker@ukmuenster.de (B.S.); jens.brockmann@ukmuenster.de (J.G.B.); andreas.pascher@ukmuesnter.de (A.P.); schmitz.volker@icloud.com (V.S.)

2 Charité – Universitätsmedizin Berlin, corporate member of Freie Universität Berlin, Humboldt-Universität zu Berlin, and Berlin Institute of Health, Department of Surgery CCM|CVK, 10117 Berlin, Germany; brigitta.globke@charite.de (B.G.); anja.selke@charite.de (A.R.-S.); marion.marksteiner@charite.de (M.M.)

3 Department of Nephrology and Internal Intensive Care Medicine, Charité Universitätsmedizin Berlin, Campus Virchow Klinikum, 10117 Berlin, Germany; natalie.otto@charite.de

* Correspondence: shadi.katou@ukmuenster.de

Abstract: The aim of this study was to analyze the value of urine α- and π-GST in monitoring and predicting kidney graft function following transplantation. In addition, urine samples from corresponding organ donors was analyzed and compared with graft function after organ donation from brain-dead and living donors. Urine samples from brain-dead ($n = 30$) and living related ($n = 50$) donors and their corresponding recipients were analyzed before and after kidney transplantation. Urine α- and π-GST values were measured. Kidney recipients were grouped into patients with acute graft rejection (AGR), calcineurin inhibitor toxicity (CNI), and delayed graft function (DGF), and compared to those with unimpaired graft function. Urinary π-GST revealed significant differences in deceased kidney donor recipients with episodes of AGR or DGF at day one after transplantation ($p = 0.0023$ and $p = 0.036$, respectively). High π-GST values at postoperative day 1 (cutoff: >21.4 ng/mg urine creatinine (uCrea) or >18.3 ng/mg uCrea for AGR or DGF, respectively) distinguished between rejection and no rejection (sensitivity, 100%; specificity, 66.6%) as well as between DGF and normal-functioning grafts (sensitivity, 100%; specificity, 62.6%). In living donor recipients, urine levels of α- and π-GST were about 10 times lower than in deceased donor recipients. In deceased donors with impaired graft function in corresponding recipients, urinary α- and π-GST were elevated. α-GST values >33.97 ng/mg uCrea were indicative of AGR with a sensitivity and specificity of 77.7% and 100%, respectively. In deceased donor kidney transplantation, evaluation of urinary α- and π-GST seems to predict different events that deteriorate graft function. To elucidate the potential advantages of such biomarkers, further analysis is warranted.

Keywords: kidney transplantation; urinary biomarkers; α-GST; π-GST; acute rejection; delayed graft function; nephrotoxicity

---

1. Introduction

Kidney transplantation is by far the best therapeutic option for patients with end-stage renal disease (ESRD). After transplantation, the main challenges, besides surgical complications, are acute graft rejection, delayed graft function, and adverse effects of immunosuppressants [1]. Acute graft rejection still occurs in up to 25% of recipients and is a significant prognostic factor for long-term graft survival [2]. The improvements of immunosuppressive drugs have turned transplantation into a safe and widely predictable therapy; however, many of the agents used today still contribute to graft failure due to their nephrotoxic potential [3]. Delayed graft function, defined by the need for dialysis within the first week after transplantation and mainly caused by acute tubular necrosis, is mostly due to long ischemia times, advanced donor age, and comorbidities [4,5]. Recognizing the cause of graft dysfunction may be challenging, yet immediate diagnosis and therapy are essential for optimal graft survival.

The signs of graft dysfunction are decreased diuresis and impaired creatinine blood levels. Monitoring immunosuppressive drugs and their toxicity through serum levels is of limited value, since the difference between therapeutic and toxic levels is not fixed [6]. In order to define the pathomechanism of graft dysfunction, a graft biopsy is required in most cases. However, this is an invasive procedure and risks associated complications endangering the transplanted kidney [7].

α- and π-GST, which are specifically present in the kidney tubules, are two isotypes of the glutathione-S-transferases. Beyond their biochemical differences, they are also located in different parts of the tubule system [8]. α-GST is found in cells of the proximal tubules, which are predominantly affected by ischemia time and nephrotoxic substances. π-GST is located in distal tubules, which are damaged during acute graft rejection [9]. Their release into the urine as a result of cell damage gives an accurate prediction of the impaired part of the tubules system and therefore the underlying cause of graft dysfunction [10,11]. Analyses of α- and π-GST have been reported to be promising for discriminating between the different causes of graft dysfunction [11–13].

The aim of our study was to determine the value of measuring α- and π-GST concentrations in urine as biomarkers for monitoring graft function and predicting postoperative events in the first week after transplantation in living and deceased donor kidney transplantation.

2. Experimental Section

2.1. Samples and Data Collection

This study was approved by the Ethics Committee of Berlin's Charité University Hospital (EA2/137/10). We prospectively analyzed blood and urine samples as well as demographic data from 160 patients: 30 brain-dead donors and their 30 corresponding recipients; and 50 living kidney donors as well as their 50 corresponding living donor kidney recipients. All surgeries were carried out at the Department of General, Visceral and Transplantation surgery of Charité University Hospital, Berlin. Machine perfusion was not performed for any kidney allograft in this study. Except for brain-dead donors, all patients were followed during the first week after surgery. Blood and urine samples were collected at the following time points: day 0, day 1, day 3, day 5, and day 7. Samples from brain-dead organ donors were obtained on day 0, the day of the organ donation surgery. Urine samples were collected from recipients after transplantation through an externalized uretero-vesico-cutaneous stent and therefore exclusively reflected the α- and π-GST content of the transplanted grafts.

2.2. Immunosuppression Events and Subgroups

All recipients received a triple immunosuppressant consisting of prednisolone, mycophenolate mofetil (MMF), and a calcineurin inhibitor. All deceased donor kidney recipients received tacrolimus, whereas living donor kidney recipients were treated with either tacrolimus or cyclosporine. Recipients were divided into subgroups according to the events in the first postoperative week: acute graft rejection (AGR, G1), calcineurin-induced nephrotoxicity (CNI, G2), both acute kidney rejection and calcineurin-induced nephrotoxicity (AGR + CNI, G3), delayed graft function (DGF, G4), and event-free (healthy, G5) subgroup (Figure 1). An acute graft rejection was confirmed by graft biopsy and classified according to the BANFF criteria. Calcineurin-induced nephrotoxicity was defined by serum levels of agents (tacrolimus >15 ng/mL, cyclosporin >250 ng/mL). It is worth noting that delayed graft function, characterized by the need for dialysis in the first week after transplantation, was not recorded in any of the living donor recipients. In case dialysis was required due to a known graft-damaging event such as AGR or CNI, those patients were enrolled in subgroups of primary cause and not defined as DGF. Recipients with no signs for any of the above events were considered healthy and were used as our control group.

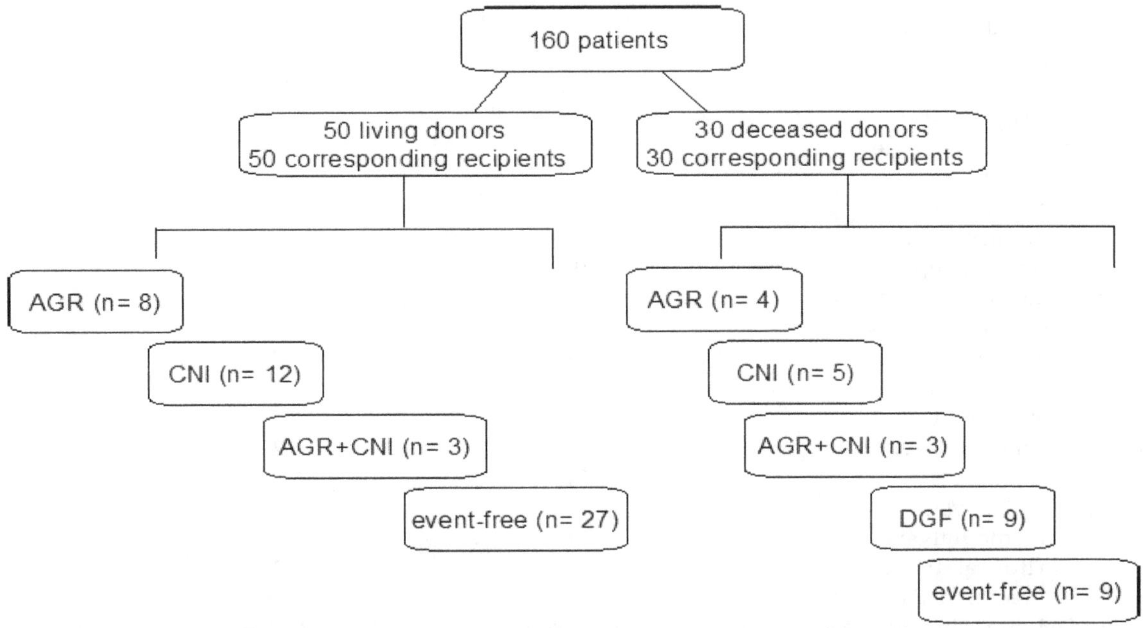

Figure 1. Patients, groups, and subgroups.

2.3. GST Analysis and Statistics

Urinary α- and π-GST values were measured using a commercially available ELISA test kit provided by Argutus Medical Ltd. (Dublin, Ireland). To consider the physiological differences in urine concentrations, α- and π-GST values were standardized to urine creatinine. The resulting unit for GST was ng/mg uCrea. Reference ranges of urinary α- and π-GST were determined as recommended from the measured GST values in the healthy population of this study group. For this purpose, the α- and π-GST values in the urine of healthy living donors were considered before donor nephrectomy. The reference interval for α-GST is 2.7–7.6 ng/mg uCrea and for π-GST 4.1–13 ng/mg uCrea in this study.

For statistical analysis, GraphPad Prism 6 (GraphPad Software, San Diego, CA, USA) was used. Quantitative data are given as the mean and standard deviation. To compare normally distributed variables, *t*-tests such as Mann-Whitney and Wilcoxon were performed. For the comparison of multiple variables, we used two-way ANOVA; here we applied Tukey and Holm-Sidak tests for post hoc analysis of the subgroups. The area under the curve was calculated in ROC analysis and a log-rank (Mantel-Cox) test was performed in survival analysis. A p-value less than 0.05 was defined as significant.

3. Results

3.1. Demographic Data

There were no differences regarding gender and BMI between the patient groups. The mean eGFR before graft recovery or transplantation (d0) did not differ between the groups. Recipients of deceased donor kidneys were significantly older than those of living donors (58 ± 13 and 48 ± 15 respectively, $p = 0.006$), whereas the donor's age was not different. Cold as well as warm ischemic time were significantly higher in the deceased donor group (both $p < 0.0001$). The demographic data of donors and recipients are given in Table 1. The increase in the eGFR of recipients after transplantation was, as expected, more noticeable in living donation scenarios (Figure 2).

Table 1. Demographic data of donors and recipients.

	Deceased Donor Grafts	Living Donor Grafts	*p* Value
Donor	30	50	
Age (years)	58 ± 15	53 ± 10	n.s.
Sex (male/female)	11/19	22/28	n.s.
BMI	27.3 ± 6.5	25.3 ± 3.2	n.s.
eGFR, d0 (mL/min)	96 ± 39	97 ± 18	n.s.
Diuresis in last hour (mL)	152 ± 81	-	
Recipient	30	50	
Age (years)	58 ± 12	47 ± 15	<0.05
Sex (male/female)	22/8	35/15	n.s.
BMI	26.4 ± 4	25.8 ± 4.9	n.s.
eGFR, d0 (mL/min)	9 ± 3	8 ± 4	n.s.
Primary disease			
Glomerulonephritis	9	24	n.s.
Hypertensive nephrosclerosis	7	9	n.s.
Polycystic kidney disease	6	2	n.s.
Autoimmune disease	2	5	n.s.
Diabetes	2	3	n.s.
Urologic disease	2	2	n.s.
Calcineurin-induced nephrotoxicity	0	2	n.s.
Others	2	3	n.s.
Dialysis			
Hemodialysis	29	28	n.s.
Peritoneal dialysis	1	3	n.s.
No dialysis	0	19	<0.05
Cold ischemia time (minutes)	613 ± 269	193 ± 62	<0.05
Warm ischemia time (minutes)	34 ± 11	23 ± 7	<0.05

BMI, body mass index; eGFR, estimated glomerular filtration rate; n.s., not significant.

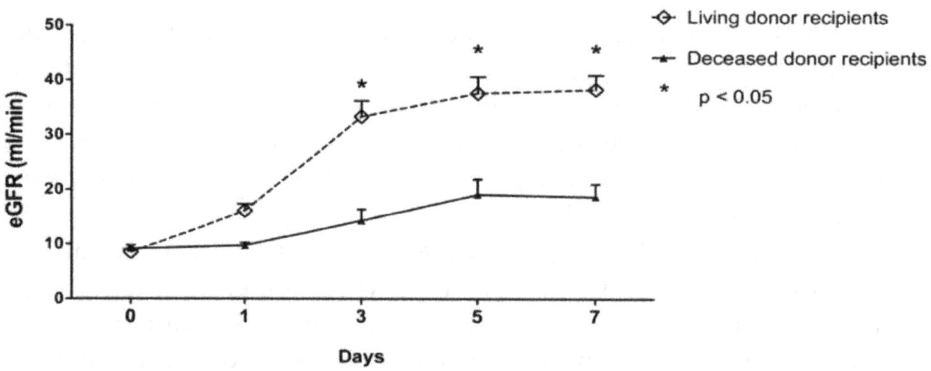

Figure 2. eGFR comparison between deceased and living donor recipients before and during the first week after transplantation.

3.2. *α- and π-GST in Recipients*

Neither α- nor π-GST correlated with age, BMI, and cold or warm ischemic time in any group. However, both GST isoenzymes correlated with renal function in living donors and in the healthy recipients subgroup. In deceased donor recipients and living donor recipients we observed acute rejection in four (13.4%) and eight patients (16%), calcineurin-induced nephrotoxicity in five (16.7%) and 12 (24%) patients, and both simultaneously in three (10%) and three (6%) patients, respectively. Delayed graft function occurred only with deceased donors (nine patients, 30%). Patients with an uneventful postoperative course in the deceased donor recipient group numbered nine (30%) and, in the living donor recipient group, 27 (54%). Both α- and π-GST were significantly elevated at 1st postoperative day (POD) in deceased donor recipients, with acute rejection when compared with the corresponding healthy subgroup (α-GST: Mean 473.5 ± 818 vs. 15.6 ± 21.2 ng/mg uCrea,

$p = 0.0094$; π-GST: mean 477.8 ± 804 vs. 8 ± 6.4 ng/mg uCrea, $p = 0.0023$). In living donor recipients, only π-GST showed an increase, reaching a peak at day 5 (mean 21.5 ± 28.2 ng/mg uCrea); however, there was no significant difference between this group and the healthy subgroup. In patients with CNI toxicity, α-GST performed better in both recipient groups; in deceased donor recipients, the mean was 316 ± 704.5 ng/mg uCrea at 1 POD and was easily discriminated from the uneventful subgroup ($p = 0.06$). Also, in the living donor group, a rise of α-GST to 68.9 ± 219 ng/mg uCrea was noted at day 5, when CNI toxicity occurred. When both acute rejection and CNI toxicity were recorded, neither α- nor π-GST was able to distinguish those patients; however, it is worth mentioning that the number of subjects in this subgroup was very low in our study. In the case of delayed graft function, present only in deceased donor recipients in our study, α- as well as π-GST were elevated in the urine, with means at 1st POD of 81.5 ± 201.3 and 151.6 ± 270.6 ng/mg uCrea, respectively. Only π-GST levels proved significant when compared to the control subgroup ($p = 0.036$) (Figure 3).

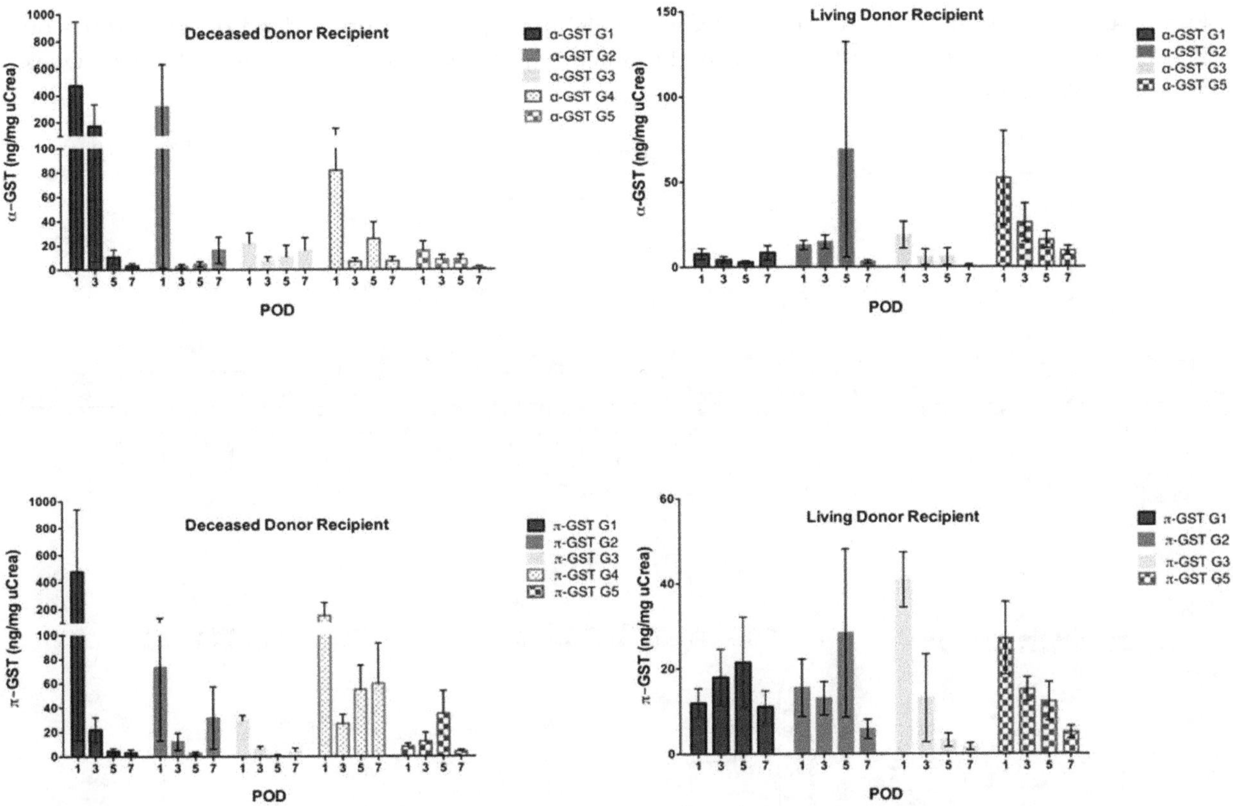

Figure 3. Urinary α- and π-GST levels in subgroups of deceased and living donor recipients during the first week after transplantation; G1: Acute graft rejection (AGR), G2: Calcineurin-induced nephrotoxicity (CNI), G3: Simultaneous acute graft rejection and calcineurin-induced nephrotoxicity (AGR + CNI), G4: Delayed graft function (DGF), G5: Event-free (control).

Furthermore, we performed ROC curve and survival analysis on the most outstanding biomarkers at a specific point in the study. π-GST showed the most promising results in deceased donor recipients with acute graft rejection and delayed graft function at day 1 after transplantation. Patients who developed a biopsy confirmed acute graft rejection within the first week after transplantation had significantly higher levels of urinary π-GST at POD 1. With an estimated cutoff of 21.4 ng/mg uCrea, π-GST was able to distinguish the occurrence of AGR from a rejection-free course with 100% and 66.6% sensitivity and specificity, respectively (Figure 4). Similar reliability for π-GST was observed in the DGF subgroup; however, the estimated cutoff at POD 1 was slightly lower at 18.3 ng/mg uCrea (sensitivity, 100%; specificity, 62.6%). Higher urinary π-GST levels could be seen in recipients with delayed graft function; this was observed at POD1, POD 3 as well as POD 7. π-GST was not able to differentiate between the causes of graft dysfunction in the early postoperative period (Figure 5).

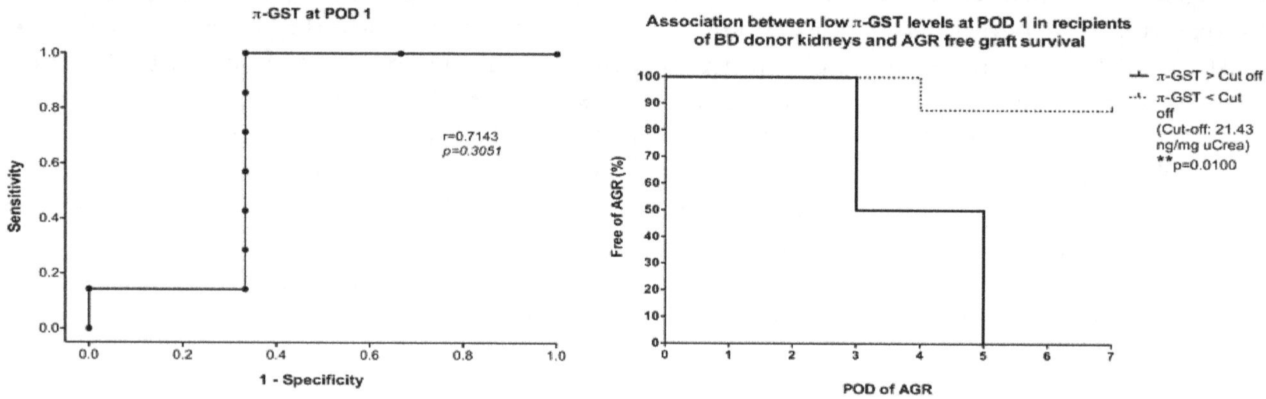

Figure 4. Correlation between urinary π-GST levels in recipients of brain-dead donors' grafts on POD 1, and probability of graft survival without acute graft rejection (AGR) during the first week after transplantation.

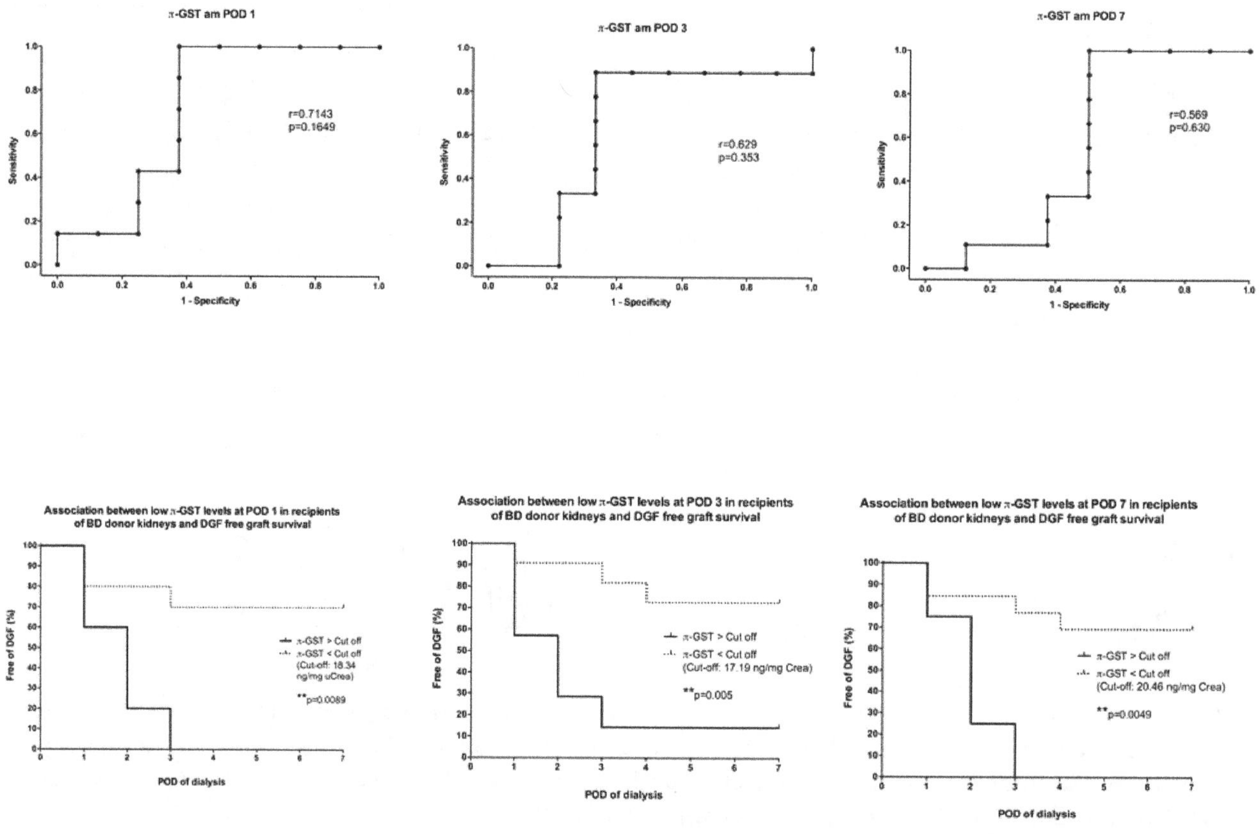

Figure 5. Correlation between urinary π-GST levels in recipients of brain-dead donors' grafts on POD 1, 3, and 7; and probability of graft survival without delayed graft function (DGF) during the first week after transplantation.

3.3. α- and π-GST in Donors

α- and π-GST showed interesting results when measured in deceased donor urine before organ harvesting as they were elevated in those with poorer graft function after transplantation, and seemed to predict a foreseeable event such as acute rejection or delayed graft function, which was 3- to 8-fold more likely to occur than in those recipients with an uneventful course of treatment. α-GST stood out in the subgroup with both acute rejection and CNI toxicity ($p = 0.02$), while α- and π-GST were remarkably higher (but not significantly so) in the DGF subgroup compared to the control group (Figure 6). As for the predictive value of GST when measured in donor urine, α-GST stood out with significant results in the AGR subgroup when ROC curve analysis was performed, and a cutoff value of >33.97 ng/mg uCrea was calculated (AUC, 0.86; sensitivity, 77.7%; specificity, 100%). Based on the donor's urinary α-GST alone, all four renal grafts from deceased donors that showed acute rejection in recipients were distinguished from those who had an AGR-free course in the survival curve analysis ($p = 0.0109$) (Figure 7).

On the other hand, urinary GST in living donors showed no differences between subgroups and the corresponding control group, and therefore failed to predict future events in recipients.

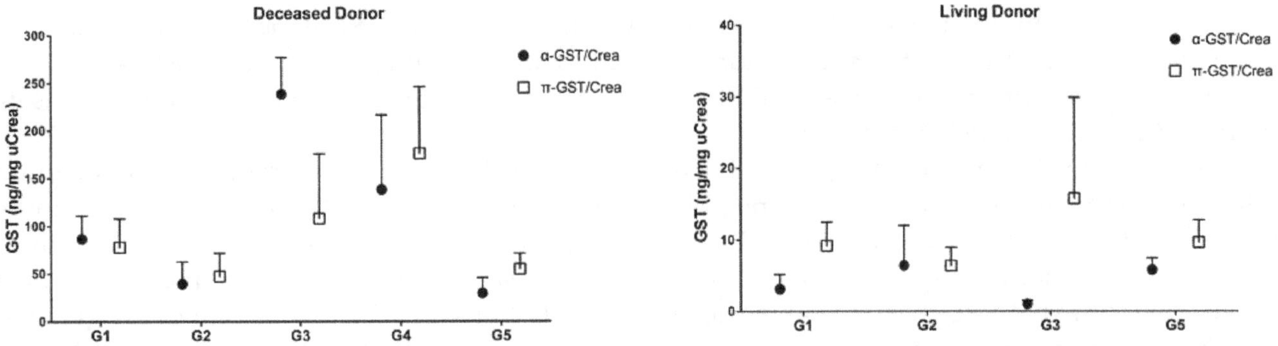

Figure 6. Urinary α- and π-GST levels in deceased donors before transplantation; G1: Acute graft rejection (AGR), G2: Calcineurin-induced nephrotoxicity (CNI), G3: Simultaneous acute graft rejection and calcineurin-induced nephrotoxicity (AGR+CNI), G4: Delayed graft function (DGF), G5: Event-free (control).

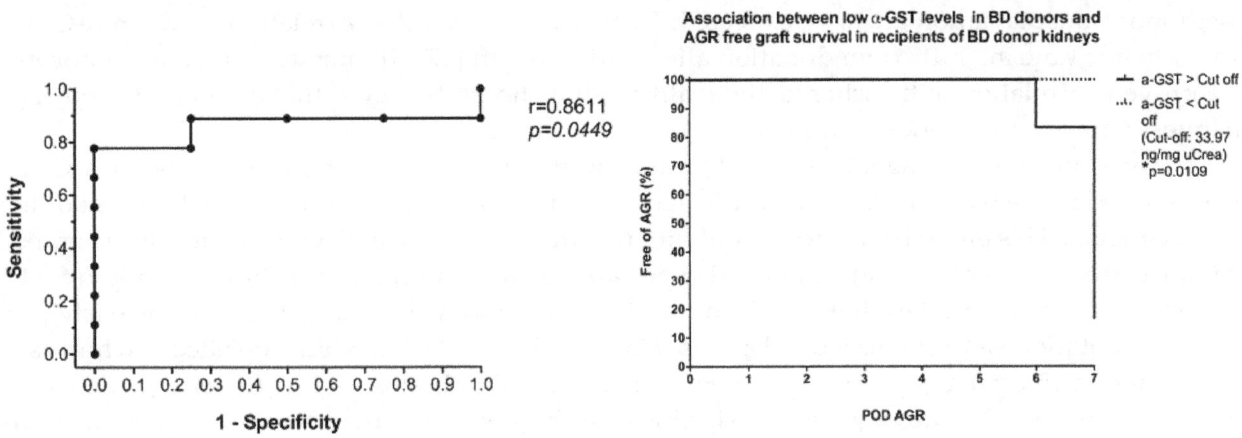

Figure 7. Correlation between urinary α-GST levels in brain-dead donors before transplantation and probability of graft survival without acute graft rejection in corresponding recipients during the first week after transplantation.

3.4. Six- and 12-Months Graft Survival

We followed up recipients of the subgroups G1 (AGR) and G4 (DGF) at six and 12 months after transplantation, as correlations of α- and π-GST in those cohorts showed the most promising results. However, in subgroup G1 only one patient out of four lost the graft due to recruiting nephritis; in subgroup G4 all three grafts were lost due to death not associated with graft function (cancer or cardiac arrest).

4. Discussion

The results of our prospective study, evaluating urinary α- and π-GST in deceased as well as living kidney donors and their corresponding recipients as biomarkers for graft quality and function, suggest the potential value of these enzymes. Previous studies showed the ability of urinary α- and π-GST to predict acute renal damage in kidney graft recipients and demonstrated a release of these enzymes in malfunctioning grafts [10–15]. However, none of these groups has compared the course of α- and π-GST in donors as well as in corresponding recipients. In addition, we investigated the differences in the markers in two settings, brain-dead/deceased and living organ donation. Our analyses reveal that the determination of urinary π-GST concentration in deceased donor recipients, especially on the first day after graft transplantation, could be valuable and indicative of kidney allograft function and survival without AGR or DGF. Secondly, we found higher concentrations of α- and π-GST in the urine of deceased kidney donors, whose grafts performed poorly in the corresponding recipients; α-GST was able to predict AGR before transplantation. A determination between the causes of impaired allograft function could not be reached by assessing urinary α- and π-GST alone, though it is unlikely that in the complex setting of transplantation a single biomarker will reliably distinguish between the pathogenesis of multifactorial elements; therefore, the proposed markers should be seen as an useful tool in addition to established methods.

Research studies investigating α- and π-GST in living donation are extremely limited: in our review of the literature we only found one publication on this issue, and this concerned liver rather than kidney transplantation [16]. Our findings showed lower concentrations of α- and π-GST in the urine of living donor kidney recipients than in that of deceased donor kidney recipients. This was observed in almost all subgroups, and especially on POD 1. Except for a notable, yet insignificant, rise of π-GST in living donor recipients with AGR when compared to the control group, our results find no further significances of urinary α- and π-GST in living donor recipients when harmful events occurred. Considering the superior organ quality and logistics in living donation transplantation, as demonstrated by over half of living donor grafts surviving the first week after transplantation event-free compared to 30% of deceased donor grafts, lower urinary concentrations of α- nor π-GST in living donor transplantation are to be expected. Daemen et al. found a correlation between α-GST and warm ischemic time in grafts from donation after cardiac death [17]. In our study neither α- nor π-GST had a proven correlation with ischemic time, although it should be noted that a different type of graft was investigated in the work mentioned.

The toxic effect of CNI agents on renal grafts and its association with the excretion of α-GST has been described in the past [10,18]. Our results failed to indicate such a correlation in deceased or living donor recipients. This might be due to our definition of the toxic range of CNI serum levels. Therapeutic and toxic serum levels of several drugs and especially immunosuppressants have been known to be inconsistent and even overlapping [6,19]. In the 1990s, serum levels of tacrolimus in the early period after transplantation were suggested to be below 20 ng/mL in order to avoid side effects, whereas later on levels above 15 ng/mg were proven to be associated with a higher risk of toxicity [20,21]. On the other hand, the risk of acute rejection is significantly higher when there are low concentrations of the agent [22]. A helpful step would be to find the toxic serum level of immunosuppressants that is agreed upon by transplant communities; currently, despite all efforts, this varies significantly between transplant centers. Another concerning factor is the design of the study, which did not include daily and therefore more precise surveillance on that matter. In order to investigate the correlation between toxic exposure to immunosuppressants and the excretion of GST into the urine, a closer observation with more frequent sample collection is required.

DGF was observed only in deceased donor recipients in our study. It occurred with an incidence of 30%, which is similar to the findings of a recent work by Willicombe et al. [23]. Risk factors and characteristics of donors and recipients associated with DGF such as cold ischemic time and donor age have been established in previous publications [4,5,24]. However, taking these factors into consideration, it is to be expected that DGF is less common in living donation. It has been demonstrated that α-GST excretion would be increased in the case of DGF due to its location in the renal tubular system and the association between DGF and proximal tubular necrosis [8,25]. On the other hand, π-GST has been shown to be of predictive value in terms of the need for dialysis in a publication by

Seabra et al. including 245 patients with acute kidney injury [26]. Hall et al. investigated α- and π-GST in a perfusate solution during machine perfusion of kidney allografts from deceased donors, and suggested an independent association between π-GST and DGF [27]. Our findings demonstrated the consistent significance of urinary π-GST in differentiating between DGF and normally functioning grafts when measured in deceased donor recipients. This was observed at several time points of the study and had a strong power of sensitivity and specificity. Little is known about the behavior of the proteins under dialysis, so it is unclear whether α-GST is more dialyzable than π-GST or the other way round. The sample collection from patients undergoing dialysis in our study did not occur with respect to dialysis time, which should be seen as another possible disturbance factor.

Further limitations of this study are the small number of patients in certain subgroups and the overall high standard deviations. We distinguished well between the causes of impaired graft function and took into consideration simultaneous events. The time frame of our observation was limited in that it focused only on the first week after transplantation. We believe that multiple serial samples and an extended study design would be beneficial in future projects.

5. Conclusions

In summary, the elevation of urinary π-GST in deceased donor kidney recipients at day 1 after kidney transplantation could be a helpful monitoring parameter, in addition to urinary output and serum creatinine, to determine graft function in recipients. It might be indicative of acute rejection or a need for dialysis. The measuring of urinary α- and π-GST should also be considered in deceased donors as this seems to be of predictive value in terms of graft outcome and might help with assessing allograft quality. Our findings reveal an association between urinary α-GST in deceased donors and AGR in corresponding recipients. Thus, further investigation of α- and π-GST in a larger population and daily sample collection should be considered. Although urinary α- and π-GST in living kidney donation showed no relevant correlation with harmful events in our analyses, this is, to the best of our knowledge, the first study demonstrating differences in biomarkers between deceased and living kidney donation, so subsequent investigations will be needed in order to confirm or contradict our findings.

Author Contributions: Conceptualization, S.K. and V.S.; methodology, S.K., V.S. and B.G.; software, S.K., A.R.-S. and B.S.; validation, B.G., M.M. and B.S.; formal analysis, S.K. and A.R.-S.; investigation, S.K., B.G. and V.S.; resources, A.P., V.S. and N.M.O.; data curation, S.K., B.G., M.M. and N.M.O.; writing—original draft preparation, S.K.; writing—review and editing, J.G.B., M.H.M. and T.V.; visualization, S.K., M.H.M. and T.V.; supervision, V.S., A.P. and J.G.B.; project administration, S.K. and V.S. All authors have read and approved the final version of the manuscript.

Acknowledgments: We acknowledge support from the Open Access Publication Fund of the University of Münster. The authors also extend their gratitude to Argutus Medical Ltd. (Dublin, Ireland) for providing the kits.

References

1. Wu, W.K.; Famure, O.; Li, Y.; Kim, S.J. Delayed graft function and the risk of acute rejection in the modern era of kidney transplantation. *Kidney Int.* **2015**, *88*, 851–858. [CrossRef]
2. Marcen, R.; Fernandez-Rodriguez, A.; Rodriguez-Mendiola, N.; Ponte, B.; Galeano, C.; Villafruela, J.J.; Teruel, J.L.; Burgos, F.J.; Ortuno, J. Evolution of rejection rates and kidney graft survival: A historical analysis. *Transplant Proc.* **2009**, *41*, 2357–2359. [CrossRef]
3. Martins, L.; Ventura, A.; Branco, A.; Carvalho, M.J.; Henriques, A.C.; Dias, L.; Sarmento, A.M.; Amil, M. Cyclosporine versus tacrolimus in kidney transplantation: Are there differences in nephrotoxicity? *Transplant Proc.* **2004**, *36*, 877–879. [CrossRef]
4. Ojo, A.O.; Wolfe, R.A.; Held, P.J.; Port, F.K.; Schmouder, R.L. Delayed graft function: Risk factors and implications for renal allograft survival. *Transplantation* **1997**, *63*, 968–974. [CrossRef]
5. Siedlecki, A.; Irish, W.; Brennan, D.C. Delayed graft function in the kidney transplant. *Am. J. Transplant.* **2011**, *11*, 2279–2296. [CrossRef]

6. Klintmalm, G.; Sawe, J.; Ringden, O.; von Bahr, C.; Magnusson, A. Cyclosporine plasma levels in renal transplant patients. Association with renal toxicity and allograft rejection. *Transplantation* **1985**, *39*, 132–137. [CrossRef]
7. Wilczek, H.E. Percutaneous needle biopsy of the renal allograft. A clinical safety evaluation of 1129 biopsies. *Transplantation* **1990**, *50*, 790–797. [CrossRef]
8. Branten, A.J.; Mulder, T.P.; Peters, W.H.; Assmann, K.J.; Wetzels, J.F. Urinary excretion of glutathione S transferases alpha and pi in patients with proteinuria: Reflection of the site of tubular injury. *Nephron* **2000**, *85*, 120–126. [CrossRef]
9. Harrison, D.J.; Kharbanda, R.; Cunningham, D.S.; McLellan, L.I.; Hayes, J.D. Distribution of glutathione S-transferase isoenzymes in human kidney: Basis for possible markers of renal injury. *J. Clin. Pathol.* **1989**, *42*, 624–628. [CrossRef]
10. Backman, L.; Appelkvist, E.L.; Ringden, O.; Dallner, G. Glutathione transferase in the urine: A marker for post-transplant tubular lesions. *Kidney Int.* **1988**, *33*, 571–577. [CrossRef]
11. Kuzniar, J.; Marchewka, Z.; Krasnowski, R.; Boratynska, M.; Dlugosz, A.; Klinger, M. Enzymuria and low molecular weight protein excretion as the differentiating marker of complications in the early post kidney transplantation period. *Int. Urol. Nephrol.* **2006**, *38*, 753–758. [CrossRef]
12. Polak, W.P.; Kosieradzki, M.; Kwiatkowski, A.; Danielewicz, R.; Lisik, W.; Michalak, G.; Paczek, L.; Lao, M.; Walaszewski, J.; Rowinski, W.A. Activity of glutathione S-transferases in the urine of kidney transplant recipients during the first week after transplantation. *Ann. Transplant.* **1999**, *4*, 42–45.
13. Sundberg, A.G.; Appelkvist, E.L.; Backman, L.; Dallner, G. Urinary Pi-Class Glutathione Transferase as an Indicator of Tubular Damage in the Human Kidney. *Nephron* **1994**, *67*, 308–316. [CrossRef]
14. Backman, L.; Appelkvist, E.L.; Ringden, O.; Dallner, G. Appearance of basic glutathione transferase in the urine during tubular complications in renal transplant recipients. *Transplant. Proc.* **1988**, *20*, 427–430.
15. Westhuyzen, J.; Endre, Z.H.; Reece, G.; Reith, D.M.; Saltissi, D.; Morgan, T.J. Measurement of tubular enzymuria facilitates early detection of acute renal impairment in the intensive care unit. *Nephrol. Dial. Transplant.* **2003**, *18*, 543–551. [CrossRef]
16. Jochum, C.; Beste, M.; Sowa, J.P.; Farahani, M.S.; Penndorf, V.; Nadalin, S.; Saner, F.; Canbay, A.; Gerken, G. Glutathione-S-transferase subtypes alpha and pi as a tool to predict and monitor graft failure or regeneration in a pilot study of living donor liver transplantation. *Eur. J. Med. Res.* **2011**, *16*, 34–40. [CrossRef]
17. Daemen, J.W.; Oomen, A.P.; Janssen, M.A.; van de Schoot, L.; van Kreel, B.K.; Heineman, E.; Kootstra, G. Glutathione S-transferase as predictor of functional outcome in transplantation of machine-preserved non-heart-beating donor kidneys. *Transplantation* **1997**, *63*, 89–93. [CrossRef]
18. Sundberg, A.; Appelkvist, E.L.; Dallner, G.; Nilsson, R. Glutathione transferases in the urine—Sensitive methods for detection of kidney damage-induced by nephrotoxic agents in humans. *Environ. Health Perspect.* **1994**, *102*, 293–296.
19. Min, D.I.; Perry, P.J.; Chen, H.Y.; Hunsicker, L.G. Cyclosporine trough concentrations in predicting allograft rejection and renal toxicity up to 12 months after renal transplantation. *Pharmacotherapy* **1998**, *18*, 282–287.
20. Bottiger, Y.; Brattstrom, C.; Tyden, G.; Sawe, J.; Groth, C.G. Tacrolimus whole blood concentrations correlate closely to side-effects in renal transplant recipients. *Br. J. Clin. Pharmacol.* **1999**, *48*, 445–448. [CrossRef]
21. Schiff, J.; Cole, E.; Cantarovich, M. Therapeutic monitoring of calcineurin inhibitors for the nephrologist. *Clin. J. Am. Soc. Nephrol.* **2007**, *2*, 374–384. [CrossRef]
22. Undre, N.A.; van Hooff, J.; Christiaans, M.; Vanrenterghem, Y.; Donck, J.; Heeman, U.; Kohnle, M.; Zanker, B.; Land, W.; Morales, J.M.; et al. Stevenson, P. Low systemic exposure to tacrolimus correlates with acute rejection. *Transplant. Proc.* **1999**, *31*, 296–298. [CrossRef]
23. Willicombe, M.; Rizzello, A.; Goodall, D.; Papalois, V.; McLean, A.G.; Taube, D. Risk factors and outcomes of delayed graft function in renal transplant recipients receiving a steroid sparing immunosuppression protocol. *World J. Transplant.* **2017**, *7*, 34–42. [CrossRef] [PubMed]
24. Irish, W.D.; Ilsley, J.N.; Schnitzler, M.A.; Feng, S.; Brennan, D.C. A risk prediction model for delayed graft function in the current era of deceased donor renal transplantation. *Am. J. Transplant.* **2010**, *10*, 2279–2286. [CrossRef]
25. Sundberg, A.G.; Nilsson, R.; Appelkvist, E.L.; Dallner, G. Immunohistochemical Localization of Alpha-Class and Pi-Class Glutathione Transferases in Normal Human Tissues. *Pharmacol. Toxicol.* **1993**, *72*, 321–331. [CrossRef]

26. Seabra, V.F.; Perianayagam, M.C.; Tighiouart, H.; Liangos, O.; dos Santos, O.F.; Jaber, B.L. Urinary alpha-GST and pi-GST for prediction of dialysis requirement or in-hospital death in established acute kidney injury. *Biomarkers* **2011**, *16*, 709–717. [CrossRef] [PubMed]
27. Hall, I.E.; Bhangoo, R.S.; Reese, P.P.; Doshi, M.D.; Weng, F.L.; Hong, K.; Lin, H.; Han, G.; Hasz, R.D.; Goldstein, M.J.; et al. Glutathione S-transferase iso-enzymes in perfusate from pumped kidneys are associated with delayed graft function. *Am. J. Transplant.* **2014**, *14*, 886–896. [CrossRef]

3

Serum Klotho in Living Kidney Donors and Kidney Transplant Recipients

Charat Thongprayoon [1,*], Javier A. Neyra [2,3,4], Panupong Hansrivijit [5], Juan Medaura [6], Napat Leeaphorn [7], Paul W. Davis [6], Wisit Kaewput [8], Tarun Bathini [9], Sohail Abdul Salim [6], Api Chewcharat [1], Narothama Reddy Aeddula [10], Saraschandra Vallabhajosyula [11], Michael A. Mao [12] and Wisit Cheungpasitporn [6,*]

1. Division of Nephrology and Hypertension, Mayo Clinic, Rochester, MN 55905, USA; chewcharat.api@mayo.edu
2. Division of Nephrology, Bone and Mineral Metabolism, Department of Internal Medicine, University of Kentucky, Lexington, KY 40506, USA; javier.neyra@uky.edu
3. Charles and Jane Pak Center for Mineral Metabolism and Clinical Research, Dallas, TX 75390, USA
4. Division of Nephrology, Department of Internal Medicine, University of Texas Southwestern Medical Center, Dallas, TX 75390, USA
5. Department of Internal Medicine, University of Pittsburgh Medical Center Pinnacle, Harrisburg, PA 17105, USA; hansrivijitp@upmc.edu
6. Division of Nephrology, Department of Medicine, University of Mississippi Medical Center, Jackson, MS 39216, USA; jmedaura@umc.edu (J.M.); pwdavis@umc.edu (P.W.D.); sohail3553@gmail.com (S.A.S.)
7. Renal Transplant Program, University of Missouri-Kansas City School of Medicine/Saint Luke's Health System, Kansas City, MO 64110, USA; napat.leeaphorn@gmail.com
8. Department of Military and Community Medicine, Phramongkutklao College of Medicine, Bangkok 10400, Thailand; wisitnephro@gmail.com
9. Department of Internal Medicine, University of Arizona, Tucson, AZ 85721, USA; tarunjacobb@gmail.com
10. Division of Nephrology, Department of Medicine, Deaconess Health System, Evansville, IN 47710, USA; dr.anreddy@gmail.com
11. Department of Cardiovascular Medicine, Mayo Clinic, Rochester, MN 55905, USA; Vallabhajosyula.Saraschandra@mayo.edu
12. Division of Nephrology and Hypertension, Mayo Clinic, Jacksonville, FL 32224, USA; mao.michael@mayo.edu

* Correspondence: charat.thongprayoon@gmail.com (C.T.); wcheungpasitporn@gmail.com (W.C.)

Abstract: α-Klotho is a known anti-aging protein that exerts diverse physiological effects, including phosphate homeostasis. Klotho expression occurs predominantly in the kidney and is significantly decreased in patients with chronic kidney disease. However, changes in serum klotho levels and impacts of klotho on outcomes among kidney transplant (KTx) recipients and kidney donors remain unclear. A literature search was conducted using MEDLINE, EMBASE, and Cochrane Database from inception through October 2019 to identify studies evaluating serum klotho levels and impacts of klotho on outcomes among KTx recipients and kidney donors. Study results were pooled and analyzed utilizing a random-effects model. Ten cohort studies with a total of 431 KTx recipients and 5 cohort studies with a total of 108 living kidney donors and were identified. After KTx, recipients had a significant increase in serum klotho levels (at 4 to 13 months post-KTx) with a mean difference (MD) of 243.11 pg/mL (three studies; 95% CI 67.41 to 418.81 pg/mL). Although KTx recipients had a lower serum klotho level with a MD of = −234.50 pg/mL (five studies; 95% CI −444.84 to −24.16 pg/mL) compared to healthy unmatched volunteers, one study demonstrated comparable klotho levels between KTx recipients and eGFR-matched controls. Among kidney donors, there was a significant decrease in serum klotho levels post-nephrectomy (day 3 to day 5) with a mean difference (MD) of −232.24 pg/mL (three studies; 95% CI −299.41 to −165.07 pg/mL). At one year following kidney donation, serum klotho levels remained lower than baseline before nephrectomy with a MD of = −110.80 pg/mL (two studies; 95% CI 166.35 to 55.24 pg/mL). Compared to healthy volunteers, living kidney donors had lower serum klotho levels with a MD of = −92.41 pg/mL (two studies; 95% CI −180.53 to −4.29 pg/mL). There is a significant reduction in serum klotho levels after living kidney donation and an increase in serum klotho levels after KTx. Future prospective studies are needed to assess the impact of changes in klotho on clinical outcomes in KTx recipients and living kidney donors.

Keywords: klotho; α-Klotho; FGF-23; kidney transplantation; kidney donor; renal transplantation; transplantation; Nephrology; CKD-MBD; CKD-Mineral and Bone Disorder

---

1. Introduction

α-Klotho (klotho) is a membrane protein that is highly expressed in the kidney, especially in the distal tubular epithelial cells [1–10]. Membrane-bound klotho regulates phosphate homeostasis by acting as a co-factor of fibroblast growth factor 23 (FGF23) [11–14]. FGF23-Klotho signaling promotes urinary phosphate excretion and suppresses the expression of renal 1α-hydroxylase, resulting in reduced vitamin D-dependent intestinal absorption of calcium and phosphate [11,15]. Altogether, FGF23-Klotho signaling regulates phosphate metabolism and prevents phosphate retention [16–20]. Soluble klotho can be detected in the circulation in two forms: (1) cleaved klotho, which is derived from cleavage of the extracellular domain of membrane klotho, and potentially (2) secreted klotho, which is derived from an alternatively spliced klotho mRNA transcript [21,22].

Soluble klotho displays diverse physiological effects and hormonal functions, including the reduction of oxidative stress and the inhibition of intracellular insulin and insulin-like growth factor 1 (IGF-1) signaling [15,23–28]. Klotho protects the kidney by suppression of apoptosis [29,30] and cell senescence [31,32], suppression of fibrosis [33–37], and upregulation of autophagy [3,38] in renal tubular cells. Klotho-deficient mice develop premature aging, hyperphosphatemia, vascular calcification and endothelial dysfunction, and have shorter lifespans, while klotho overexpressing mice have 20–30% longer lifespans than wild type mice [2,24,39]. Since klotho expression is the most abundant in the kidney [40], patients with kidney diseases, including acute kidney injury (AKI) and chronic kidney disease (CKD), are found to have a significant reduction in klotho expression and soluble levels [41–51]. Studies have demonstrated that serum klotho declines in progressive human CKD with the lowest serum klotho levels among patients with end-stage kidney disease (ESKD) on dialysis [41,48]. Low serum klotho is associated with increased mortality and cardiovascular events among patients with ESKD [52].

When compared to treatment with chronic dialysis, kidney transplantation (KTx) is the best therapeutic option for patients with ESKD and is associated with increased survival and better quality of life [53–56]. In addition, living donor KTx provides greater allograft longevity than those transplanted from a deceased donor [57]. However, changes in serum klotho levels and the impact of klotho on outcomes among KTx recipients and kidney donors remain unclear [58–75]. Thus, we conducted this systematic review and meta-analysis to assess serum klotho levels and the impact of klotho on outcomes among KTx recipients and kidney donors.

2. Methods

2.1. Search Strategy and Literature Review

A systematic literature search of MEDLINE (1946 to October 2019), EMBASE (1988 to October 2019), and the Cochrane Database of Systematic Reviews (database inception to October 2019) was conducted (1) to assess studies evaluating serum klotho levels and effects of klotho on outcomes among KTx recipients and kidney donors. The systematic literature review was undertaken independently by two investigators (C.T. and W.C.) using a search strategy that combined the terms of ("klotho" OR "klotho protein" OR "klotho gene") AND ("kidney transplantation" OR "renal transplantation" OR "kidney donor") which is provided in online Supplementary Materials (Table S1). No language limitation was applied. A manual search for conceivably relevant studies using references of the included articles was also performed. This study was conducted by the PRISMA (Preferred Reporting Items for Systematic Reviews and Meta-Analysis) statement [76]. The data for this meta-analysis are publicly available through the Open Science Framework (URL: https://osf.io/kx9we/).

2.2. Selection Criteria

Eligible studies must have been (1) clinical trials or observational studies (cohort, case-control, or cross-sectional studies) that evaluated serum klotho levels and effects of klotho on outcomes among KTx recipients or kidney donors, and (2) studies that presented data to calculate mean differences (MDs) with 95% confidence intervals (CIs) that evaluated changes in serum klotho before and after KTx/kidney donation or compared serum klotho between KTx patients/donors and a control group composed of non-KTx or non-donor controls. Retrieved articles were individually reviewed for eligibility by the two investigators (C.T. and W.C.). Discrepancies were addressed and solved by joint consensus. Inclusion was not limited by the size of the study.

2.3. Data Abstraction

A structured data collecting form was used to obtain the following information from each study including the title, name of the first author, publication year, year of the study, country where the study was conducted, demographic data of kidney transplant recipients and donors, methods used to measure serum klotho, serum klotho levels, estimated glomerular filtration rate (eGFR), control group, and adjusted effect estimates with 95% CI and covariates that were adjusted for in the multivariable analysis. This data extraction process was independently performed by two investigators (C.T. and W.C.).

2.4. Statistical Analysis

Analyses were performed utilizing the Comprehensive Meta-Analysis 3.3 software (version 3; Biostat Inc., Englewood, NJ, USA). Adjusted point estimates from each study were consolidated by the generic inverse variance approach of DerSimonian and Laird, which designated the weight of each study based on its variance [77]. The summary statistics for each outcome were the mean change from baseline and standard deviation (SD) of the mean change. The mean change in each group was obtained by subtracting the final mean from the baseline mean. The MDs were preferred since all studies use the same continuous outcome and unit of measure (pg/mL) of serum klotho and FGF-23 levels. The SD of mean change was computed, assuming a conservative correlation coefficient of 0.5 [78]. Effects sizes of 0.2 were interpreted as small, those of 0.5 as moderate, and of 0.8 as large [79]. Given the possibility of between-study variance, we used a random-effect model rather than a fixed-effect model. Cochran's Q test and I^2 statistics were applied to determine between-study heterogeneity. A value of I^2 of 0% to 25% represents insignificant heterogeneity, 26% to 50% low heterogeneity, 51% to 75% moderate heterogeneity and 76–100% high heterogeneity [80]. The presence of publication bias was assessed by the Egger test [81].

3. Results

A total of 132 potentially eligible articles were identified using our search strategy. After the exclusion of 93 articles based on title and abstract for clearly not fulfilling inclusion criteria on the basis of the type of article, study design, population or outcome of interest, or due to being duplicates,

39 articles were left for full-length review. Eighteen of these were excluded from the full-length review as they did not report the outcome of interest, while six articles were excluded because they were not observational studies. Thus, 15 studies (10 cohort studies [58–67] with a total of 431 KTx recipients and 5 cohort studies [68–72] with a total of 108 living kidney donors) were included. The literature retrieval, review, and selection process are demonstrated in Figure 1.

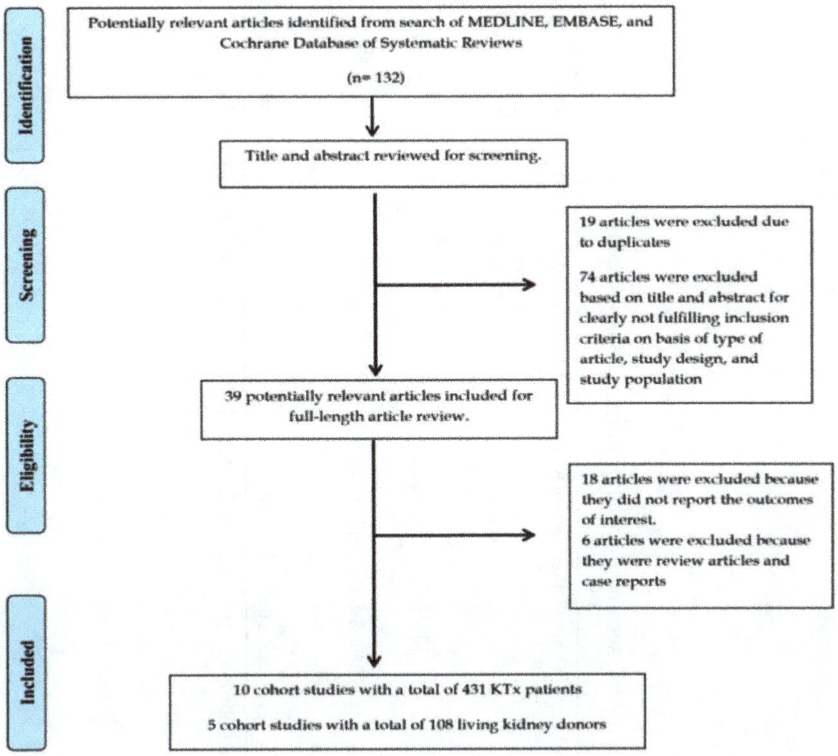

Figure 1. Outline of our search methodology. Abbreviation: KTx, kidney transplant.

3.1. Serum Klotho after Kidney Transplantation

The characteristics of the included studies assessing serum klotho after kidney transplantation are presented in Tables 1 and 2. After KTx, there was a significant increase in serum klotho levels in recipients (at 4 to 13 months post-KTx) in reference to baseline levels before KTx with a mean difference (MD) of 243.11 pg/mL (three studies; 95% CI 67.41 to 418.81 pg/mL, $I^2 = 93\%$), Figure 2A. There were significant reductions in serum PTH and phosphate levels with MDs of −134.65 pg/mL (95% CI −176.09 to −93.21 pg/mL, $I^2 = 0\%$) and −2.81 mg/dL (95% CI −3.46 to −2.16 mg/dL, $I^2 = 97\%$), respectively. There was no significant change in serum calcium levels with a MD of 0.37 mg/dL (95% CI, −0.05 to 0.79 mg/dL, $I^2 = 83\%$). Although KTx recipients had lower serum klotho levels with a MD of = −234.50 pg/mL (five studies; 95% CI −444.84 to −24.16 pg/mL, $I^2 = 93\%$, Figure 2B) compared to healthy unmatched volunteers, one study demonstrated comparable klotho level between KTx recipients and eGFR-matched controls [66]. Two studies demonstrated high serum klotho levels in deceased donors as a prognostic marker for good allograft function within one year after KTx ($p < 0.05$) [59,60].

Table 1. Characteristics of the included studies assessing serum klotho after kidney transplantation.

Study	Year	Country	N-KTx	Characteristics-KTx	Klotho before KTx (pg/mL)	Other Markers before KTx	Kloth after KTx (pg/mL)	Other Markers after KTx
Kubota et al.		Japan	20	Age 6.9 ± 4.5 years Male 12 (60%)	988 ± 122	FGF23 5343 ± 1350 pg/mL	At 4 months 1405 ± 125	N/A
Tan et al.	2017	Australia	29	Age 49 (35–55) years Male 17 (59%)	307 (279–460)	iFGF23 2060 (825–5075) pg/mL eGFR 7.4 (6.5–8.7) mL/min/1.73 m^2	At 52 weeks 460 (311–525)	At 52 weeks iFGF23 64 (34–88) pg/mL eGFR 60.4 (50.5–71.6) mL/min/1.73 m^2
Mizusaki et al.	2019	Japan	36	Age 38.1 ± 14 years Male 15 (42%)	211.8	eGFR 3.8 ± 0.8 mL/min/1.73 m^2	At 1 year 369.3	At 1 year eGFR 49 ± 17 mL/min/1.73 m^2

Abbreviations: eGFR, estimated glomerular filtration rate; iFGF23, intact fibroblast growth factor-23; KTx, kidney transplant; N/A, not available.

Table 2. Characteristics of the included studies comparing serum klotho between KTx recipients and healthy volunteers.

Study	Year	Country	N-KTx	Characteristics-KTx	Klotho-KTx (pg/mL)	Other Markers-KTx	N-Control	Klotho-Control (pg/mL)	Other Markers-Control
Balogu et al.		Turkey	40	N/A	153 ± 170	FGF23 47.4 ± 61 pg/mL	20 healthy subjects	641 ± 1797	FGF23 1.6 ± 1.3 pg/mL
Malyszko et al.	2014	Poland	84	Median time from KTx 37 (13–72) months Age 47.9 ± 12.0 years Male 64 (76%)	228 (161–384)	eGFR 56.3 ± 1.6 mL/min/1.73 m^2 FGF23 16.7 (13.8–21.2) pg/mL	22 healthy subjects	757 (632–839)	eGFR 97.3 ± 13.5 mL/min/1.73 m^2 FGF23 11.7 (10.8–17.2) pg/mL
Bleskestad et al.	2015	Norway	40	Median time from KTx 18.3 (IQR 12.2–26.2) years Age 61.3 ± 11.8 years Male 29 (73%)	605 (506–784)	eGFR 62 (52–72) mL/min/1.73 m^2 iFGF23 75 (53–108) pg/mL	39 GFR-matched controls 20 healthy subjects	GFR-matched controls 660 (536–847) Healthy volunteers 692 (618–866)	GFR-matched control eGFR 62 (57–73) mL/min/1.73 m^2 iFGF23 63 (52–87) pg/mL Healthy volunteer eGFR 99.5 (89.5–110.8) mL/min/1.73 m^2 iFGF23 51 (36–68) pg/mL
Tartaglione et al.	2017	Italy	80	Time for KTx 77.6 (37.6–119.5) months Age 54.7 ± 10.3 years Male 49 (61%)	449 (388–534)	eGFR 46.3 (36.2–58.3) mL/min/1.73 m^2 FGF23 41 (25–59) pg/mL	30 healthy subjects	795 (619–901)	eGFR 109.1 ± 14.1 mL/min/1.73 m^2 FGF23 34 (28–441) pg/mL
Nahandi et al.	2017	Iran	30	Time from KTx 6.42 ± 2.44 years Age 30.9 ± 5.3 years	276 ± 241	eGFR 64.53 ± 17.83 mL/min/1.73 m^2	27 healthy subjects	N/A	N/A

Abbreviations: eGFR, estimated glomerular filtration rate; FGF23, fibroblast growth factor-23; KTx, kidney transplant; N/A, not available.

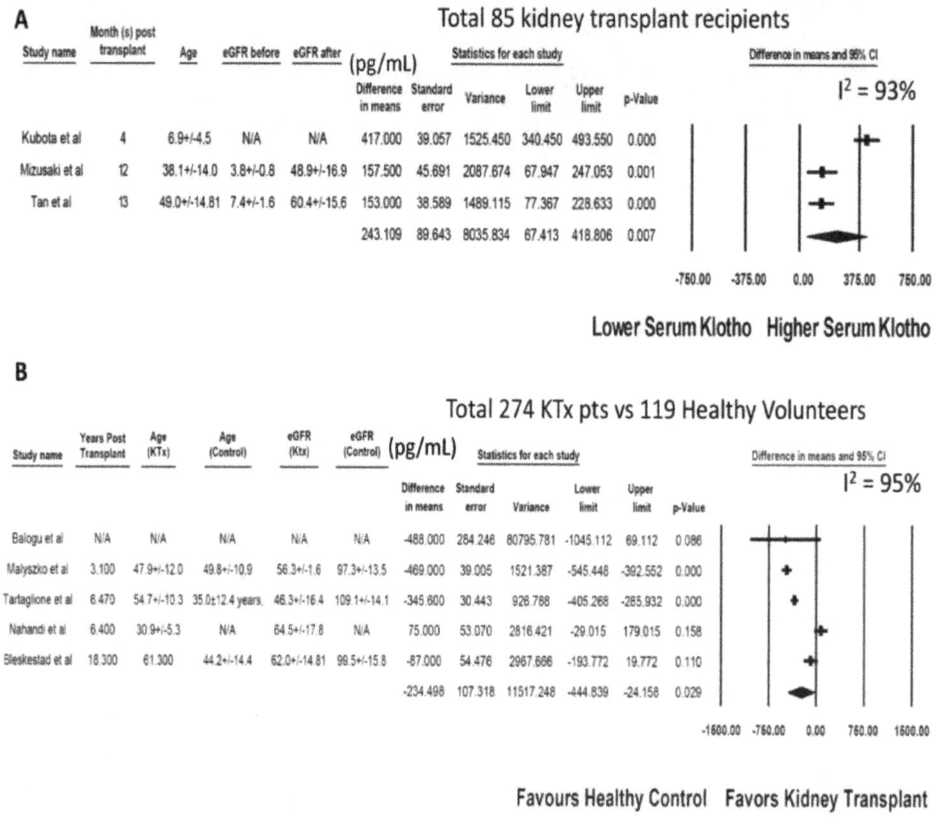

Figure 2. (**A**) Change in Serum Klotho in KTx Recipients after Kidney Transplant. (**B**) Serum Klotho in KTx Recipients Compared to Unmatched Healthy Volunteers.

3.2. *Serum Klotho after Living Kidney Donation*

The characteristics of the included studies assessing serum klotho after kidney transplantation are presented in Tables 3 and 4. A total of 108 living kidney donors were identified from five cohort studies. After kidney donation, there was a significant decrease in serum klotho levels post-nephrectomy (day 3 to day 5) with a mean difference (MD) of −232.24 pg/mL (three studies; 95% CI −299.41 to −165.07 pg/mL, $I^2 = 0$), Figure 3A. At one year following the kidney donation, serum klotho levels remained lower than baseline before nephrectomy with a MD of = −110.80 pg/mL (two studies; 95% CI −166.35 to −55.24 pg/mL, $I^2 = 5$), Figure 3B.

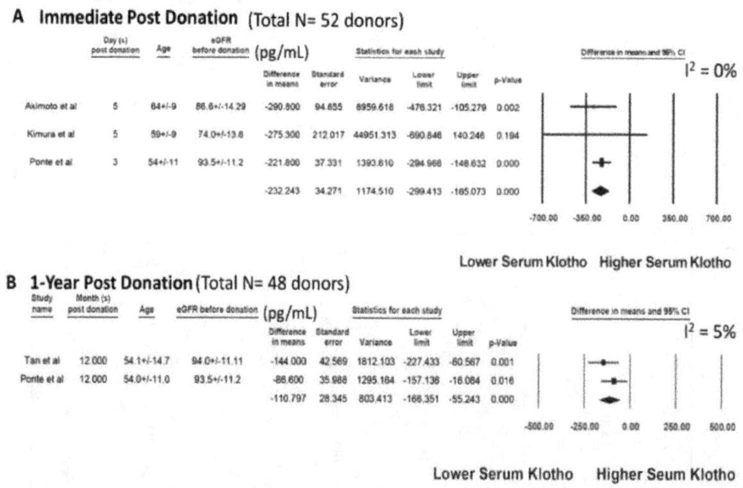

Figure 3. Changes in serum klotho after living kidney donation: (**A**) immediate post-donation and (**B**) one year post-donation.

Table 3. Characteristics of the included studies evaluating serum klotho after living kidney donation.

Study	Year	Country	N-Donor	Characteristics-Donor	Klotho before Donor Nephrectomy (pg/mL)	Other Markers before Donor Nephrectomy	Klotho after Donor Nephrectomy (pg/mL)	Other Markers after Donor Nephrectomy
Akimoto et al.	2013	Japan	10	Age 64 ± 9 years Male 4 (40%) Living donor	910 (755–1132)	eGFR 87 (72–92) mL/min/1.73 m^2	At day 5 619 (544.6–688.5)	N/A
Ponte et al.	2014	Switzerland	27	Age 54 ± 11 years Male 15 (57%) Living donor	526 (482–615)	eGFR 95 ± 11 mL/min/1.73 m^2 FGF23 48.1 (37.4–60.0) pg/mL	At day 3 304 (266–491) At day 360 440 (398–613)	At day 3 FGF23 26.9 (22.1–38.0) pg/mL At day 360 eGFR 63 ± 13 mL/min/1.73 m^2 FGF23 45.2 (37.7–56.4) pg/mL
Kimura et al.	2015	Japan	15	Age 59 ± 9 years Male 8 (53%) Living donor	1084 (795–1638)	eGFR 74 ± 14 mL/min/1.73 m^2	At day 5 809 (638–1357)	N/A
Tan et al.	2017	Australia	21	Age 54.1 ± 14.7 Male 13 (62%) Living donor	564 (468–663)	eGFR 94 (82–97) mL/min/1.73 m^2 iFGF23 52 ± 15 pg/mL	At 12 months 420 (378–555)	At 12 months eGFR 61 (49–69) mL/min/1.73 m^2 iFGF23 72 ± 22 pg/mL

Abbreviations: eGFR, estimated glomerular filtration rate; FGF23, fibroblast growth factor-23; N/A, not available.

Table 4. Characteristics of the included studies comparing serum klotho between living kidney donors and healthy volunteers.

Study	Year	Country	N-Donor	Characteristics-Donor	Klotho-Donor (pg/mL)	Other Markers-Donor	N-Control	Klotho-Control (pg/mL)	Other Markers-Control
Thorsen et al.	2016	Norway	35	Age 56.5 ± 9.4 years	669 (409–1161)	FGF23	35 healthy subjects	725 (458–1222)	FGF23
				Male 21 (60%)		62.6 (6.6–112) pg/mL			51.8 (25.9–90) pg/mL
				Living donor					
				Time from donor nephrectomy		eGFR			eGFR
				Median 15 years		75.8 ± 12.3 mL/min/1.73 m^2			99.0 ± 13.1 mL/min/1.73 m^2
Tan et al.	2017	Australia	21	Age 54.1 ± 14.7 years	420 (378–555)	eGFR	20 healthy subjects	517 (434–667)	eGFR
				Male 13 (62%)		61 (49–69) mL/min/1.73 m^2			97 (89–102) mL/min/1.73 m^2
				Living donor		iFGF23			iFGF
				Time from donor nephrectomy 1 year		72 ± 22 pg/mL			52 ± 15 pg/mL

Abbreviations: eGFR, estimated glomerular filtration rate; FGF23, fibroblast growth factor-23.

There was no significant change in serum FGF-23 at one year post-donation with a MD of = 8.19 pg/mL (two studies; 95% CI −14.24 to 30.62 pg/mL, I^2 = 85%), Figure 4A. Compared to unmatched healthy volunteers, living kidney donors had lower serum klotho levels with a MD of = −92.41 pg/mL (two studies; 95% CI −180.53 to −4.29 pg/mL, I^2 = 44%), Figure 4B.

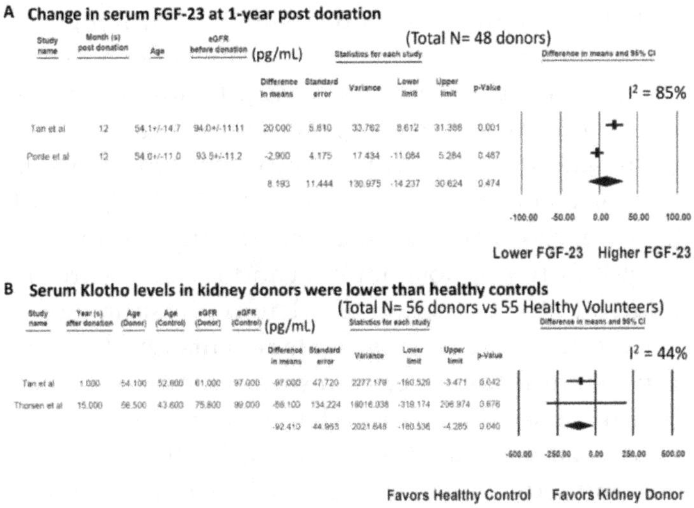

Figure 4. (**A**) Changes in Serum FGF-23 at one year post-donation and (**B**) Serum klotho levels in kidney donors compared to unmatched healthy controls.

3.3. Evaluation for Publication Bias

A funnel plot was not drawn because of the limited number of studies in each analysis. Generally, tests for funnel plot asymmetry should be used only when there are at least ten study groups, because the power of the test is too low to distinguish chance from real asymmetry [82]. Egger's regression test demonstrated no significant publication bias in all analyses ($p > 0.05$).

4. Discussion

In this meta-analysis, we demonstrated that serum klotho levels were significantly increased after successful KTx. While KTx recipients had lower serum klotho levels compared to unmatched healthy volunteers, serum klotho levels in kidney transplant recipients were comparable to those in eGFR-matched controls. Among kidney donors, we found a significant decrease in serum klotho levels post-nephrectomy at day 3 to day 5, which remained lower than baseline before nephrectomy at one year following kidney donation. Compared to healthy volunteers, living kidney donors had lower serum klotho levels.

The findings from our meta-analysis support that klotho is primarily synthesized in the kidneys [40], and transplanting a new kidney into ESKD patients would result in an increase in renal klotho and serum klotho levels post-KTx. In addition to the oligo-anuric state, patients with advanced CKD/ESKD have a significant reduction in klotho and progressively lose the ability to prevent phosphate retention, resulting in hyperphosphatemia, vascular calcification, and cardiovascular disease [83,84]. After successful KTx, in addition to improvement in eGFR, there is also a significant increase in klotho, altogether leading to an improvement in phosphate homeostasis. Recent studies have demonstrated that post-transplant hypophosphatemia after KTx is associated with good kidney allograft function [85,86]. Although the actual underlying mechanisms remain unclear, this is likely because excellent quality transplanted kidneys have higher eGFR and klotho expression, resulting in a reduction in phosphate levels post-KTx.

We identified two cohorts of KTx patients who received their kidneys from deceased donors; higher serum klotho levels in these donors were prognostic for good allograft function at one year after KTx [59,60]. In the ischemia-reperfusion injury (IRI), which is unavoidable to a certain degree in all KTx surgeries, soluble klotho protects renal tubular cells from oxidative damage by inhibiting the insulin/IGF-1 signaling pathway and by inhibition of TGF-β1 for decreasing renal fibrosis [87,88], and upregulation of autophagy in renal tubular cells [3,89]. In addition, klotho is also involved in the inhibition of Wnt pathway-associated β-catenin activation, thus improving renal fibrosis [87]. Compared to patients with early graft function, a lower level of klotho is observed in implantation biopsies among patients with delayed graft function (DGF) [90]. Although data on the effects of klotho on long-term allograft outcomes are limited, it is well known that poor allograft function at one year after KTx and DGF is associated with renal allograft loss [91,92]. Following successful KTx, patients regain functions of klotho via FGF23-Klotho signaling, and with the previously accumulated FGF23, residual hyperparathyroidism, and the use of calcineurin inhibitors (especially cyclosporine) [93–95], post-KTx hypophosphatemia can commonly occur up to 86% [85,96,97]. Post-KTx hypophosphatemia is known to be associated with lower risks of death-censored graft failure and cardiovascular mortality [85]. The association between post-KTx hypophosphatemia and reduced cardiovascular mortality among KTx recipients could be related to the reduction of calcium phosphate product, an important factor associated with vascular calcification and cardiovascular events [98,99]. Our study demonstrated that successful KTx can result in a significant increase in serum klotho levels among KTx recipients [85]. In addition, previous literature has demonstrated trending towards normal FGF-23 levels after successful KTx [42,100]. Thus, regaining function in FGF23-Klotho signaling after KTx helps promote urinary phosphate excretion and reduced vitamin D-dependent intestinal absorption of calcium and phosphate [11,15], which might explain the association between post-KTx hypophosphatemia and reduced cardiovascular mortality. Future studies are needed to assess the impact of klotho levels on long-term cardiovascular health in KTx recipients, allograft, and patient survival.

Living donors supply approximately 40% of kidney allografts in the United States [101]. Overall, living kidney donation is considered safe and does not appear to increase long-term mortality compared with controls [102–107]. A recent systematic review of 52 studies comprising 118,426 living kidney donors reassured the safety of living kidney donations with the finding of no difference in all-cause mortality among donors and controls [108]. In addition, a large retrospective population-based matched cohort study of 2028 kidney donors in comparison with 20,280 matched non-donor controls (followed for a median of 6.5 years) demonstrated no difference in the rate of cardiovascular events between the two groups [109]. Although the findings of our study showed a significant reduction in serum klotho at post-operative day 3 to 5 and at one year following kidney donation, the degree of klotho reduction seemed to be attenuated at one year post-donation compared to the early post-operative period. In addition, we found no significant change in serum FGF-23 at one year post-donation. It is possible that after living kidney donation serum klotho is not severely reduced enough to stimulate the rise in serum FGF-23, which occurred in patients with advanced CKD [41,110]. Elevated FGF-23 levels have been shown to be associated with increased mortality and cardiovascular events [111–113]. Thus, no significant increase in FGF-23 levels after living kidney donation is consistent with the findings of no difference in all-cause mortality among donors and controls in previous literature [108,109].

Despite these published reassuring findings of donor safety [108,109], a recent small multicenter study of living kidney donors and healthy controls (n = 124) demonstrated an association between living kidney donation and a significant increase in left ventricular mass and reduced aortic distensibility [114]. In addition to functions of klotho via FGF23-Klotho signaling, soluble klotho also has FGF23-independent effects, including endothelial protection from senescence, anti-fibrotic properties, cardioprotection, and prevention of vascular calcifications [84,115,116]. Klotho-deficient CKD mice have significant left ventricular hypertrophy (LVH) and cardiac fibrosis compared with wild-type mice [117]. Soluble klotho also provides cardioprotection against stress-induced exaggerated cardiac remodeling through downregulation of transient receptor potential cation channel 6 (TRPC6) [118]. Although an increased LVH and reduced aortic distensibility in living kidney donors could be related to an increased risk of hypertension post living kidney donation [102,103], future studies are required to assess whether a reduction in serum klotho levels after living kidney donation may play a role in the higher risk of LVH, and reduced aortic distensibility observed among living kidney donors.

Our meta-analysis is subject to certain limitations. First, although there were comparative groups, all studies are observational, making them susceptible to selection bias. Second, many variables may influence klotho levels in the post-transplant period that may contribute to the heterogeneity between the included studies evaluating changes in serum klotho levels among KTx recipients. Data on medications that may affect endogenous klotho expression in the kidney and soluble levels such as angiotensin II inhibitors and hydroxymethylglutaryl-CoA (HMG-CoA) reductase inhibitors [17,21,119,120] as well as data on immunosuppression were limited in included studies. Lifestyle, diet, psychological stress, and activities such as exercises may also affect serum klotho levels [121–124]. Thus, future prospective studies are needed to assess the impact of changes in klotho on clinical outcomes in KTx recipients and living kidney donors. Third, the follow-up duration of included studies was limited to only one year, and future studies are required to evaluate the impacts of serum klotho levels on long-term clinical outcomes. Fourth, serum klotho is also affected by the aging process and declines with older age [125]. However, we demonstrated an increase in serum klotho levels after KTx at one year and a decrease in klotho levels at immediate postoperative (which is less likely to be affected by the aging process). Lastly, all included studies measured serum klotho levels by ELISA. Recently, immunoprecipitation-immunoblot (IP-IB) assay is shown to be superior to the ELISA and highly correlated with eGFR [126]. However, this technique requires the labor-intensive nature of the IP-IB assay, and further research is needed to evaluate the use of the IP-IB assay in KTx patients.

In conclusion, compared to patients' baseline, serum klotho levels increase early after successful KTx and decrease after living kidney donation, respectively. Future studies are required to assess the impact of serum klotho levels on risk-stratification and patient-centered outcomes in both living donors and KTx recipients.

Author Contributions: Conceptualization, C.T., J.A.N., J.M., N.L., P.W.D., W.K., T.B., S.A.S., A.C., N.R.A., S.V., M.A.M. and W.C.; Data curation, C.T., N.L. and W.C.; Formal analysis, C.T. and W.C.; Funding acquisition, J.M.; Investigation, C.T., P.H., N.L., W.K. and W.C.; Methodology, C.T., J.A.N., P.H., W.K. and W.C.; Project administration, C.T. and T.B.; Resources, T.B.; Software, T.B.; Supervision, J.A.N., J.M., P.W.D., S.A.S., A.C., S.V., M.A.M. and W.C.; Validation, C.T., P.W.D., W.K., N.R.A. and W.C.; Visualization, J.A.N., P.H., J.M. and N.L.; Writing—original draft, C.T. and W.C.; Writing—review and editing, J.A.N., P.H., J.M., N.L., P.W.D., W.K., T.B., S.A.S., A.C., N.R.A., S.V., M.A.M. and W.C. All authors have read and agreed to the published version of the manuscript.

Acknowledgments: None. All authors had access to the data and played essential roles in writing of the manuscript. Neyra is currently supported by an Early Career Pilot Grant from the National Center for Advancing Translational Sciences (NCATS), National Institutes of Health (NIH), through Grant UL1 TR001998.

References

1. Hu, M.C.; Shi, M.; Zhang, J.; Pastor, J.; Nakatani, T.; Lanske, B.; Razzaque, M.S.; Rosenblatt, K.P.; Baum, M.G.; Kuro-o, M.; et al. Klotho: A novel phosphaturic substance acting as an autocrine enzyme in the renal proximal tubule. *FASEB J.* **2010**, *24*, 3438–3450. [CrossRef]
2. Kuro-o, M. Klotho and aging. *Biochim. Biophys. Acta* **2009**, *1790*, 1049–1058. [CrossRef]
3. Bian, A.; Neyra, J.A.; Zhan, M.; Hu, M.C. Klotho, stem cells, and aging. *Clin. Interv. Aging* **2015**, *10*, 1233–1243. [PubMed]
4. Hu, M.C.; Shi, M.; Cho, H.J.; Adams-Huet, B.; Paek, J.; Hill, K.; Shelton, J.; Amaral, A.P.; Faul, C.; Taniguchi, M.; et al. Klotho and phosphate are modulators of pathologic uremic cardiac remodeling. *J. Am. Soc. Nephrol.* **2015**, *26*, 1290–1302. [CrossRef] [PubMed]

5. Henao Agudelo, J.S.; Baia, L.C.; Ormanji, M.S.; Santos, A.R.P.; Machado, J.R.; Saraiva Câmara, N.O.; Navis, G.J.; de Borst, M.H.; Heilberg, I.P. Fish Oil Supplementation Reduces Inflammation but Does Not Restore Renal Function and Klotho Expression in an Adenine-Induced CKD Model. *Nutrients* **2018**, *10*, 1283. [CrossRef]
6. Huang, X.; Liu, T.; Zhao, M.; Fu, H.; Wang, J.; Xu, Q. Protective Effects of Moderate Ca Supplementation against Cd-Induced Bone Damage under Different Population-Relevant Doses in Young Female Rats. *Nutrients* **2019**, *11*, 849. [CrossRef] [PubMed]
7. Muñoz-Castañeda, J.R.; Rodelo-Haad, C.; Pendon-Ruiz de Mier, M.V.; Martin-Malo, A.; Santamaria, R.; Rodriguez, M. Klotho/FGF23 and Wnt Signaling as Important Players in the Comorbidities Associated with Chronic Kidney Disease. *Toxins (Basel)* **2020**, *12*, 185.
8. Buendía, P.; Carracedo, J.; Soriano, S.; Madueño, J.A.; Ortiz, A.; Martín-Malo, A.; Aljama, P.; Ramírez, R. Klotho Prevents NFκB Translocation and Protects Endothelial Cell From Senescence Induced by Uremia. *J. Gerontol. A Biol. Sci. Med. Sci.* **2015**, *70*, 1198–1209. [CrossRef] [PubMed]
9. Carracedo, J.; Buendía, P.; Merino, A.; Madueño, J.A.; Peralbo, E.; Ortiz, A.; Martín-Malo, A.; Aljama, P.; Rodríguez, M.; Ramírez, R. Klotho modulates the stress response in human senescent endothelial cells. *Mech. Ageing Dev.* **2012**, *133*, 647–654. [CrossRef] [PubMed]
10. Donate-Correa, J.; Martín-Núñez, E.; Ferri, C.; Hernández-Carballo, C.; Tagua, V.G.; Delgado-Molinos, A.; López-Castillo, Á.; Rodríguez-Ramos, S.; Cerro-López, P.; López-Tarruella, V.C.; et al. FGF23 and Klotho Levels are Independently Associated with Diabetic Foot Syndrome in Type 2 Diabetes Mellitus. *J. Clin. Med.* **2019**, *8*. [CrossRef] [PubMed]
11. Shimada, T.; Hasegawa, H.; Yamazaki, Y.; Muto, T.; Hino, R.; Takeuchi, Y.; Fujita, T.; Nakahara, K.; Fukumoto, S.; Yamashita, T. FGF-23 is a potent regulator of vitamin D metabolism and phosphate homeostasis. *J. Bone Miner. Res.* **2004**, *19*, 429–435. [CrossRef] [PubMed]
12. Komaba, H.; Fukagawa, M. FGF23-parathyroid interaction: Implications in chronic kidney disease. *Kidney Int.* **2010**, *77*, 292–298. [CrossRef] [PubMed]
13. Rodelo-Haad, C.; Santamaria, R.; Muñoz-Castañeda, J.R.; Pendón-Ruiz de Mier, M.V.; Martin-Malo, A.; Rodriguez, M. FGF23, Biomarker or Target? *Toxins (Basel)* **2019**, *11*, 175. [CrossRef] [PubMed]
14. Liu, Y.C.; Tsai, J.P.; Wang, L.H.; Lee, M.C.; Hsu, B.G. Positive correlation of serum fibroblast growth factor 23 with peripheral arterial stiffness in kidney transplantation patients. *Clin. Chim. Acta* **2020**, *505*, 9–14. [CrossRef]
15. Razzaque, M.S. The FGF23-Klotho axis: Endocrine regulation of phosphate homeostasis. *Nat. Rev. Endocrinol.* **2009**, *5*, 611–619. [CrossRef]
16. Shimada, T.; Kakitani, M.; Yamazaki, Y.; Hasegawa, H.; Takeuchi, Y.; Fujita, T.; Fukumoto, S.; Tomizuka, K.; Yamashita, T. Targeted ablation of Fgf23 demonstrates an essential physiological role of FGF23 in phosphate and vitamin D metabolism. *J. Clin. Investig.* **2004**, *113*, 561–568. [CrossRef]
17. Zou, D.; Wu, W.; He, Y.; Ma, S.; Gao, J. The role of klotho in chronic kidney disease. *BMC Nephrol.* **2018**, *19*, 285. [CrossRef] [PubMed]
18. Erben, R.G.; Andrukhova, O. FGF23-Klotho signaling axis in the kidney. *Bone* **2017**, *100*, 62–68. [CrossRef] [PubMed]
19. Olauson, H.; Lindberg, K.; Amin, R.; Jia, T.; Wernerson, A.; Andersson, G.; Larsson, T.E. Targeted deletion of Klotho in kidney distal tubule disrupts mineral metabolism. *J. Am. Soc. Nephrol.* **2012**, *23*, 1641–1651. [CrossRef] [PubMed]
20. Martin, A.; David, V.; Quarles, L.D. Regulation and function of the FGF23/klotho endocrine pathways. *Physiol. Rev.* **2012**, *92*, 131–155. [CrossRef] [PubMed]
21. Hu, M.C.; Kuro-o, M.; Moe, O.W. Secreted klotho and chronic kidney disease. *Adv. Exp. Med. Biol.* **2012**, *728*, 126–157. [PubMed]
22. Takeshita, A.; Kawakami, K.; Furushima, K.; Miyajima, M.; Sakaguchi, K. Central role of the proximal tubular αKlotho/FGF receptor complex in FGF23-regulated phosphate and vitamin D metabolism. *Sci. Rep.* **2018**, *8*, 6917. [CrossRef] [PubMed]
23. Mencke, R.; Olauson, H.; Hillebrands, J.L. Effects of Klotho on fibrosis and cancer: A renal focus on mechanisms and therapeutic strategies. *Adv. Drug Deliv. Rev.* **2017**, *121*, 85–100. [PubMed]
24. Kuro-o, M.; Matsumura, Y.; Aizawa, H.; Kawaguchi, H.; Suga, T.; Utsugi, T.; Ohyama, Y.; Kurabayashi, M.; Kaname, T.; Kume, E.; et al. Mutation of the mouse klotho gene leads to a syndrome resembling ageing. *Nature* **1997**, *390*, 45–51. [PubMed]

25. Maekawa, Y.; Ishikawa, K.; Yasuda, O.; Oguro, R.; Hanasaki, H.; Kida, I.; Takemura, Y.; Ohishi, M.; Katsuya, T.; Rakugi, H. Klotho suppresses TNF-alpha-induced expression of adhesion molecules in the endothelium and attenuates NF-kappaB activation. *Endocrine* **2009**, *35*, 341–346.
26. Nabeshima, Y. Toward a better understanding of Klotho. *Sci. Aging Knowl. Environ.* **2006**, *2006*, pe11.
27. Jin, M.; Lv, P.; Chen, G.; Wang, P.; Zuo, Z.; Ren, L.; Bi, J.; Yang, C.W.; Mei, X.; Han, D. Klotho ameliorates cyclosporine A-induced nephropathy via PDLIM2/NF-kB p65 signaling pathway. *Biochem. Biophys. Res. Commun.* **2017**, *486*, 451–457. [PubMed]
28. Wang, Y.; Kuro-o, M.; Sun, Z. Klotho gene delivery suppresses Nox2 expression and attenuates oxidative stress in rat aortic smooth muscle cells via the cAMP-PKA pathway. *Aging Cell* **2012**, *11*, 410–417. [CrossRef] [PubMed]
29. Panesso, M.C.; Shi, M.; Cho, H.J.; Paek, J.; Ye, J.; Moe, O.W.; Hu, M.C. Klotho has dual protective effects on cisplatin-induced acute kidney injury. *Kidney Int.* **2014**, *85*, 855–870.
30. Hu, M.C.; Shi, M.; Zhang, J.; Quinones, H.; Griffith, C.; Kuro-o, M.; Moe, O.W. Klotho deficiency causes vascular calcification in chronic kidney disease. *J. Am. Soc. Nephrol.* **2011**, *22*, 124–136.
31. Kuro-o, M. Klotho as a regulator of oxidative stress and senescence. *Biol. Chem.* **2008**, *389*, 233–241. [CrossRef]
32. Liu, F.; Wu, S.; Ren, H.; Gu, J. Klotho suppresses RIG-I-mediated senescence-associated inflammation. *Nat. Cell Biol.* **2011**, *13*, 254–262. [CrossRef] [PubMed]
33. Doi, S.; Zou, Y.; Togao, O.; Pastor, J.V.; John, G.B.; Wang, L.; Shiizaki, K.; Gotschall, R.; Schiavi, S.; Yorioka, N.; et al. Klotho inhibits transforming growth factor-beta1 (TGF-beta1) signaling and suppresses renal fibrosis and cancer metastasis in mice. *J. Biol. Chem.* **2011**, *286*, 8655–8665. [PubMed]
34. Zhou, L.; Li, Y.; Zhou, D.; Tan, R.J.; Liu, Y. Loss of Klotho contributes to kidney injury by derepression of Wnt/beta-catenin signaling. *J. Am. Soc. Nephrol.* **2013**, *24*, 771–785. [CrossRef]
35. Sugiura, H.; Yoshida, T.; Shiohira, S.; Kohei, J.; Mitobe, M.; Kurosu, H.; Kuro-o, M.; Nitta, K.; Tsuchiya, K. Reduced Klotho expression level in kidney aggravates renal interstitial fibrosis. *Am. J. Physiol. Renal Physiol.* **2012**, *302*, F1252–F1264. [CrossRef]
36. Guan, X.; Nie, L.; He, T.; Yang, K.; Xiao, T.; Wang, S.; Huang, Y.; Zhang, J.; Wang, J.; Sharma, K.; et al. Klotho suppresses renal tubulo-interstitial fibrosis by controlling basic fibroblast growth factor-2 signalling. *J. Pathol.* **2014**, *234*, 560–572. [PubMed]
37. Huang, J.S.; Chuang, C.T.; Liu, M.H.; Lin, S.H.; Guh, J.Y.; Chuang, L.Y. Klotho attenuates high glucose-induced fibronectin and cell hypertrophy via the ERK1/2-p38 kinase signaling pathway in renal interstitial fibroblasts. *Mol. Cell Endocrinol.* **2014**, *390*, 45–53.
38. Shi, M.; Flores, B.; Gillings, N.; Bian, A.; Cho, H.J.; Yan, S.; Liu, Y.; Levine, B.; Moe, O.W.; Hu, M.C. AlphaKlotho Mitigates Progression of AKI to CKD through Activation of Autophagy. *J. Am. Soc. Nephrol.* **2016**, *27*, 2331–2345. [CrossRef]
39. Wang, Y.; Sun, Z. Current understanding of klotho. *Ageing Res. Rev.* **2009**, *8*, 43–51. [CrossRef]
40. Olauson, H.; Mencke, R.; Hillebrands, J.L.; Larsson, T.E. Tissue expression and source of circulating αKlotho. *Bone* **2017**, *100*, 19–35. [CrossRef]
41. Hu, M.C.; Kuro-o, M.; Moe, O.W. The emerging role of Klotho in clinical nephrology. *Nephrol. Dial. Transplant.* **2012**, *27*, 2650–2657. [CrossRef] [PubMed]
42. Amiri, F.S.; Khatami, M.R. Fibroblast Growth Factor 23 in Postrenal Transplant: An Often Forgotten Hormone. *Exp. Clin. Transplant.* **2016**, *14*, 606–616. [PubMed]
43. Neyra, J.A.; Li, X.; Mescia, F.; Ortiz-Soriano, V.; Adams-Huet, B.; Pastor, J.; Hu, M.C.; Toto, R.D.; Moe, O.W. Urine Klotho Is Lower in Critically Ill Patients With Versus Without Acute Kidney Injury and Associates With Major Adverse Kidney Events. *Crit. Care Explor.* **2019**, *1*, e0016. [CrossRef]
44. Sanchez-Niño, M.D.; Fernandez-Fernandez, B.; Ortiz, A. Klotho, the elusive kidney-derived anti-ageing factor. *Clin. Kidney J.* **2019**, *13*, 125–127.
45. Christov, M.; Neyra, J.A.; Gupta, S.; Leaf, D.E. Fibroblast Growth Factor 23 and Klotho in AKI. *Semin. Nephrol.* **2019**, *39*, 57–75. [CrossRef] [PubMed]
46. Neyra, J.A.; Hu, M.C. αKlotho and Chronic Kidney Disease. *Vitam. Horm.* **2016**, *101*, 257–310. [PubMed]
47. Hu, M.C.; Kuro-o, M.; Moe, O.W. Klotho and chronic kidney disease. *Contrib. Nephrol.* **2013**, *180*, 47–63. [PubMed]
48. Barker, S.L.; Pastor, J.; Carranza, D.; Quiñones, H.; Griffith, C.; Goetz, R.; Mohammadi, M.; Ye, J.; Zhang, J.; Hu, M.C.; et al. The demonstration of αKlotho deficiency in human chronic kidney disease with a novel synthetic antibody. *Nephrol. Dial. Transplant.* **2015**, *30*, 223–233. [CrossRef]

49. Seiler, S.; Rogacev, K.S.; Roth, H.J.; Shafein, P.; Emrich, I.; Neuhaus, S.; Floege, J.; Fliser, D.; Heine, G.H. Associations of FGF-23 and sKlotho with cardiovascular outcomes among patients with CKD stages 2–4. *Clin. J. Am. Soc. Nephrol.* **2014**, *9*, 1049–1058. [CrossRef]
50. Wang, Q.; Su, W.; Shen, Z.; Wang, R. Correlation between Soluble α-Klotho and Renal Function in Patients with Chronic Kidney Disease: A Review and Meta-Analysis. *Biomed. Res. Int.* **2018**, *2018*, 9481475. [CrossRef]
51. Sari, F.; Inci, A.; Dolu, S.; Ellidag, H.Y.; Cetinkaya, R.; Ersoy, F.F. High serum soluble α-Klotho levels in patients with autosomal dominant polycystic kidney disease. *J. Investig. Med.* **2017**, *65*, 358–362. [CrossRef]
52. Memmos, E.; Sarafidis, P.; Pateinakis, P.; Tsiantoulas, A.; Faitatzidou, D.; Giamalis, P.; Vasilikos, V.; Papagianni, A. Soluble Klotho is associated with mortality and cardiovascular events in hemodialysis. *BMC Nephrol.* **2019**, *20*, 217. [CrossRef] [PubMed]
53. Thongprayoon, C.; Hansrivijit, P.; Leeaphorn, N.; Acharya, P.; Torres-Ortiz, A.; Kaewput, W.; Kovvuru, K.; Kanduri, S.R.; Bathini, T.; Cheungpasitporn, W. Recent Advances and Clinical Outcomes of Kidney Transplantation. *J. Clin. Med.* **2020**, *9*, 1193. [CrossRef]
54. Thongprayoon, C.; Kaewput, W.; Kovvuru, K.; Hansrivijit, P.; Kanduri, S.R.; Bathini, T.; Chewcharat, A.; Leeaphorn, N.; Gonzalez-Suarez, M.L.; Cheungpasitporn, W. Promises of Big Data and Artificial Intelligence in Nephrology and Transplantation. *J. Clin. Med.* **2020**, *9*, 1107. [CrossRef]
55. Cheungpasitporn, W.; Thongprayoon, C.; Vaitla, P.K.; Chewcharat, A.; Hansrivijit, P.; Koller, F.L.; Mao, M.A.; Bathini, T.; Salim, S.A.; Katari, S.; et al. Degree of Glomerulosclerosis in Procurement Kidney Biopsies from Marginal Donor Kidneys and Their Implications in Predicting Graft Outcomes. *J. Clin. Med.* **2020**, *9*, 1469. [CrossRef]
56. Leeaphorn, N.; Thongprayoon, C.; Chon, W.J.; Cummings, L.S.; Mao, M.A.; Cheungpasitporn, W. Outcomes of kidney retransplantation after graft loss as a result of BK virus nephropathy in the era of newer immunosuppressant agents. *Am. J. Transplant.* **2020**, *20*, 1334–1340. [CrossRef] [PubMed]
57. Davis, C.L.; Delmonico, F.L. Living-donor kidney transplantation: a review of the current practices for the live donor. *J. Am. Soc. Nephrol.* **2005**, *16*, 2098–2110. [CrossRef] [PubMed]
58. Mizusaki, K.; Hasuike, Y.; Kimura, T.; Nagasawa, Y.; Kuragano, T.; Yamada, Y.; Nojima, M.; Yamamoto, S.; Nakanishi, T.; Ishihara, M. Inhibition of the Mammalian Target of Rapamycin May Augment the Increase in Soluble Klotho Levels in Renal Transplantation Recipients. *Blood Purif.* **2019**, *47* (Suppl. 2), 12–18. [CrossRef] [PubMed]
59. Deng, G.; Yang, A.; Wu, J.; Zhou, J.; Meng, S.; Zhu, C.; Wang, J.; Shen, S.; Ma, J.; Liu, D. The Value of Older Donors' Klotho Level in Predicting Recipients' Short-Term Renal Function. *Med. Sci. Monit.* **2018**, *24*, 7936–7943. [CrossRef] [PubMed]
60. Kim, S.M.; Kim, S.J.; Ahn, S.; Min, S.-I.; Min, S.-K.; Ha, J. The Potential Role of Klotho as a Prognostic Biomarker in Deceased Donor Kidney Transplantation. *Transplantation* **2018**, *102*, S539. [CrossRef]
61. Kubota, M.; Hamasaki, Y.; Masuda, T.; Hashimoto, J.; Takahashi, Y.; Saito, A.; Yuasa, R.; Muramatsu, M.; Sakai, K.; Shishido, S. Fgf 23-Aklotho axis and phosphate metabolism in the early post-kidney transplantation period. In *Pediatric Transplantation*; Wiley: Hoboken, NJ, USA, 2019.
62. Tan, S.J.; Crosthwaite, A.; Langsford, D.; Obeysekere, V.; Ierino, F.L.; Roberts, M.A.; Hughes, P.D.; Hewitson, T.D.; Dwyer, K.M.; Toussaint, N.D. Mineral adaptations following kidney transplantation. *Transpl. Int.* **2017**, *30*, 463–473. [CrossRef] [PubMed]
63. Baloglu, İ.; Turkmen, K.; Selçuk, N.Y.; Tonbul, H.Z.; Erdur, F.M. Fgf-23 and Klotho Levels in Renal Transplant Patients and Comparison with Hemodialysis Patients. In *Nephrology Dialysis Transplantation*; Oxford University Press: Oxford, UK, 2017.
64. Tartaglione, L.; Pasquali, M.; Rotondi, S.; Muci, M.L.; Leonangeli, C.; Farcomeni, A.; Fassino, V.; Mazzaferro, S. Interactions of sclerostin with FGF23, soluble klotho and vitamin D in renal transplantation. *PLoS ONE* **2017**, *12*, e0178637. [CrossRef] [PubMed]
65. Zaare Nahandi, M.; Ardalan, M.R.; Banagozar Mohamadi, A.; Ghorbani Haghjo, A.; Jabbarpor Bonyadi, M.; Mohamadian, T. Relationship of Serum Klotho Level With ACE Gene Polymorphism in Stable Kidney Allograft Recipients. *Iran. J. Kidney Dis.* **2017**, *11*, 151–156. [PubMed]
66. Bleskestad, I.H.; Thorsen, I.S.; Jonsson, G.; Skadberg, Ø.; Bergrem, H.; Gøransson, L.G. Soluble Klotho and intact fibroblast growth factor 23 in long-term kidney transplant patients. *Eur. J. Endocrinol.* **2015**, *172*, 343–350. [CrossRef]

67. Malyszko, J.; Koc-Zorawska, E.; Matuszkiewicz-Rowinska, J. FGF23 and Klotho in relation to markers of endothelial dysfunction in kidney transplant recipients. *Transplant. Proc.* **2014**, *46*, 2647–2650. [CrossRef]
68. Akimoto, T.; Kimura, T.; Watanabe, Y.; Ishikawa, N.; Iwazu, Y.; Saito, O.; Muto, S.; Yagisawa, T.; Kusano, E. The impact of nephrectomy and renal transplantation on serum levels of soluble Klotho protein. *Transplant. Proc.* **2013**, *45*, 134–136. [CrossRef]
69. Kimura, T.; Akimoto, T.; Watanabe, Y.; Kurosawa, A.; Nanmoku, K.; Muto, S.; Kusano, E.; Yagisawa, T.; Nagata, D. Impact of Renal Transplantation and Nephrectomy on Urinary Soluble Klotho Protein. *Transplant. Proc.* **2015**, *47*, 1697–1699. [CrossRef]
70. Ponte, B.; Trombetti, A.; Hadaya, K.; Ernandez, T.; Fumeaux, D.; Iselin, C.; Martin, P.Y.; de Seigneux, S. Acute and long term mineral metabolism adaptation in living kidney donors: A prospective study. *Bone* **2014**, *62*, 36–42. [CrossRef]
71. Tan, S.J.; Hewitson, T.D.; Hughes, P.D.; Holt, S.G.; Toussaint, N.D. Changes in Markers of Mineral Metabolism After Living Kidney Donation. *Transplant. Direct* **2017**, *3*, e150. [CrossRef]
72. Thorsen, I.S.; Bleskestad, I.H.; Jonsson, G.; Skadberg, Ø.; Gøransson, L.G. Neutrophil Gelatinase-Associated Lipocalin, Fibroblast Growth Factor 23, and Soluble Klotho in Long-Term Kidney Donors. *Nephron Extra* **2016**, *6*, 31–39. [CrossRef]
73. Hong, Y.A.; Choi, D.E.; Lim, S.W.; Yang, C.W.; Chang, Y.K. Decreased parathyroid Klotho expression is associated with persistent hyperparathyroidism after kidney transplantation. *Transplant. Proc.* **2013**, *45*, 2957–2962. [CrossRef]
74. Ozdem, S.; Yılmaz, V.T.; Ozdem, S.S.; Donmez, L.; Cetinkaya, R.; Suleymanlar, G.; Ersoy, F.F. Is Klotho F352V Polymorphism the Missing Piece of the Bone Loss Puzzle in Renal Transplant Recipients? *Pharmacology* **2015**, *95*, 271–278. [CrossRef]
75. Krajisnik, T.; Olauson, H.; Mirza, M.A.; Hellman, P.; Akerström, G.; Westin, G.; Larsson, T.E.; Björklund, P. Parathyroid Klotho and FGF-receptor 1 expression decline with renal function in hyperparathyroid patients with chronic kidney disease and kidney transplant recipients. *Kidney Int.* **2010**, *78*, 1024–1032. [CrossRef] [PubMed]
76. Moher, D.; Liberati, A.; Tetzlaff, J.; Altman, D.G. Preferred reporting items for systematic reviews and meta-analyses: The PRISMA statement. *PLoS Med.* **2009**, *6*, e1000097. [CrossRef]
77. DerSimonian, R.; Laird, N. Meta-analysis in clinical trials. *Control. Clin. Trials* **1986**, *7*, 177–188. [CrossRef]
78. Follmann, D.; Elliott, P.; Suh, I.; Cutler, J. Variance imputation for overviews of clinical trials with continuous response. *J. Clin. Epidemiol.* **1992**, *45*, 769–773. [CrossRef]
79. Cohen, J. Statistical power analysis. *Curr. Dir. Psychol. Sci.* **1992**, *1*, 98–101. [CrossRef]
80. Higgins, J.P.; Thompson, S.G.; Deeks, J.J.; Altman, D.G. Measuring inconsistency in meta-analyses. *BMJ* **2003**, *327*, 557–560. [CrossRef] [PubMed]
81. Easterbrook, P.J.; Berlin, J.A.; Gopalan, R.; Matthews, D.R. Publication bias in clinical research. *Lancet* **1991**, *337*, 867–872. [CrossRef]
82. Egger, M.; Davey Smith, G.; Schneider, M.; Minder, C. Bias in meta-analysis detected by a simple, graphical test. *BMJ* **1997**, *315*, 629–634. [CrossRef]
83. John, G.B.; Cheng, C.Y.; Kuro-o, M. Role of Klotho in aging, phosphate metabolism, and CKD. *Am. J. Kidney Dis.* **2011**, *58*, 127–134. [CrossRef] [PubMed]
84. Kalaitzidis, R.G.; Duni, A.; Siamopoulos, K.C. Klotho, the Holy Grail of the kidney: from salt sensitivity to chronic kidney disease. *Int. Urol. Nephrol.* **2016**, *48*, 1657–1666. [CrossRef] [PubMed]
85. Van Londen, M.; Aarts, B.M.; Deetman, P.E.; van der Weijden, J.; Eisenga, M.F.; Navis, G.; Bakker, S.J.L.; de Borst, M.H. Post-Transplant Hypophosphatemia and the Risk of Death-Censored Graft Failure and Mortality after Kidney Transplantation. *Clin. J. Am. Soc. Nephrol.* **2017**, *12*, 1301–1310. [CrossRef] [PubMed]
86. Nakai, K.; Mitsuiki, K.; Kuroki, Y.; Nishiki, T.; Motoyama, K.; Nakano, T.; Kitazono, T. Relative hypophosphatemia early after transplantation is a predictor of good kidney graft function. *Clin. Exp. Nephrol.* **2019**, *23*, 1161–1168. [CrossRef]
87. Hu, M.C.; Moe, O.W. Klotho as a potential biomarker and therapy for acute kidney injury. *Nat. Rev. Nephrol.* **2012**, *8*, 423–429. [CrossRef] [PubMed]
88. Aiello, S.; Noris, M. Klotho in acute kidney injury: Biomarker, therapy, or a bit of both? *Kidney Int.* **2010**, *78*, 1208–1210. [CrossRef] [PubMed]

89. Li, P.; Shi, M.; Maique, J.; Shaffer, J.; Yan, S.; Moe, O.W.; Hu, M.C. Beclin 1/Bcl-2 complex-dependent autophagy activity modulates renal susceptibility to ischemia-reperfusion injury and mediates renoprotection by Klotho. American journal of physiology. *Am. J. Physiol. Renal Physiol.* **2020**, *318*, F772–F792. [CrossRef] [PubMed]
90. Castellano, G.; Intini, A.; Stasi, A.; Divella, C.; Gigante, M.; Pontrelli, P.; Franzin, R.; Accetturo, M.; Zito, A.; Fiorentino, M.; et al. Complement Modulation of Anti-Aging Factor Klotho in Ischemia/Reperfusion Injury and Delayed Graft Function. *Am. J. Transplant.* **2016**, *16*, 325–333. [CrossRef]
91. De Sandes-Freitas, T.V.; Felipe, C.R.; Aguiar, W.F.; Cristelli, M.P.; Tedesco-Silva, H.; Medina-Pestana, J.O. Prolonged Delayed Graft Function Is Associated with Inferior Patient and Kidney Allograft Survivals. *PLoS ONE* **2015**, *10*, e0144188. [CrossRef] [PubMed]
92. Weber, S.; Dienemann, T.; Jacobi, J.; Eckardt, K.U.; Weidemann, A. Delayed graft function is associated with an increased rate of renal allograft rejection: A retrospective single center analysis. *PLoS ONE* **2018**, *13*, e0199445. [CrossRef] [PubMed]
93. Lee, C.H.; Kim, G.H. Electrolyte and Acid-base disturbances induced by clacineurin inhibitors. *Electrolyte Blood Press* **2007**, *5*, 126–130. [PubMed]
94. Demeule, M.; Béliveau, R. Cyclosporin inhibits phosphate transport and stimulates alkaline phosphatase activity in renal BBMV. *Am. J. Physiol.* **1991**, *260*, F518–F524. [PubMed]
95. Falkiewicz, K.; Nahaczewska, W.; Boratynska, M.; Owczarek, H.; Klinger, M.; Kaminska, D.; Wozniak, M.; Szepietowski, T.; Patrzalek, D. Tacrolimus decreases tubular phosphate wasting in renal allograft recipients. *Transplant. Proc.* **2003**, *35*, 2213–2215.
96. Messa, P.; Cafforio, C.; Alfieri, C. Calcium and phosphate changes after renal transplantation. *J. Nephrol.* **2010**, *23* (Suppl. 16), S175–S181. [PubMed]
97. Sakhaee, K. Post-renal transplantation hypophosphatemia. *Pediatr. Nephrol.* **2010**, *25*, 213–220.
98. Cheungpasitporn, W.; Thongprayoon, C.; Hansrivijit, P.; Medaura, J.; Chewcharat, A.; Bathini, T.; Mao, M.; Erickson, S. Impact of admission calcium-phosphate product on 1-year mortality among hospitalized patients. *Adv. Biomed. Res.* **2020**, *9*, 14.
99. Thongprayoon, C.; Cheungpasitporn, W.; Mao, M.A.; Erickson, S.B. Calcium-phosphate product and its impact on mortality in hospitalized patients. *Nephrology (Carlton)* **2020**, *25*, 22–28. [PubMed]
100. Pichler, G.; Haller, M.C.; Kainz, A.; Wolf, M.; Redon, J.; Oberbauer, R. Prognostic value of bone- and vascular-derived molecular biomarkers in hemodialysis and renal transplant patients: A systematic review and meta-analysis. *Nephrol. Dial. Transplant.* **2017**, *32*, 1566–1578.
101. Lentine, K.L.; Patel, A. Risks and outcomes of living donation. *Adv. Chronic Kidney Dis.* **2012**, *19*, 220–228.
102. Ommen, E.S.; Winston, J.A.; Murphy, B. Medical risks in living kidney donors: absence of proof is not proof of absence. *Clin. J. Am. Soc. Nephrol.* **2006**, *1*, 885–895.
103. Asgari, E.; Hilton, R.M. One size does not fit all: Understanding individual living kidney donor risk. *Pediatr. Nephrol.* **2020**. [CrossRef] [PubMed]
104. Fehrman-Ekholm, I.; Elinder, C.G.; Stenbeck, M.; Tydén, G.; Groth, C.G. Kidney donors live longer. *Transplantation* **1997**, *64*, 976–978. [CrossRef]
105. Okamoto, M.; Akioka, K.; Nobori, S.; Ushigome, H.; Kozaki, K.; Kaihara, S.; Yoshimura, N. Short- and long-term donor outcomes after kidney donation: analysis of 601 cases over a 35-year period at Japanese single center. *Transplantation* **2009**, *87*, 419–423. [CrossRef] [PubMed]
106. Ibrahim, H.N.; Foley, R.; Tan, L.; Rogers, T.; Bailey, R.F.; Guo, H.; Gross, C.R.; Matas, A.J. Long-term consequences of kidney donation. *N. Engl. J. Med.* **2009**, *360*, 459–469. [CrossRef] [PubMed]
107. Segev, D.L.; Muzaale, A.D.; Caffo, B.S.; Mehta, S.H.; Singer, A.L.; Taranto, S.E.; McBride, M.A.; Montgomery, R.A. Perioperative mortality and long-term survival following live kidney donation. *JAMA* **2010**, *303*, 959–966. [CrossRef] [PubMed]
108. O'Keeffe, L.M.; Ramond, A.; Oliver-Williams, C.; Willeit, P.; Paige, E.; Trotter, P.; Evans, J.; Wadström, J.; Nicholson, M.; Collett, D.; et al. Mid- and Long-Term Health Risks in Living Kidney Donors: A Systematic Review and Meta-analysis. *Ann. Intern. Med.* **2018**, *168*, 276–284. [CrossRef] [PubMed]
109. Garg, A.X.; Meirambayeva, A.; Huang, A.; Kim, J.; Prasad, G.V.; Knoll, G.; Boudville, N.; Lok, C.; McFarlane, P.; Karpinski, M.; et al. Cardiovascular disease in kidney donors: Matched cohort study. *BMJ* **2012**, *344*, e1203. [CrossRef]
110. Musgrove, J.; Wolf, M. Regulation and Effects of FGF23 in Chronic Kidney Disease. *Annu. Rev. Physiol.* **2020**, *82*, 365–390. [CrossRef]

111. Wolf, M. Forging forward with 10 burning questions on FGF23 in kidney disease. *J. Am. Soc. Nephrol.* **2010**, *21*, 1427–1435. [CrossRef]
112. Marthi, A.; Donovan, K.; Haynes, R.; Wheeler, D.C.; Baigent, C.; Rooney, C.M.; Landray, M.J.; Moe, S.M.; Yang, J.; Holland, L.; et al. Fibroblast Growth Factor-23 and Risks of Cardiovascular and Noncardiovascular Diseases: A Meta-Analysis. *J. Am. Soc. Nephrol.* **2018**, *29*, 2015–2027. [CrossRef]
113. Grabner, A.; Amaral, A.P.; Schramm, K.; Singh, S.; Sloan, A.; Yanucil, C.; Li, J.; Shehadeh, L.A.; Hare, J.M.; David, V.; et al. Activation of Cardiac Fibroblast Growth Factor Receptor 4 Causes Left Ventricular Hypertrophy. *Cell Metab.* **2015**, *22*, 1020–1032. [CrossRef] [PubMed]
114. Moody, W.E.; Ferro, C.J.; Edwards, N.C.; Chue, C.D.; Lin, E.L.; Taylor, R.J.; Cockwell, P.; Steeds, R.P.; Townend, J.N. Cardiovascular Effects of Unilateral Nephrectomy in Living Kidney Donors. *Hypertension* **2016**, *67*, 368–377. [CrossRef] [PubMed]
115. Vervloet, M.G.; Massy, Z.A.; Brandenburg, V.M.; Mazzaferro, S.; Cozzolino, M.; Ureña-Torres, P.; Bover, J.; Goldsmith, D. Bone: A new endocrine organ at the heart of chronic kidney disease and mineral and bone disorders. *Lancet Diabetes Endocrinol.* **2014**, *2*, 427–436. [CrossRef]
116. Hum, J.M.; O'Bryan, L.M.; Tatiparthi, A.K.; Cass, T.A.; Clinkenbeard, E.L.; Cramer, M.S.; Bhaskaran, M.; Johnson, R.L.; Wilson, J.M.; Smith, R.C.; et al. Chronic Hyperphosphatemia and Vascular Calcification Are Reduced by Stable Delivery of Soluble Klotho. *J. Am. Soc. Nephrol.* **2017**, *28*, 1162–1174. [CrossRef] [PubMed]
117. Xie, J.; Yoon, J.; An, S.W.; Kuro-o, M.; Huang, C.L. Soluble Klotho Protects against Uremic Cardiomyopathy Independently of Fibroblast Growth Factor 23 and Phosphate. *J. Am. Soc. Nephrol.* **2015**, *26*, 1150–1160. [CrossRef] [PubMed]
118. Xie, J.; Cha, S.K.; An, S.W.; Kuro, O.M.; Birnbaumer, L.; Huang, C.L. Cardioprotection by Klotho through downregulation of TRPC6 channels in the mouse heart. *Nat. Commun.* **2012**, *3*, 1238. [CrossRef] [PubMed]
119. Leone, F.; Lofaro, D.; Gigliotti, P.; Perri, A.; Vizza, D.; Toteda, G.; Lupinacci, S.; Armentano, F.; Papalia, T.; Bonofiglio, R. Soluble Klotho levels in adult renal transplant recipients are modulated by recombinant human erythropoietin. *J. Nephrol.* **2014**, *27*, 577–585. [CrossRef]
120. Donate-Correa, J.; Henríquez-Palop, F.; Martín-Núñez, E.; Pérez-Delgado, N.; Muros-de-Fuentes, M.; Mora-Fernández, C.; Navarro-González, J.F. Effect of Paricalcitol on FGF-23 and Klotho in Kidney Transplant Recipients. *Transplantation* **2016**, *100*, 2432–2438. [CrossRef]
121. Prather, A.A.; Epel, E.S.; Arenander, J.; Broestl, L.; Garay, B.I.; Wang, D.; Dubal, D.B. Longevity factor klotho and chronic psychological stress. *Transl. Psychiatry* **2015**, *5*, e585. [CrossRef]
122. Jurado-Fasoli, L.; Amaro-Gahete, F.J.; De-la, O.A.; Gutiérrez, Á.; Castillo, M.J. Alcohol consumption and S-Klotho plasma levels in sedentary healthy middle-aged adults: A cross sectional study. *Drug Alcohol Depend.* **2019**, *194*, 107–111. [CrossRef]
123. Amaro-Gahete, F.J.; De-la, O.A.; Jurado-Fasoli, L.; Ruiz, J.R.; Castillo, M.J.; Gutiérrez, Á. Role of Exercise on S-Klotho Protein Regulation: A Systematic Review. *Curr. Aging Sci.* **2018**, *11*, 100–107. [CrossRef] [PubMed]
124. Jurado-Fasoli, L.; Amaro-Gahete, F.J.; De-la, O.A.; Martinez-Tellez, B.; Ruiz, J.R.; Gutiérrez, Á.; Castillo, M.J. Adherence to the Mediterranean diet, dietary factors, and S-Klotho plasma levels in sedentary middle-aged adults. *Exp. Gerontol.* **2019**, *119*, 25–32. [CrossRef] [PubMed]
125. Deng, G.; Liu, D. Klotho: A Promising Biomarker Closely Related to Kidney Transplant. *Exp. Clin. Transplant.* **2018**, *16*, 253–258. [PubMed]
126. Neyra, J.A.; Moe, O.W.; Pastor, J.; Gianella, F.; Sidhu, S.S.; Sarnak, M.J.; Ix, J.H.; Drew, D.A. Performance of soluble Klotho assays in clinical samples of kidney disease. *Clin. Kidney J.* **2020**, *13*, 235–244. [CrossRef] [PubMed]

4

Proton-Pump Inhibitors and Hypomagnesaemia in Kidney Transplant Recipients

Rianne M. Douwes [1,*], António W. Gomes-Neto [1], Joëlle C. Schutten [1], Else van den Berg [1], Martin H. de Borst [1], Stefan P. Berger [1], Daan J. Touw [2], Eelko Hak [3], Hans Blokzijl [4], Gerjan Navis [1] and Stephan J. L. Bakker [1]

1 Department of Internal Medicine, Division of Nephrology, University Medical Center Groningen, University of Groningen, 9700 RB Groningen, The Netherlands; a.w.gomes.neto@umcg.nl (A.W.G.-N.); j.c.schutten@umcg.nl (J.C.S); e.van.den.berg@umcg.nl (E.v.d.B.); m.h.de.borst@umcg.nl (M.H.d.B.); s.p.berger@umcg.nl (S.P.B.); g.j.navis@umcg.nl (G.N.); s.j.l.bakker@umcg.nl (S.J.L.B.)

2 Department of Clinical Pharmacy and Pharmacology, University Medical Center Groningen, University of Groningen, 9700 RB Groningen, The Netherlands; d.j.touw@umcg.nl

3 Unit PharmacoTherapy, -Epidemiology and -Economics, Groningen Research Institute of Pharmacy, University of Groningen, 9713 AV Groningen, The Netherlands; e.hak@rug.nl

4 Department of Gastroenterology and Hepatology, University Medical Center Groningen, University of Groningen, 9700 RB Groningen, The Netherlands; h.blokzijl@umcg.nl

* Correspondence: r.m.douwes@umcg.nl

Abstract: Proton-pump inhibitors (PPIs) are commonly used after kidney transplantation and there is rarely an incentive to discontinue treatment. In the general population, PPI use has been associated with hypomagnesaemia. We aimed to investigate whether PPI use is associated with plasma magnesium, 24-h urinary magnesium excretion and hypomagnesaemia, in kidney transplant recipients (KTR). Plasma magnesium and 24-h urinary magnesium excretion were measured in 686 stable outpatient KTR with a functioning allograft for ≥1 year from the TransplantLines Food and Nutrition Biobank and Cohort-Study (NCT02811835). PPIs were used by 389 KTR (56.6%). In multivariable linear regression analyses, PPI use was associated with lower plasma magnesium (β: −0.02, $P = 0.02$) and lower 24-h urinary magnesium excretion (β: −0.82, $P < 0.001$). Moreover, PPI users had a higher risk of hypomagnesaemia (plasma magnesium <0.70 mmol/L), compared with non-users (Odds Ratio (OR): 2.12; 95% confidence interval (CI) 1.43–3.15, $P < 0.001$). This risk tended to be highest among KTR taking high PPI dosages (>20 mg omeprazole Eq/day) and was independent of adjustment for potential confounders (OR: 2.46; 95% CI 1.32–4.57, $P < 0.005$). No interaction was observed between PPI use and the use of loop diuretics, thiazide diuretics, tacrolimus, or diabetes ($P_{interaction} > 0.05$). These results demonstrate that PPI use is independently associated with lower magnesium status and hypomagnesaemia in KTR. The concomitant decrease in urinary magnesium excretion indicates that this likely is the consequence of reduced intestinal magnesium absorption. Based on these results, it might be of benefit to monitor magnesium status periodically in KTR on chronic PPI therapy.

Keywords: proton-pump inhibitors; magnesium; hypomagnesaemia; kidney transplantation

---

1. Introduction

Proton-pump inhibitors (PPIs) are frequently used after kidney transplantation for their gastro- protective properties in the setting of immunosuppressive therapy, which usually includes glucocorticoids. Since their first introduction in the late 1980s, numerous case reports and observational studies have been published that associate PPI use with unfavorable clinical outcomes, including an increased risk of hypomagnesaemia [1–8]. Recently, this observation has been strengthened by a large population based cohort study which demonstrated a two times higher risk of hypomagnesaemia among subjects from the general populations on chronic PPI therapy compared to non-users [9].

Magnesium homeostasis depends mainly on the balance between intestinal Mg^{2+} uptake, storage and resorption from bones and urinary excretion of Mg^{2+} via the kidneys [10]. It is postulated that PPIs induce hypomagnesaemia through inhibition of pH-dependent active magnesium absorption via transient receptor potential melastatin (TRPM) 6 and 7 channels in the intestine [11,12]. Moreover, increased renal magnesium retention has been observed in magnesium depleted subjects using chronic PPI therapy, indicating a defect in intestinal magnesium absorption or increased losses into the gastrointestinal tract, rather than renal magnesium wasting [1,7,13].

Hypomagnesaemia is very common after kidney transplantation and it is generally thought to be a side effect of immunosuppressive therapy, especially of calcineurin inhibitors (CNI) which are known to induce renal magnesium wasting [14]. It has been shown that hypomagnesaemia is not only present in the immediate post transplantation period, but persists in about 20% of kidney transplant recipients (KTR) for many years after transplantation [15,16]. Importantly, hypomagnesaemia has been associated with onset of post-transplant diabetes mellitus (PTDM) in KTR [17,18] and has also been associated with increased risk of cardiovascular morbidity [19,20] and mortality [21] in the general population. Whether use of PPIs contributes to hypomagnesaemia in KTR has not been well established. To our knowledge only one cohort study investigated the association between PPI use and hypomagnesaemia in 512 KTR, with negative results [22]. Reasons for absence of an association were unclear, but may have included a low prevalence of PPI use of 20%, which could have led to low statistical power of the study. Thus, whether PPI use negatively affects magnesium status after transplantation remains to be determined. We aimed to investigate whether PPI use is associated with magnesium status and hypomagnesaemia in a large single center cohort of stable outpatient KTR, in which plasma magnesium measurements were not part of routine clinical care but were assessed from samples that had been stored in a biobank.

2. Methods

2.1. Study Design and Population

This is a cross-sectional analysis using data from a previously described prospective cohort study registered at clinicaltrials.gov as 'TransplantLines Food and Nutrition Biobank and Cohort-study', NCT02811835 [23]. In summary, all adult KTR with a functioning graft beyond the first year after transplantation and without known or apparent systemic illnesses (i.e., malignancies other than cured skin cancer, opportunistic infections, overt congestive heart failure) who visited the outpatient clinic of the University Medical Center Groningen (UMCG) between November 2008 and March 2011, were asked to participate. A total of 707 out of the initially 817 invited KTR signed informed consent. We excluded KTR with missing biomaterial (n = 8), missing data on PPI dosage (n = 1), with on-demand PPI use (n = 3) or using magnesium supplements (n = 6) from statistical analyses, leaving 689 cases eligible for analysis. Study measurements were performed during a single study visit at the outpatient clinic. All study procedures were conducted in adherence with the Declaration of Helsinki and Declaration of Istanbul. The institutional review board of the UMCG approved the study protocol (METC 2008/186, approved on 17 September 2008).

2.2. Exposure Definition

PPI type and daily dosage were obtained from electronic patient records and are demonstrated in Table S1. KTR using any PPI on a daily basis during a period of at least 3 months prior to the study visit were defined as chronic PPI users as described previously [24]. To investigate a potential dose–response relationship, KTR were divided into three groups based on daily PPI dose defined in omeprazole equivalents: no PPI, low PPI dose (≤20 mg omeprazole equivalents/day (Eq/day)) and high PPI dose (>20 mg omeprazole Eq/day) [24,25].

2.3. Assessement of Plasma and Urinary Magnesium

Plasma magnesium was measured in samples containing lithium heparin, using a xylidyl blue method (Roche Modular analyzer, Roche Diagnostics, Mannheim, Germany). Urinary magnesium excretion was assessed in 24 h-urine samples and measured on a MEGA clinical chemistry analyzer (Merck, Darmstadt, Germany). Hypomagnesaemia was defined as plasma magnesium <0.70 mmol/L.

2.4. Assessment of Dietary Magnesium Intake

Dietary magnesium intake was calculated using a validated semi quantitative food frequency questionnaire (FFQ) developed and updated at the Wageningen University, which was filled out at home [26,27]. Dietary data were converted into daily nutrient intake using the Dutch Food Composition Table of 2006 [28].

2.5. Assessment of Covariates

Medical history was obtained from electronic patient records as described previously [23]. History of cardiovascular disease was classified according to the International Classification of Diseases, 10th revision (ICD-10) code Z86.7. Body mass index (BMI) was calculated as weight in kilograms divided by height in meters squared. Blood pressure was measured as described in detail previously [29]. Information on alcohol use and smoking behavior was obtained using a questionnaire. Medication use, including the use of PPIs, H2-receptor antagonists, diuretics, prednisolone, mycophenolate mofetil (MMF), tacrolimus, cyclosporine, and sirolimus was recorded at baseline. Routine immunosuppressive therapy consisted of: A combination of azathioprine and prednisolone from 1968 to 1989; a combination of cyclosporine and prednisolone from 1989 to 1996. In 1997 mycophenolate motefil was added to the standard immunosuppressive regimen and cyclosporine was slowly withdrawn after the first year in KTR without complications. In 2012 cyclosporine was replaced by tacrolimus, and KTR received triple-immunosuppressive therapy with prednisolone, tacrolimus and mycophenolate mofetil. PPIs were routinely prescribed after kidney transplantation for their gastro-protective properties with concurrent use of prednisolone. Blood samples were collected after an 8–12 h fasting period. Serum creatinine was measured using an enzymatic, isotope dilution mass spectrometry-traceable assay (P-Modular automated analyzer, Roche Diagnostics, Mannheim, Germany). Estimated glomerular filtration rate (eGFR) was calculated using the serum creatinine based Chronic Kidney Disease Epidemiology Collaboration (CKD-EPI) equation. Serum potassium, calcium, parathyroid hormone (PTH), glucose and hemoglobin A1c (HbA1c), were determined using standard laboratory methods. Proteinuria was defined as urinary protein excretion ≥0.5 g/24 h.

2.6. Statistical Analyses

Statistical analyses were performed using SPSS, version 23.0 (IBM corp., Armonk, NY, USA). Data are presented as mean ± SD for normally distributed data, median with interquartile range (IQR) for skewed data and number with percentage for nominal data. Differences between PPI users versus PPI non-users were tested using independent sample *T*-tests, Mann–Whitney U-tests and Chi-square tests or Fishers exact tests when appropriate.

To study the effect of PPI use on plasma magnesium linear regression analyses were performed with adjustment for potential confounders of magnesium status including: age, sex, BMI, eGFR, proteinuria, time since transplantation, alcohol use, diabetes, history of cardiovascular disease, use of loop diuretics, thiazide diuretics, tacrolimus, cyclosporine, MMF, and dietary magnesium intake. To investigate the association between PPI use and hypomagnesaemia we performed logistic regression analyses with adjustment for the same potential confounders used in multivariable linear regression analyses. Effect modification by loop diuretics, thiazide diuretics, tacrolimus and diabetes was tested by inclusion of interaction terms. To investigate a potential dose–response relationship we performed additional analyses in which KTR were divided into three groups based on daily PPI dose defined in omeprazole equivalents: No PPI, low PPI dose (≤20 mg omeprazole Eq/day) and high PPI dose (>20 mg omeprazole Eq/day) [24,25]. Tests of linear trend were conducted by assigning the median of daily PPI dose equivalents in subgroups treated as a continuous variable. We performed sensitivity analyses in which H2-receptor antagonist (H2RA) users (n = 18) were excluded to assess the robustness of the association between PPI use and hypomagnesaemia. Lastly, we investigated which KTR are at increased risk of developing hypomagnesaemia. A two-sided P-value < 0.05 was considered statistically significant in all analyses.

3. Results

3.1. Baseline Characteristics

Baseline characteristics are shown in Table 1. PPIs were used by a small majority of 389 (56.5%) KTR and omeprazole was the most often prescribed PPI (n = 340). Other PPIs used were esomeprazole (n = 30), pantoprazole (n = 16), and rabeprazole (n = 3). KTR who used PPIs were older than KTR who did not use PPIs, had a higher BMI and had shorter time between transplantation and baseline measurements. Diabetes was significantly more prevalent in PPI users compared with non-users (28.3% vs. 18.3%, P < 0.002). Plasma magnesium and 24-h urinary magnesium excretion were significantly lower in PPI users and 102 (26.2%) PPI users had hypomagnesaemia compared with 43 (14.3%) non-users (P < 0.001). Dietary magnesium intake was not significantly different between PPI users and non-users. Loop diuretics, cyclosporine and MMF, were more often used by PPI users compared with non-users. Triple immunosuppressive therapy consisting of MMF, cyclosporine and prednisolone, was more common in PPI users compared with non-users. Duo therapy consisting of MMF-prednisolone, MMF-cyclosporine, and cyclosporine-prednisolone was more common in PPI users compared with non-users.

Table 1. Baseline characteristics of 689 kidney transplant recipients.

Characteristics	Total Population	Non-PPI Users	PPI Users	P
Number of subjects, n (%)	689 (100)	300 (43.5)	389 (56.5)	n/a
Demographics				
Age, year	53 ± 13	51 ± 13	54 ± 12	0.001
Men, n (%)	395 (57.3)	177 (59.0)	218 (56.0)	0.4
BMI, kg/m^2	26.6 ± 4.8	25.9 ± 4.6	27.1 ± 4.8	0.002
Diabetes Mellitus, n (%)	165 (23.9)	55 (18.3)	110 (28.3)	0.002
History of CV disease, n (%)	274 (39.8)	92 (30.7)	182 (46.8)	<0.001
Time since transplantation, year	5.5 (1.9–12.1)	9.6 (4.1–15.0)	4.2 (1.1–8.7)	<0.001
Lifestyle parameters				
Current smoker, n (%)	84 (13.0)	35 (12.4)	49 (13.6)	0.7
Alcohol consumer, n (%)	436 (70.3)	198 (72.8)	238 (68.4)	0.2
Magnesium intake, mg/day	329.9 ± 88.7	333.0 ± 89.2	327.6 ± 88.4	0.5
Renal function parameters				
eGFR, mL/min/1.73 m^2	52.3 ± 20.2	55.1 ± 19.9	50.2 ± 20.1	0.002
Serum creatinine, μmol/L	124 (100–160)	119 (98–152)	128 (101–168)	0.03
Proteinuria (≥0.5 g/24 h), n (%)	157 (22.9)	71 (23.7)	86 (22.2)	0.7
Laboratory parameters				
Hypomagnesaemia, n (%)	145 (21.0)	43 (14.3)	102 (26.2)	<0.001
Plasma magnesium, mmol/L	0.77 ± 0.11	0.79 ± 0.09	0.76 ± 0.11	<0.001
24-h urinary magnesium excretion, mmol/24 h	3.3 (2.3–3.3)	3.8 (2.8–4.8)	3.1 (2.0–3.9)	<0.001
Serum potassium, mmol/L	3.98 ± 0.46	3.97 ± 0.47	3.99 ± 0.46	0.6
Serum calcium, mmol/L	2.40 ± 0.15	2.40 ± 0.15	2.40 ± 0.15	0.8
PTH, pmol/L	9.0 (6.0–14.8)	8.7 (6.0–13.6)	9.2 (5.9–16.3)	0.2
Glucose, mmol/L	5.3 (4.8–6)	5.2 (4.7–5.8)	5.3 (4.8–6.2)	0.01
HbA1c, mmol/mol	40 (37–44)	39 (36–42)	41 (38–45)	<0.001

Table 1. *Cont.*

Characteristics	Total Population	Non-PPI Users	PPI Users	*P*
Medication use				
Mycophenolate mofetil, *n* (%)	452 (65.6)	178 (59.3)	274 (70.4)	0.002
Tacrolimus, *n* (%)	124 (18.0)	49 (16.3)	75 (19.3)	0.3
Cyclosporine, *n* (%)	272 (39.5)	97 (32.3)	175 (45.0)	0.001
Sirolimus, *n* (%)	13 (2.0)	8 (2.8)	5 (1.4)	0.3
Prednisolone, *n* (%)	682 (99.0)	298 (99.3)	384 (98.7)	0.7
Loop diuretics, *n* (%)	160 (23.2)	41 (13.7)	119 (30.6)	<0.001
Thiazide diuretics, *n* (%)	120 (17.4)	53 (17.7)	67 (17.4)	0.9
H2-receptor antagonists, *n* (%)	18 (2.6)	17 (5.7)	1 (0.3)	<0.001
Combination therapy				
MMF + Tac + pred, *n* (%)	78 (11.3)	32 (10.7)	46 (11.8)	0.6
MMF + Cyclo + pred, *n* (%)	175 (25.4)	51 (17.0)	124 (31.9)	<0.001
MMF + Tac, *n* (%)	81 (11.8)	33 (11.0)	48 (12.3)	0.6
MMF + Pred, *n* (%)	447 (64.9)	176 (58.7)	271 (69.7)	0.003
MMF + Cyclo, *n* (%)	177 (25.7)	52 (17.3)	125 (32.1)	<0.001
Cyclo + Pred, *n* (%)	269 (39.0)	96 (32.0)	173 (44.5)	0.001
Tac + Pred, *n* (%)	120 (17.4)	48 (16.0)	72 (18.5)	0.4

Data are presented as mean ± SD, median with interquartile ranges (IQR) or number with percentages (%). Abbreviations: BMI, body mass index; eGFR, estimated glomerular filtration rate; HbA1c, hemoglobin A1c; PTH, Parathyroid hormone; MMF, mycophenolate mofetil; Tac, tacrolimus; Pred, prednisolone.

3.2. *Association of PPI Use with Plasma Magnesium and 24-h urinary Magnesium Excretion*

PPI use was significantly associated with lower plasma magnesium (β = −0.03; 95% CI −0.04; −0.01 mmol/L, *P* = 0.001) and lower urinary magnesium excretion (β = −0.86; 95% CI −1.10; −0.06 mmol/24 h, *P* < 0.001) as compared to non-users, Table 2. After adjustment for potential confounders, PPI use remained significantly associated with lower plasma magnesium levels (β = −0.02, 95% CI −0.04; −0.003, *P* = 0.02) and 24-h urinary magnesium excretion (β = −0.82, 95% CI −1.07; −0.57, *P* < 0.001).

Table 2. Association of proton-pump inhibitor (PPI) use with plasma magnesium and 24-h urinary magnesium excretion in 689 kidney transplant recipients.

	Plasma Magnesium, mmol/L			Urinary Magnesium Excretion, mmol/24 h		
	β	95% CI	*P*	β	95% CI	*P*
Crude	−0.03	−0.04; −0.01	0.001	−0.86	−1.10; −0.06	<0.001
Multivariable model	−0.02	−0.04; −0.003	0.02	−0.82	−1.07; −0.57	<0.001

Multivariable analyses were adjusted for age, sex, BMI, eGFR, proteinuria, time since transplantation, alcohol use, diabetes, history of CV disease, loop diuretics, thiazide diuretics, tacrolimus use, cyclosporine use, MMF use and dietary magnesium intake. Abbreviations: CI, confidence interval.

3.3. *Association of PPI Use with Hypomagnesaemia*

In crude logistic regression analysis, PPI use was associated with a more than two times higher risk of hypomagnesaemia compared with no use (OR: 2.12; 95% CI 1.43–3.15, *P* < 0.001), as shown in Table 3. The association remained independent of adjustment for potential confounders including age, sex, eGFR, proteinuria, time since transplantation, alcohol use, diabetes, history of cardiovascular disease, medication use (loop diuretics, thiazide diuretics, tacrolimus, cyclosporine and MMF) and dietary magnesium intake (OR: 2.00; 95% CI 1.21–3.31, *P* = 0.007). No significant interaction was observed between PPI use and the use of loop diuretics, thiazide diuretics, tacrolimus, or diabetes for the association with hypomagnesaemia ($P_{interaction} = 0.2$, $P_{interaction} = 0.7$, $P_{interaction} = 0.7$, $P_{interaction} = 0.9$, respectively).

Table 3. Logistic regression analyses investigating the association of PPI use with hypomagnesaemia in 689 kidney transplant recipients.

	Hypomagnesaemia		
N = 689	**Odds Ratio**	**95% CI**	***P***
Crude	2.12	1.43–3.15	<0.001
Multivariable model	2.00	1.21–3.31	0.007

Multivariable analyses were adjusted for age, sex, BMI, eGFR, proteinuria, time since transplantation, alcohol use, diabetes, history of CV disease, loop diuretics, thiazide diuretics, tacrolimus use, cyclosporine use, MMF use and dietary magnesium intake. Abbreviations: CI, confidence interval.

3.4. Dose–Response Analyses

Based on daily dose equivalents of omeprazole, 251 KTR received a low PPI dose (≤20 mg omeprazole Eq/day) and 138 KTR received a high PPI dose (>20 mg omeprazole Eq/day). As shown in Table 4 and Figure 1, risk of hypomagnesaemia tended to be highest among KTR taking a high PPI dose (OR: 2.53; 95% CI 1.55–4.11, $P < 0.001$). The association remained materially unchanged after multivariable adjustment (OR: 2.46; 95% CI 1.32–4.57, $P < 0.005$), Table 4. Moreover, a significant trend between PPI dose and risk of hypomagnesaemia was observed ($P_{trend} = 0.004$).

Table 4. Subgroup analyses of the association of PPI use with hypomagnesaemia in 689 kidney transplant recipients.

	Categories of PPI Use						
	No PPI		**Low PPI Dose**		**High PPI Dose**		
Number of subjects	300		251		138		
	Odds ratio (95% CI)	*P*	Odds ratio (95% CI)	*P*	Odds ratio (95% CI)	*P*	*P*-Trend
Hypomagnesaemia							
Crude	1.00 (reference)	n/a	1.92 (1.25–2.96)	0.003	2.53 (1.55–4.11)	<0.001	<0.001
Multivariable model	1.00 (reference)	n/a	1.79 (1.04–3.08)	0.04	2.46 (1.32–4.57)	0.005	0.004

Multivariable analyses were adjusted for age, sex, BMI, eGFR, proteinuria, time since transplantation, alcohol use, diabetes, history of CV disease, loop diuretics, thiazide diuretics, tacrolimus use, cyclosporine use, MMF use, dietary magnesium intake. Low PPI dose (≤20 mg omeprazole Eq/day), High PPI dose (>20 mg omeprazole Eq/day). Abbreviations: CI, confidence interval.

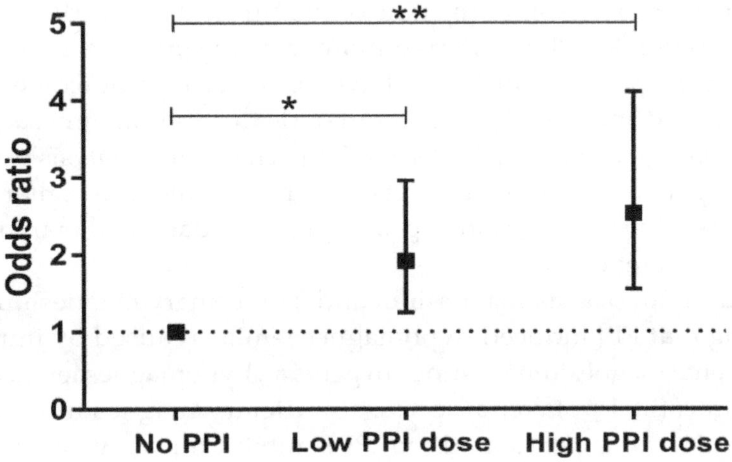

Figure 1. Crude association between PPI use and risk of hypomagnesaemia stratified by subgroups of PPI use. No PPI, Low PPI dose (≤20 mg omeprazole Eq/day), High PPI dose (>20 mg omeprazole Eq/day). Presented are odds ratio's with 95% confidence intervals. * $P = 0.004$; ** $P < 0.001$; $P_{trend} < 0.001$.

3.5. Sensitivity Analyses for Risk of Hypomagnesaemia

To account for the use of other important gastric acid reducing medication, we performed sensitivity analyses in which H2RA users ($N = 18$) were excluded form statistical analyses (Table S2). The association between PPI use and hypomagnesaemia remained materially unchanged when H2RA users were excluded (OR: 2.17, 95% CI 1.29–3.67, $P = 0.004$). We also performed analyses to investigate which KTR are at increased risk of developing hypomagnesaemia. These analyses are presented in Table S3. We found that patients with a history of cardiovascular disease, patients at shorter time after transplantation, not consuming alcohol, PPI users, thiazide diuretic users and patients using tacrolimus based immunosuppressive regimens were at increased risk of developing hypomagnesaemia. Moreover, KTR with hypomagnesaemia had higher fasting glucose levels, HbA1c and lower serum calcium levels compared with KTR without hypomagnesaemia.

4. Discussion

The present study is to our knowledge the largest cohort study to date exploring the association between PPI use and hypomagnesaemia in a cohort of KTR. Our results demonstrate a higher risk of hypomagnesaemia among KTR using PPIs, with subsequently lower plasma magnesium levels in combination with lower renal magnesium excretion. The association between PPI use and risk of hypomagnesaemia remained significant after adjustment for important potential confounders and tended to be highest among KTR taking high PPI dosages.

Our results confirm previous case-series and cohort studies investigating the association between PPI use and increased risk of hypomagnesaemia [1,2,7,9]. In a large cohort study ($N = 9818$) among subjects from the general population, it was shown that PPI users had significantly lower serum magnesium levels and had a two times higher risk of hypomagnesaemia compared with non-users [9]. Our results are in line with observations from this large cohort study and show a similar increased risk of hypomagnesaemia (OR 2.12).

So far, only one other study by van Ende et al. investigating the association between PPI use and magnesium status in KTR has been published [22]. Contrary to our findings, van Ende et al. found no association between PPI use and serum magnesium levels. Reasons for the lower proportion of PPI users in the study by van Ende et al. are unclear, though underreporting may have played a role, given that it was not specified how data regarding PPI use was obtained. It was also unclear whether the data of van Ende et al. were derived from routine outpatient assessment of plasma magnesium concentrations, which may have provided an incentive for stopping PPI use in KTR with low magnesium concentrations. This could have biased their results and could possibly also explain the large difference in PPI use between our study and their study, because in our center no plasma magnesium data were available at the time of the study. It was furthermore unclear whether it concerned on-demand or chronic PPI use. Furthermore, data regarding PPI dose, type and magnesium supplementation were not reported, which may have influenced the outcome.

In a recently published meta-analysis, a similar risk of hypomagnesaemia among KTR was demonstrated (pooled OR = 1.56, 95% CI 1.19–2.05) [30]. This meta-analysis by Boonpheng et al. was based on one published paper and seven abstracts presented at medical conferences. Our study adds that it investigated a dose–response relationship, and provides data on dietary magnesium intake and 24-h urinary magnesium excretion.

In the present study, both plasma magnesium and 24-h urinary magnesium excretion were lower in PPI users, suggesting that PPI induced hypomagnesaemia is caused by impaired gastrointestinal absorption rather than renal magnesium wasting. In general, hypomagnesaemia can be the consequence of either a decreased intestinal uptake, a decrease in dietary magnesium intake or an increase in renal magnesium excretion. It is postulated that PPIs inhibit the active magnesium absorption via the TRPM 6 and 7 channels in the intestine [11,12]. In KTR other contributing factors than PPI use may add to the risk of hypomagnesaemia. For example, decreased intestinal magnesium absorption can also be the consequence of chronic post-transplant diarrhea, which is highly prevalent and often complicated by hypomagnesaemia [10,31]. Data regarding symptoms of severe diarrhea were unfortunately unavailable in this study, therefore we could not correct for this potential confounder. Likewise, hypomagnesaemia can be the result of insufficient intake of foods rich in magnesium. In our study, mean dietary magnesium intake was 329.9 ± 88.7 mg/day, which was slightly lower than the mean habitual intake of magnesium among the general Dutch population, as reported in the Dutch National Food Consumption Survey 2007–2010 [32]. A low dietary magnesium intake can also be a reflection of an overall poor diet. Nonetheless, when we adjusted for dietary magnesium intake in our logistic regression analyses, the relationship between PPI use and risk of hypomagnesaemia remained materially unchanged, indicating that the observed risk associated with PPI use was not confounded by dietary magnesium intake.

The main strength of this study is measurement of three important pillars of magnesium status: plasma magnesium, 24-h urinary magnesium excretion and dietary magnesium intake. Because of this, we were able to confirm that PPI use does not lead to increased renal magnesium wasting but very likely impairs intestinal magnesium absorption. Furthermore, we only included KTR who were using PPIs for at least 3 months before blood sampling. It is previously noted that hypomagnesaemia occurs mainly in patients on prolonged PPI therapy suggesting that it takes time before magnesium stores are meaningfully depleted [6,7,33]. Moreover, we excluded KTR using magnesium supplements and adjusted for potential confounders, including CNI use, which did not alter the association.

A limitation of our study is its cross-sectional design. Therefore, a causal relationship between PPI use and hypomagnesaemia remains to be determined and changes over time in magnesium status parameters were unknown. Furthermore, no information regarding compliance to PPI treatment was available, which may have led to underestimation of effect sizes. PPI users had a shorter time between transplantation and baseline measurements. However, adjustment for time since transplantation did not alter the association between PPI use and hypomagnesaemia. Lastly, the possibility of residual confounding or bias by indication remains, which may have led to overestimation of the role of PPIs since on average PPI users were less healthy than non-users. A strength of the current study is, that no routine outpatient monitoring of plasma magnesium was performed and that we measured plasma and urine magnesium in samples that had been stored in a biobank, which reduces the change of selection bias in our cohort.

Our findings may be of clinical importance. KTR with low magnesium levels seem to develop post-transplant diabetes mellitus (PTDM) more frequently [17]. In this study we also found that KTR with hypomagnesaemia had higher fasting glucose levels and HbA1c. Next to that, a higher degree of arterial stiffness, as assessed by a carotid-femoral pulse wave velocity (PWV) measurement, has been found in KTR with low magnesium levels [34]. This same PWV measurement was found to be an independent predictor of cardiovascular events in KTR [35]. Moreover, hypomagnesaemia has been associated with cardiovascular morbidity [19,20] and mortality [21] in the general population. However, whether this association is also present in KTR is currently unknown. Another clinical significance lies in the association with lower calcium levels, which potentially points to an increased risk of developing osteoporosis. Long-term PPI use has indeed been associated with decreased bone mineral density and increased risk of fractures [36]. Because many patients use PPIs without evidence based indication [37–39], we believe that reevaluation of treatment indication in KTR on chronic PPI therapy might be of benefit. In situations in which PPIs are clinically needed, it would be judicious to assess and follow-up magnesium levels periodically during treatment, as recommended by the US Food and Drug administration and stated in the summary of product characteristics of all PPIs.

5. Conclusions

This study demonstrates that PPI use is associated with lower magnesium status and hypomagnesaemia in KTR. Moreover, risk of hypomagnesaemia was higher among KTR taking a high PPI dosage. Healthcare professionals should be aware of this additional risk and should consider regular monitoring of magnesium levels, especially in this patient population at high risk of hypomagnesaemia.

Author Contributions: Data curation, R.M.D., A.W.G.-N., E.v.d.B., and S.J.L.B.; Formal analysis, R.M.D., A.W.G.-N., J.C.S. and S.J.L.B.; Methodology, R.M.D, A.W.G.-N., J.C.S., E.v.d.B., M.H.d.B., S.P.B., D.J.T., E.H., H.B., G.J.N. and S.J.L.B. writing—original draft preparation, R.M.D., A.W.G.-N.; writing—review and editing, R.M.D., A.W.G.-N., J.C.S., M.H.d.B., E.v.d.B., S.P.B., D.J.T., E.H., H.B., G.J.N. and S.J.L.B. Supervision, H.B., G.N., S.J.L.B.; Funding acquisition, R.M.D., E.v.d.B. and S.J.L.B.

References

1. Cundy, T.; Dissanayake, A. Severe hypomagnesaemia in long-term users of proton-pump inhibitors. *Clin. Endocrinol. (Oxf.)* **2008**, *69*, 338–341. [CrossRef] [PubMed]
2. Danziger, J.; William, J.H.; Scott, D.J.; Lee, J.; Lehman, L.W.; Mark, R.G.; Howell, M.D.; Celi, L.A.; Mukamal, K.J. Proton-pump inhibitor use is associated with low serum magnesium concentrations. *Kidney Int.* **2013**, *83*, 692–699. [CrossRef] [PubMed]
3. Hess, M.W.; Hoenderop, J.G.; Bindels, R.J.; Drenth, J.P. Systematic review: Hypomagnesaemia induced by proton pump inhibition. *Aliment. Pharmacol. Ther.* **2012**, *36*, 405–413. [CrossRef] [PubMed]
4. Park, C.H.; Kim, E.H.; Roh, Y.H.; Kim, H.Y.; Lee, S.K. The association between the use of proton pump inhibitors and the risk of hypomagnesemia: A systematic review and meta-analysis. *PLoS ONE* **2014**, *9*, e112558. [CrossRef]
5. Cheungpasitporn, W.; Thongprayoon, C.; Kittanamongkolchai, W.; Srivali, N.; Edmonds, P.J.; Ungprasert, P.; O'Corragain, O.A.; Korpaisarn, S.; Erickson, S.B. Proton pump inhibitors linked to hypomagnesemia: A systematic review and meta-analysis of observational studies. *Ren. Fail.* **2015**, *37*, 1237–1241. [CrossRef]
6. Regolisti, G.; Cabassi, A.; Parenti, E.; Maggiore, U.; Fiaccadori, E. Severe hypomagnesemia during long-term treatment with a proton pump inhibitor. *Am. J. Kidney Dis.* **2010**, *56*, 168–174. [CrossRef]
7. Hoorn, E.J.; van der Hoek, J.; de Man, R.A.; Kuipers, E.J.; Bolwerk, C.; Zietse, R. A case series of proton pump inhibitor-induced hypomagnesemia. *Am. J. Kidney Dis.* **2010**, *56*, 112–116. [CrossRef]
8. Lindner, G.; Funk, G.-C.; Leichtle, A.B.; Fiedler, G.M.; Schwarz, C.; Eleftheriadis, T.; Pasch, A.; Mohaupt, M.G.; Exadaktylos, A.K.; Arampatzis, S. Impact of proton pump inhibitor use on magnesium homoeostasis: A cross-sectional study in a tertiary emergency department. *Int. J. Clin. Pract.* **2014**, *68*, 1352–1357. [CrossRef]
9. Kieboom, B.C.; Jong, J.C.K.; Eijgelsheim, M.; Franco, O.H.; Kuipers, E.J.; Hofman, A.; Zietse, R.; Stricker, B.H.; Hoorn, E.J. Proton pump inhibitors and hypomagnesemia in the general population: A population-based cohort study. *Am. J. Kidney Dis.* **2015**, *66*, 775–782. [CrossRef]
10. de Baaij, J.H.F.; Hoenderop, J.G.J.; Bindels, R.J.M. Magnesium in Man: Implications for Health and Disease. *Physiol. Rev.* **2015**, *95*, 1–46. [CrossRef]
11. William, J.H.; Danziger, J. Proton-pump inhibitor-induced hypomagnesemia: Current research and proposed mechanisms. *World J. Nephrol.* **2016**, *5*, 152–157. [CrossRef] [PubMed]
12. Schlingmann, K.P.; Waldegger, S.; Konrad, M.; Chubanov, V.; Gudermann, T. TRPM6 and TRPM7—Gatekeepers of human magnesium metabolism. *Biochim. Biophys. Acta Mol. Basis Dis.* **2007**, *1772*, 813–821. [CrossRef] [PubMed]
13. William, J.H.; Nelson, R.; Hayman, N.; Mukamal, K.J.; Danziger, J. Proton-pump inhibitor use is associated with lower urinary magnesium excretion. *Nephrology (Carlton)* **2014**, *19*, 798–801. [CrossRef] [PubMed]
14. Barton, C.H.; Vaziri, N.D.; Martin, D.C.; Choi, S.; Alikhani, S. Hypomagnesemia and renal magnesium wasting in renal transplant recipients receiving cyclosporine. *Am. J. Med.* **1987**, *83*, 693–699. [CrossRef]
15. Vannini, S.D.; Mazzola, B.L.; Rodoni, L.; Truttmann, A.C.; Wermuth, B.; Bianchetti, M.G.; Ferrari, P. Permanently reduced plasma ionized magnesium among renal transplant recipients on cyclosporine. *Transpl. Int.* **1999**, *12*, 244–249. [CrossRef]
16. Van de Cauter, J.; Sennesael, J.; Haentjens, P. Long-term evolution of the mineral metabolism after renal transplantation: A prospective, single-center cohort study. *Transplant. Proc.* **2011**, *43*, 3470–3475. [CrossRef]
17. Van Laecke, S.; Van Biesen, W.; Verbeke, F.; De Bacquer, D.; Peeters, P.; Vanholder, R. Posttransplantation hypomagnesemia and its relation with immunosuppression as predictors of new-onset diabetes after transplantation. *Am. J. Transplant.* **2009**, *9*, 2140–2149. [CrossRef]

18. Augusto, J.-F.; Subra, J.-F.; Duveau, A.; Rakotonjanahary, J.; Dussaussoy, C.; Picquet, J.; Croue, A.; Villemain, F.; Onno, C.; Sayegh, J. Relation between pretransplant magnesemia and the risk of new onset diabetes after transplantation within the first year of kidney transplantation. *Transplantation* **2014**, *97*, 1155–1160. [CrossRef]
19. Joosten, M.M.; Gansevoort, R.T.; Mukamal, K.J.; van der Harst, P.; Geleijnse, J.M.; Feskens, E.J.; Navis, G.; Bakker, S.J.; Group, P.S. Urinary and plasma magnesium and risk of ischemic heart disease. *Am. J. Clin. Nutr.* **2013**, *97*, 1299–1306. [CrossRef]
20. Joosten, M.M.; Gansevoort, R.T.; Mukamal, K.J.; Kootstra-Ros, J.E.; Feskens, E.J.; Geleijnse, J.M.; Navis, G.; Bakker, S.J.; Group, P.S. Urinary magnesium excretion and risk of hypertension: The prevention of renal and vascular end-stage disease study. *Hypertension* **2013**, *61*, 1161–1167. [CrossRef]
21. Xu, T.; Sun, Y.; Xu, T.; Zhang, Y. Magnesium intake and cardiovascular disease mortality: A meta-analysis of prospective cohort studies. *Int. J. Cardiol.* **2013**, *167*, 3044–3047. [CrossRef] [PubMed]
22. Van Ende, C.; Van Laecke, S.; Marechal, C.; Verbeke, F.; Kanaan, N.; Goffin, E.; Vanholder, R.; Jadoul, M. Proton-pump inhibitors do not influence serum magnesium levels in renal transplant recipients. *J. Nephrol.* **2014**, *27*, 707–711. [CrossRef] [PubMed]
23. van den Berg, E.; Engberink, M.F.; Brink, E.J.; van Baak, M.A.; Joosten, M.M.; Gans, R.O.; Navis, G.; Bakker, S.J. Dietary acid load and metabolic acidosis in renal transplant recipients. *Clin. J. Am. Soc. Nephrol.* **2012**, *7*, 1811–1818. [CrossRef] [PubMed]
24. Douwes, R.M.; Gomes-Neto, A.W.; Eisenga, M.F.; Vinke, J.S.J.; de Borst, M.H.; van den Berg, E.; Berger, S.P.; Touw, D.J.; Hak, E.; Blokzijl, H.; et al. Chronic Use of Proton-Pump Inhibitors and Iron Status in Renal Transplant Recipients. *J. Clin. Med.* **2019**, *8*, 1382. [CrossRef]
25. Kirchheiner, J.; Glatt, S.; Fuhr, U.; Klotz, U.; Meineke, I.; Seufferlein, T.; Brockmoller, J. Relative potency of proton-pump inhibitors-comparison of effects on intragastric pH. *Eur. J. Clin. Pharmacol.* **2009**, *65*, 19–31. [CrossRef]
26. van den Berg, E.; Engberink, M.F.; Brink, E.J.; van Baak, M.A.; Gans, R.O.B.; Navis, G.; Bakker, S.J.L. Dietary protein, blood pressure and renal function in renal transplant recipients. *Br. J. Nutr.* **2013**, *109*, 1463–1470. [CrossRef]
27. Feunekes, I.J.; Van Staveren, W.A.; Graveland, F.; De Vos, J.; Burema, J. Reproducibility of a semiquantitative food frequency questionnaire to assess the intake of fats and cholesterol in The Netherlands. *Int. J. Food Sci. Nutr.* **1995**, *46*, 117–123. [CrossRef]
28. The Netherlands Nutrition Centre. *Dutch Food Composition Table 2006 NEVO-Tabel: Nederlands Voedingsstoffenbestand*; The Netherlands Nutrition Centre: The Hague, The Netherlands, 2006.
29. van den Berg, E.; Geleijnse, J.M.; Brink, E.J.; van Baak, M.A.; van der Heide, J.J.H.; Gans, R.O.; Navis, G.; Bakker, S.J. Sodium intake and blood pressure in renal transplant recipients. *Nephrol. Dial. Transplant.* **2012**, *27*, 3352–3359. [CrossRef]
30. Boonpheng, B.; Thongprayoon, C.; Bathini, T.; Sharma, K.; Mao, M.A.; Cheungpasitporn, W. Proton pump inhibitors and adverse effects in kidney transplant recipients: A meta-analysis. *World J. Transplant.* **2019**, *9*, 35–47. [CrossRef]
31. Aulagnon, F.; Scemla, A.; DeWolf, S.; Legendre, C.; Zuber, J. Diarrhea After Kidney Transplantation. *Transplantation* **2014**, *98*, 806–816. [CrossRef]
32. van Rossum, C.T.M.; Fransen, H.; Verkaik-Kloosterman, J.; Buurma-Rethans, E.; Ocke, M. Micronutrients. In *Dutch National Food Consumption Survey 2007–2010: Diet of Children and Adults Aged 7 to 69 Years*; National Institute for Public Health and the Environment (RIVM): Bilthoven, The Netherlands, 2011; pp. 61–76.
33. Bai, J.P.F.; Hausman, E.; Lionberger, R.; Zhang, X. Modeling and simulation of the effect of proton pump inhibitors on magnesium homeostasis. 1. Oral absorption of magnesium. *Mol. Pharm.* **2012**, *9*, 3495–3505. [CrossRef] [PubMed]
34. Van Laecke, S.; Maréchal, C.; Verbeke, F.; Peeters, P.; Van Biesen, W.; Devuyst, O.; Jadoul, M.; Vanholder, R. The relation between hypomagnesaemia and vascular stiffness in renal transplant recipients. *Nephrol. Dial. Transplant.* **2011**, *26*, 2362–2369. [CrossRef] [PubMed]
35. Verbeke, F.; Maréchal, C.; Van Laecke, S.; Van Biesen, W.; Devuyst, O.; Van Bortel, L.M.; Jadoul, M.; Vanholder, R. Aortic stiffness and central wave reflections predict outcome in renal transplant recipients. *Hypertension* **2011** *58*, 833–838. [CrossRef] [PubMed]

36. Thong, B.K.S.; Ima-Nirwana, S.; Chin, K.Y. Proton pump inhibitors and fracture risk: A review of current evidence and mechanisms involved. *Int. J. Environ. Res. Public Health* **2019**, *16*, 1571. [CrossRef]
37. Zink, D.A.; Pohlman, M.; Barnes, M.; Cannon, M.E. Long-term use of acid suppression started inappropriately during hospitalization. *Aliment. Pharmacol. Ther.* **2005**, *21*, 1203–1209. [CrossRef]
38. Batuwitage, B.T.; Kingham, J.G.; Morgan, N.E.; Bartlett, R.L. Inappropriate prescribing of proton pump inhibitors in primary care. *Postgrad. Med. J.* **2007**, *83*, 66–68. [CrossRef]
39. Nardino, R.J.; Vender, R.J.; Herbert, P.N. Overuse of acid-suppressive therapy in hospitalized patients. *Am. J. Gastroenterol.* **2000**, *95*, 3118–3122. [CrossRef]

5

Conversion to Everolimus was Beneficial and Safe for Fast and Slow Tacrolimus Metabolizers after Renal Transplantation

Gerold Thölking [1,2,*], Nils Hendrik Gillhaus [2], Katharina Schütte-Nütgen [2], Hermann Pavenstädt [2], Raphael Koch [3], Barbara Suwelack [2] and Stefan Reuter [2]

[1] Department of Internal Medicine and Nephrology, University Hospital of Münster Marienhospital Steinfurt, 48565 Steinfurt, Germany

[2] Department of Medicine D, Division of General Internal Medicine, Nephrology and Rheumatology, University Hospital of Münster, 48149 Münster, Germany; nilshendrik.gillhaus@ukmuenster.de (N.H.G.); katharina.schuette-nuetgen@ukmuenster.de (K.S.-N.); hermann.pavenstaedt@ukmuenster.de (H.P.); barbara.suwelack@ukmuenster.de (B.S.); stefan.reuter@ukmuenster.de (S.R.)

[3] Institute of Biostatistics and Clinical Research, University of Münster, 48149 Münster, Germany; raphael.koch@ukmuenster.de

* Correspondence: gerold.thoelking@ukmuenster.de

Abstract: Fast tacrolimus (TAC) metabolism (concentration/dose (C/D) ratio <1.05 ng/mL/mg) is a risk factor for inferior outcomes after renal transplantation (RTx) as it fosters, e.g., TAC-related nephrotoxicity. TAC minimization or conversion to calcineurin-inhibitor free immunosuppression are strategies to improve graft function. Hence, we hypothesized that especially patients with a low C/D ratio profit from a switch to everolimus (EVR). We analyzed data of 34 RTx recipients (17 patients with a C/D ratio <1.05 ng/mL/mg vs. 17 patients with a C/D ratio ≥1.05 ng/mL/mg) who were converted to EVR within 24 months after RTx. The initial immunosuppression consisted of TAC, mycophenolate, prednisolone, and basiliximab induction. During an observation time of 36 months after changing immunosuppression from TAC to EVR, renal function, laboratory values, and adverse effects were compared between the groups. Fast TAC metabolizers were switched to EVR 4.6 (1.5–21.9) months and slow metabolizers 3.3 (1.8–23.0) months after RTx ($p = 0.838$). Estimated glomerular filtration rate (eGFR) did not differ between the groups at the time of conversion (baseline). Thereafter, the eGFR in all patients increased noticeably (fast metabolizers eGFR 36 months: + 11.0 ± 11.7 ($p = 0.005$); and slow metabolizers eGFR 36 months: + 9.4 ± 15.9 mL/min/1.73 m^2 ($p = 0.049$)) vs. baseline. Adverse events were not different between the groups. After the switch, eGFR values of all patients increased statistically noticeably with a tendency towards a higher increase in fast TAC metabolizers. Since conversion to EVR was safe in a three-year follow-up for slow and fast TAC metabolizers, this could be an option to protect fast metabolizers from TAC-related issues.

Keywords: tacrolimus; C/D ratio; tacrolimus metabolism; everolimus; conversion; kidney transplantation

1. Introduction

Tarolimus (TAC)-based therapy is the recommended immunosuppressive standard therapy after renal transplantation (RTx), although its numerous adverse effects include the development of acute and chronic nephrotoxicity [1]. Unfortunately, TAC has a narrow therapeutic window and a high inter- and intraindividual variable pharmacokinetics, which requires therapeutic drug monitoring (TDM). TAC metabolism is subject to several non-modifiable factors such as age, sex, and CYP3A4/5 genotype of the RTx recipient as well as parameters that may vary, e.g., hematocrit, serum albumin, and steroid doses [2]. In view of the variety of impacting factors, transplant physicians are waiting for a stratification method to identify individuals with a high risk to develop TAC-related adverse effects.

Recently, we and others described a simple and cost-effective tool, the TAC concentration/dose ratio (C/D ratio), to address this problem [3,4]. The C/D ratio is calculated by dividing the TAC trough level by the daily TAC dose. To keep the tool as simple and practical as possible for clinical application, we decided to use only two different C/D ratio categories, although our first approach involved three [4]. A TAC C/D ratio < 1.05 ng/mL/mg assessed three months after RTx indicates fast TAC metabolism, whereas a C/D ratio ≥ 1.05 ng/mL/mg is suggestive of individuals with slow Tac clearance [5]. Using this C/D ratio cut off, we and others showed that the renal function of fast metabolizers is inferior to that of slow metabolizers after RTx and liver transplantation (cut off 1.09 ng/mL/mg), which is due to, e.g., higher incidences of TAC-related nephrotoxicity and rejections [4–10]. This resulted in decreased graft and patient survival [5,7]. In view of the data, modifications of the immunosuppressive regime of patients with a C/D ratio < 1.05 ng/mL/mg should be considered.

The ZEUS study showed that conversion of RTx recipients from calcineurin inhibitor (CNI) to everolimus (EVR) 4.5 months posttransplant is associated with a significant improvement in renal function, which is maintained for at least five years after RTx [11]. Despite increased rates of early mild acute rejections, long-term graft function was not affected in patients who switched to EVR. A positive effect of conversion from CNI to EVR on renal function was even shown for late conversion after RTx (after a mean of 82.6 months) [12]. However, in none of these studies was a C/D ratio-based stratification investigated in this regard.

Due to the negative impact of TAC on the outcomes of fast metabolizers, we hypothesized that these patients, after conversion to EVR, might have greater benefits than slow metabolizers.

2. Patients and Methods

2.1. Patients

This retrospective study included 17 fast metabolizers and 17 slow metabolizers undergoing RTx at the University Hospital of Münster, Germany, between December 2007 and November 2013. The inclusion criteria comprised: age ≥ 18 years of age, intake of immediate release TAC since RTx, and switch from TAC to EVR within 24 months after RTx. All patients received an initial immunosuppression with TAC (Prograf®), mycophenolate mofetil (CellCept®), prednisolone (Decortin H®/Soludecortin H®), and an induction therapy with basiliximab (Simulect®) at Days 0 and 4. TAC target trough levels were 7–12 ng/mL until the end of Month 1, 6–10 ng/mL for Months 2–3, and 3–8 ng/mL subsequently. The starting dose of mycophenolate mofetil 1 g twice a day (b.i.d). was adjusted in case of adverse effects. Prednisolone was started with 250 mg before and directly after RTx and tapered to a maintenance dosage of 5 mg once daily (q.d.) after six months. The recipient's data were taken from the electronic health records of the hospital information system. Patients were switched from TAC to EVR with a target trough level of 3–8 ng/mL.

Renal function and complications were observed in a 36-month follow-up after conversion to EVR. Renal function was expressed as the estimated glomerular filtration rate (eGFR) calculated by the CKD-EPI formula [13]. Creatinine was analyzed in a whole blood sample (enzymatic assay; Creatinine-Pap, Roche Diagnostics, Mannheim, Germany). Proteinuria was assessed using spot urine. TAC levels were determined using the automated tacrolimus (TACR) assay (Dimension Clinical Chemistry System, Siemens Healthcare Diagnostic GmbH, Eschborn, Germany). EVR levels were measured by LC-MS/MS. Only 12-h TAC and EVR trough levels were used for analysis. Donor-specific antibodies (DSA) were assessed by single beat antigen assay (Luminex).

The C/D ratio was calculated using the following formula:

$$C/D\ ratio\ (\text{ng/mL} * 1/\text{mg}) = \frac{blood\ TAC\ trough\ level\ (\text{ng/mL})}{daily\ TAC\ dose\ (\text{mg})} \quad (1)$$

The TAC C/D ratio was calculated one month after RTx and used for grouping [14]. RTx recipients with a C/D ratio <1.05 ng/mL/mg were defined as fast and with a C/D ratio ≥1.05 ng/mL/mg as slow metabolizers.

Histologic results on rejections were obtained only from indication biopsies. All biopsy specimens had been reviewed by two pathologists in the local Institute of Pathology according to the revised Banff criteria [15].

The data of all RTx recipients were anonymized prior to analysis. The study was approved by the local ethics committee (Ethik Kommission der Ärztekammer Westfalen-Lippe und der Medizinischen Fakultät der Westfälischen Wilhelms-Universität, No. 2014-381-f-N). All participants in this study had given written informed consent to record their clinical data and to use it in anonymized analyses at the time of transplantation.

2.2. Statistical Analyses

IBM SPSS Statistics 26 for Windows (IBM Corporation, Somers, NY, USA) were used for statistical analyses of all data. All p-values were two-sided and were intended to be exploratory, not confirmatory. Exploratory p-values ≤0.05 were denoted as statistically noticeable. Absolute and relative frequencies are given for categorical variables. Normally-distributed continuous variables are shown as mean ± standard deviation and not normally-distributed continuous variables as median (minimum–maximum). The corresponding pairwise comparisons between fast and slow metabolizers were performed using Welch's t-tests for normally distributed data, exact Mann–Whitney U tests for skewed distributed continuous variables, and Fisher's exact tests for categorical variables without adjusting for multiple testing. Intra-group changes between two points in time were analyzed using Wilcoxon signed-rank tests for related samples. Boxplots were used for graphical representation.

3. Results

3.1. Descriptive Statistics

Patient characteristics, transplantation data, and immunosuppression after the first month are given in Table 1. Slow metabolizers tended to be older and had a lighter body weight, but all characteristics did not differ noticeably between groups. Fast metabolizers were converted from TAC to EVR after a median of 4.6 (1.5–21.9) months, slow metabolizers 3.3 (1.8–23.0) months after RTx (p = 0.832). Despite similar TAC trough levels after the first month (M1), TAC doses were noticeably higher and C/D ratio values were lower for fast metabolizers than for slow metabolizers (both $p < 0.001$), due to group classification.

Table 1. Patient characteristics and immunosuppression.

	Fast Metabolizers (n = 17)	Slow Metabolizers (n = 17)	p-Values
	Recipient Characteristics		
Sex (m/f)	11 (65%)/6 (35%)	10 (59%)/7 (41%)	1 [a]
Age (year)	48.0 ± 15.7	54.6 ± 12.8	0.187 [b]
Height (cm)	175.0 ± 10.7	171.4 ± 10.2	0.317 [b]
Weight (kg)	79.0 ± 20.6	69.0 ± 11.9	0.095 [b]
BMI (kg/m^2)	24.7 (18.7–35.8)	22.3 (18.9–32.6)	0.114 [c]
	Transplant characteristics		
Number of RTx			
1	15 (88%)	13 (77%)	
2	2 (12%)	3 (18%)	0.511 [a]
3	0	1 (6%)	

Table 1. *Cont.*

	Fast Metabolizers (n = 17)	Slow Metabolizers (n = 17)	p-Values
	Transplant characteristics		
Living donor transplantation	6 (35%)	7 (41%)	1 [a]
ABOi	0	2 (12%)	0.485 [a]
ESP	1 (6%)	2 (12%)	1 [a]
CIT (h)	6.8 (1.6–17.4)	5.5 (1.6–19.3)	0.838 [c]
WIT (min)	35 (20–45)	30 (25–50)	0.858 [c]
CMV risk			
Low	6 (35%)	2 (12%)	
Intermediate	7 (41%)	13 (77%)	0.139 [a]
High	4 (24%)	2 (12%)	
	Donor characteristics		
Donor sex (m/f)	10 (59%)/7 (41%)	6 (35%)/11 (66%)	0.303 [a]
Donor age (year)	56.8 ± 8.8	57.4 ± 10.9	0.877 [b]
	Immunosuppression at M1		
TAC dose (mg)	12 (7–23)	7 (4–12)	<0.001 [c]
TAC trough level (ng/mL)	8.5 (4.6–17.6)	10.0 (5.6–14.1)	0.208 [c]
TAC C/D ratio (ng/mL*1/mg)	0.77 (0.40–1.00)	1.35 (1.05–2.56)	<0.001 [b]
Prednisolone dose (mg)	20 (15–40)	20 (15–50)	0.422 [c]
Mycophenolate mofetil dose (mg)	1000 (750–2000)	1000 (1000–2000)	0.501 [c]

BMI, body mass index; RTx, renal transplantation; ABOi, ABO incompatible transplantation; ESP, European senior program; CIT, cold ischemia time; WIT, warm ischemia time; CMV, cytomegalovirus; TAC, tacrolimus; C/D, concentration/dose. Statistics: Variables are reported as absolute and relative frequencies, mean ± standard deviation or median (minimum–maximum). [a] Fisher's exact test; [b] Welch's t-test; [c] Mann–Whitney U-test.

The main reason for a conversion from TAC to EVR was CNI-nephrotoxicity in both metabolism groups (Table 2).

Table 2. Reasons for the conversion to everolimus.

	Fast Metabolizers (n = 17)	Slow Metabolizers (n = 17)	p-Value
CNI-nephrotoxicity	13 (77%)	10 (59%)	
chronic rejection	0	2 (12%)	
DGF	1 (6%)	2 (12%)	
NODAT	2 (12%)	0	
BKV-infection	0	1 (6%)	0.277
neutropenia	0	1 (6%)	
neurotoxicity	0	1 (6%)	
study	1 (6%)	0	

CNI, calcineurin inhibitor; DGF, delayed graft function; NODAT, new onset diabetes mellitus after transplantation; BKV, BK virus. Statistics: Fisher's exact test.

3.2. Renal Function

The renal function of fast and slow metabolizers was similar ten days after RTx (39.2 ± 19.7 vs. 33.7 ± 22.5 mL/min/1.73 m^2, p = 0.456), one month after RTx (39.4 ± 18.8 vs. 34.2 ± 13.5 mL/min/1.73 m^2, p = 0.367), and at the time of conversion of TAC to EVR (35.1 ± 15.2 vs. 34.2 ± 13.2 mL/min/1.73 m^2, p = 0.850, Figure 1A). Figure 1B provides the renal function at different time points minus the baseline eGFR (eGFR at the time of conversion, Month 0 (M0)). At the end of the follow-up, the eGFR of the fast TAC metabolizers increased considerably by 11.0 ± 11.7 mL/min/1.73 m^2 (p = 0.005, Figure 1B) compared to 9.4 ± 15.9 mL/min/1.73 m^2 in slow metabolizers (p = 0.049). These changes were not statistically noticeably different between both groups (p = 0.691), but more homogenous in fast metabolizers.

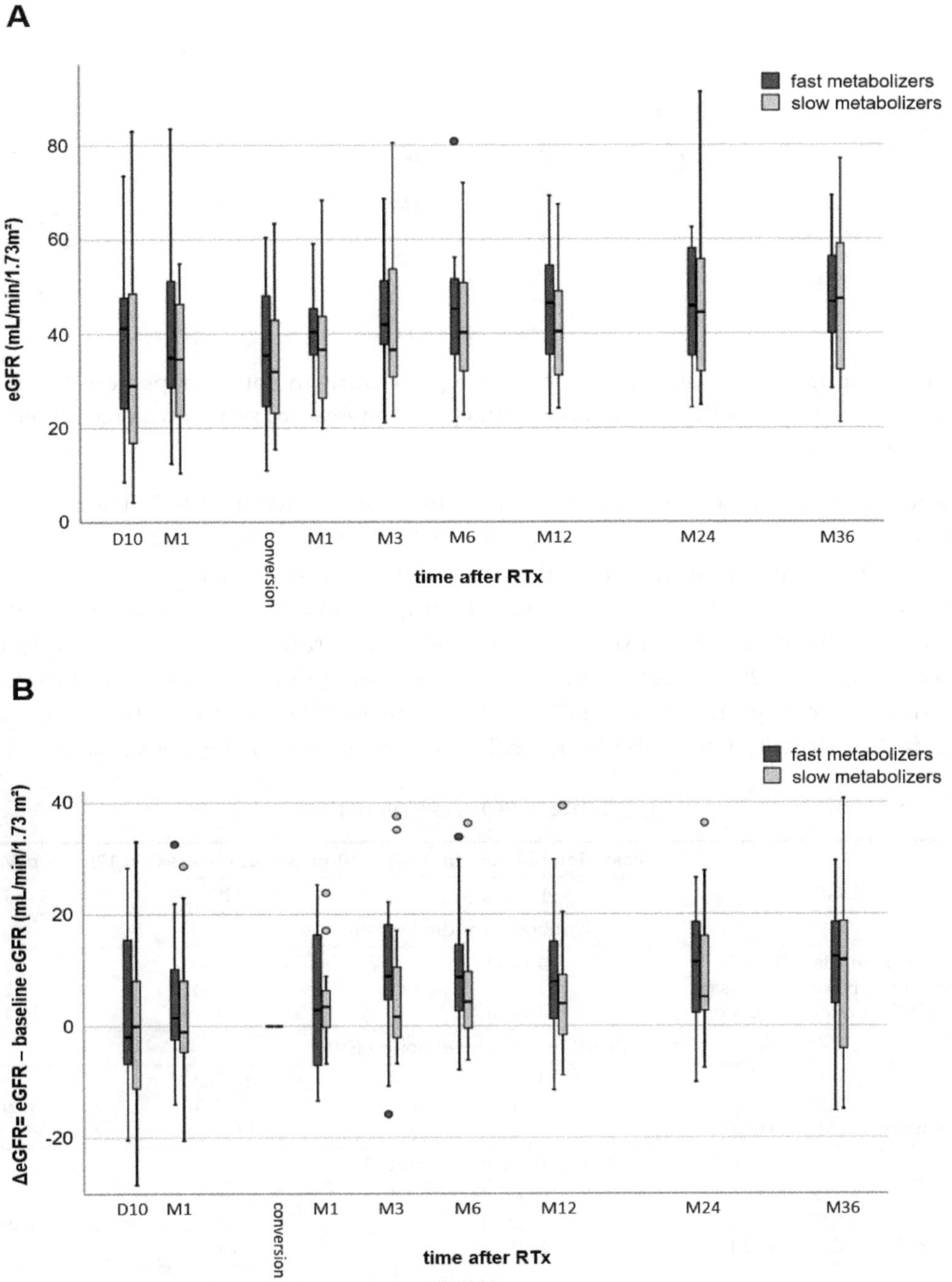

Figure 1. Comparison of renal function (eGFR values) of fast and slow TAC metabolizers. Both groups showed a considerable increase in renal function from Day 10 after kidney transplantation to 36 months after conversion from TAC to EVR (no differences between the groups) (**A**). Comparison of eGFR values to baseline eGFR (time of conversion from TAC to EVR) (**B**). Thirty-six months after transplantation, renal function of slow metabolizers showed a noticeable increase ($p = 0.049$), while fast metabolizers a highly noticeable increase ($p = 0.005$).

3.3. Adverse Events

The median proteinuria value of fast metabolizers was 193 (19–665) mg/g creatinine at M1 after RTx and 361 (97–831) mg/g creatinine at M6 (maximum values) after conversion (Figure 2). The proteinuria in slow metabolizers was 218 (137–664) mg/g creatinine at M1 after RTx and 344 (167–665) mg/g creatinine at M6 (maximum values). At M36, proteinuria had declined to the baseline values without difference between the groups at all time points.

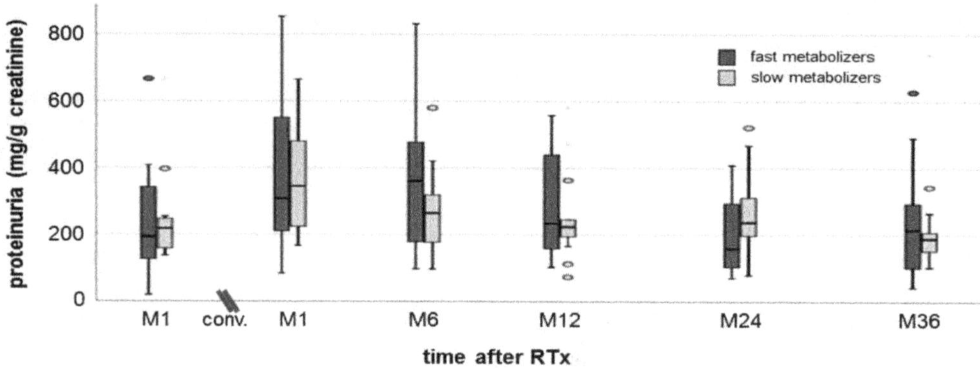

Figure 2. Proteinuria. There was a slight increase in proteinuria in both groups from M1 after RTx to M1 after conversion. At a follow-up of 36 months post-conversion, proteinuria recovered to values measured at M1 after RTx.

Table 3 shows the adverse events before and after conversion to EVR. There was no graft loss and no differences in outcomes such as delayed graft function (DGF) or overall survival between the groups. The DSA number in all patient groups before and after conversion was low and did not change noticeably. Although it was 9 vs. 6 biopsy-proven acute rejection (BPAR) cases in fast vs. slow metabolizers before conversion to EVR, BPAR rates were considerably lower during follow-up (two episodes (12%) in fast metabolizers and one episode (6%) in slow metabolizer) than before conversion. Cytomegalovirus (CMV) and BK virus (BKV) infections did not occur at different frequencies in fast or slow TAC metabolizers and were uncommon after conversion to EVR.

Table 3. Adverse events.

	Fast Metabolizers (n = 17)	Slow Metabolizers (n = 17)	p-Value
DGF	4 (24%)	5 (29%)	1 [a]
	Antibodies and rejection		
Preformed Class II DSA	1 (6%)	1 (6%)	1 [a]
Class II DSA before conversion	1 (6%)	1 (6%)	1 [a]
Class I DSA after conversion	1 (6%)	0	1 [a]
	BPAR before conversion to EVR		
AMR	1 (6%)	1 (6%)	
TCMR	1 (6%)	2 (12%)	0.490 [b]
Combined AMR + TCMR	7 (41%)	3 (18%)	
	BPAR after conversion to EVR		
AMR	0	0	
TCMR	2 (12%)	0	0.485 [a]
Combined AMR + TCMR	0	1 (6%)	
	Infections		
CMV infection before conversion	2 (12%)	4 (24%)	0.656 [a]
CMV infection after conversion	1 (6%)	0	1 [a]
BKV infection before conversion	2 (12%)	1 (6%)	1 [a]
BKV infection after conversion	0	0	-
Death	0	1 (6%)	1 [a]

DGF, delayed graft function; DSA, donor-specific antibody; BPAR, biopsy-proven acute rejection; AMR, antibody-mediated rejection; TCMR, T-cell mediated rejection; EVR, everolimus. Statistics: Adverse events are reported as absolute and relative frequencies. [a] Fisher's exact test.

Cholesterol and triglycerides tended to be higher in fast than slow metabolizers (no noticeable differences, Figure 3A,B) and increased to a similar extent (approximately 20 mg/dL) in both groups after conversion to EVR. Platelets slightly increased after RTx but without differences between fast and slow metabolizers (Figure 3C). Hemoglobin levels decreased by 1 g/dL on average in both groups one month after RTx, but increased from 10.8 ± 1.7 g/dL (M1) to 12.5 ± 1.4 g/dL (M36 after conversion) in fast metabolizers and from 10.6 ± 1.6 g/dL (M1) to 13.9 ± 1.1 g/dL (M36 after conversion) in slow metabolizers (Figure 3D). Three years after conversion, hemoglobin levels were noticeably higher in slow metabolizers ($p = 0.019$). None of the RTx recipients needed erythropoiesis-stimulating agents. HbA1c levels increased slightly from 5.3% (4.5–6.4%) at RTx to 6.3% (5.3–9.1%) at M6 after conversion in fast metabolizers and from 5.3% (4.6–6.0%) at RTx to 5.5% (5.0–7.1%) at M6 in slow metabolizers (Figure 3E). HbA1c values decreased only slightly in both groups to a comparable extent until M36.

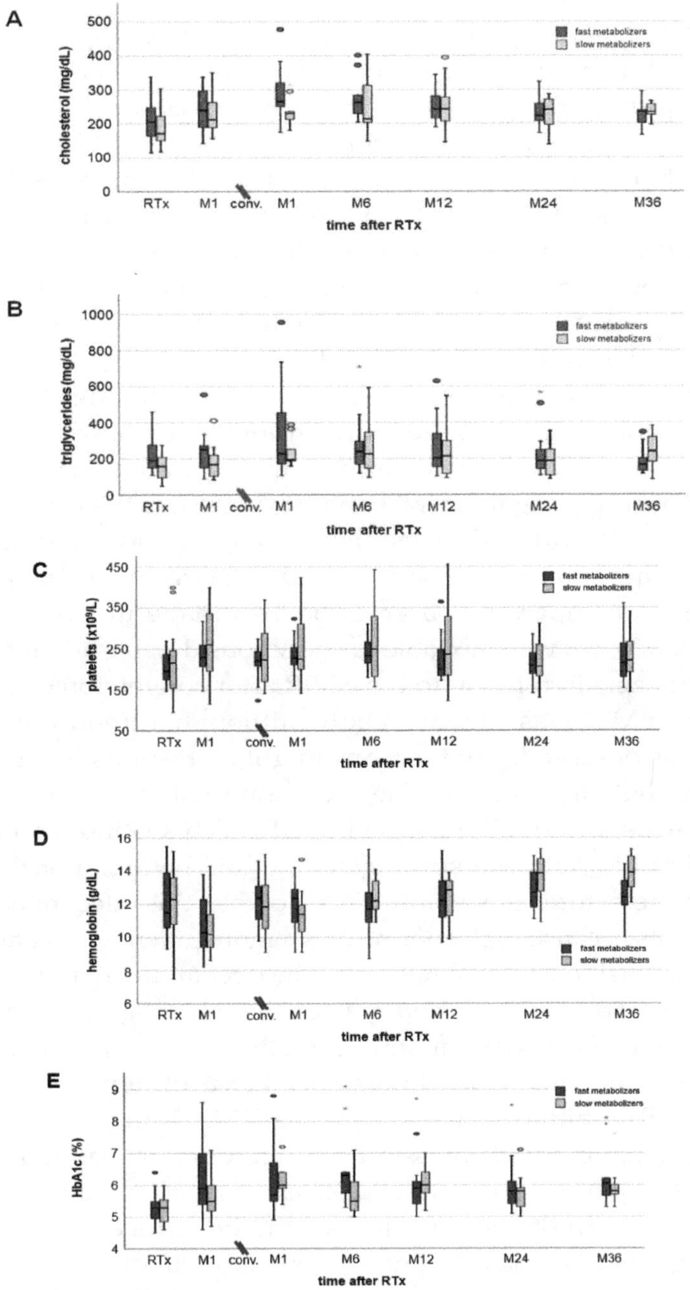

Figure 3. Courses of laboratory values. Cholesterol (**A**) and triglyceride (**B**) levels showed an increase after transplantation, but in a 36-month follow-up values decreased close to values measured at RTx (no noticeable differences between fast and slow metabolizers at any time). Mean platelets (**C**) and hemoglobin (**D**) remained in the normal range at all times without noticeable differences between the groups. Hemoglobin values dropped more than 1 g/dL at M1 after RTx, but had recovered already at the time of conversion from TAC to EVR (no noticeable differences between fast and slow metabolizers at all times). HbA1c levels (**E**) showed an increase one month after RTx without a relevant recovery during a 36-month follow-up after conversion. There were no noticeable differences in HbA1c values between the groups.

4. Discussion

The outcome of fast TAC metabolizers was shown to be inferior compared to the outcomes of slow TAC metabolizers when standard immunosuppression (immediate-release TAC, mycophenolate mofetil (MMF), and prednisolone) is used after RTx [4,5]. This finding was confirmed by others, even when higher C/D ratios were used for group definitions or when including patients receiving extended-release TAC [7,16]. In addition to increased rejection rates in patients with a low C/D ratio, increased rates of BK virus infection, CNI-related nephrotoxicity, and IF/TA were responsible for the lower eGFR of fast metabolizers [4,5,7–10]. In accordance with these data, Stegall et al. recently demonstrated in a large prospective cohort study using TAC-based immunosuppression that almost all kidney allografts have developed severe histological damage within ten years of RTx. However, the most frequently observed histological pathologies were arterial hyalinosis and glomerulosclerosis [17]. Both injuries can be linked to, e.g., CNI exposure [18]. Thus, CNI-induced nephrotoxicity remains a serious problem during CNI treatment [19]. Since only small case studies with patients who had CNI nephrotoxicity have investigated this conversion approach before and did not provide information regarding the TAC metabolism type of their patients, we herein investigated whether a conversion from TAC to EVR could be beneficial and safe for these patients [20,21].

In previous studies, we observed that as early as one month after RTx the kidney function of fast metabolizers is noticeably inferior to the kidney function of slow metabolizers [4]. Since TAC trough level and doses are usually higher within the first year after RTx and both can contribute to CNI nephrotoxicity, it is not surprising that CNI nephrotoxicity was the main reason for the conversion of TAC to EVR in our study cohort [10]. This disadvantage of fast metabolizers with respect to a lower eGFR persists over time and can still be observed to a large extent many years after Tx leading to inferior outcomes [5]. A comparable observation was made in liver transplanted patients [6]. However, in our present study, we were not able to show considerable advantages in fast metabolizers compared to slow metabolizers in relation to the eGFR after conversion of TAC to EVR. The change in eGFR from switching to M36 was similar in both, although a trend toward a higher increase in fast TAC metabolizers was observed. Two reasons might be responsible for this observation. First, the small number of cases could have masked the effect, especially when considering that a conversion of CNI to EVR usually leads to a small increase in eGRF. (This is independent of the type of TAC metabolism, although that has not been specifically studied before. For the first time, we present data relating to the C/D ratio before conversion.) [22] Notably, this effect may be more pronounced in cyclosporine-treated patients because cyclosporine A is a more potent vasoconstrictor than TAC [23,24]. Second, the time of the conversion could be relevant. Since renal function usually improves within the first year after transplantation due to the recovery from the transplant procedure and due to adaption of the kidney, these effects could also have an impact on the outcomes after conversion, since one may speculate that these processes might develop differently when using antiproliferative acting mechanistic target of rapamycin (mTOR)-inhibitors instead of CNIs [25–27]. In contrast to sirolimus-containing regimens [28,29], EVR-based immunosuppression was not found to lead to increased rates of delayed graft function or to poor results in terms of eGFR recovery after transplantation [30–33]. It was even postulated that progression of allograft fibrosis can be reduced by using mTOR-inhibition to down-regulate TGF-β signaling that is relevant for development of fibrosis [34]. However, even the large ELEVATE trial, which compared early conversion from TAC to EVR after RTx vs. CNI therapy, was not able to show differences between TAC- and EVR-treated patients in regards to the eGFR 12 months after RTx [35].

Nevertheless, we were able to show that conversion from TAC to EVR can improve eGFR even in RTx patients who had developed already CNI-induced side effects such as CNI nephrotoxcity—the main reason for conversion to EVR in our study. These data are in line with data from a small case series and a study showing reduced loss or even improvement of renal function after conversion to EVR in patients with CNI nephrotoxicity or chronic allograft nephropathy [20,21,36].

The overall rejection rate was low after conversion and not different between groups. No antibody-mediated rejection was observed until M36 and only one T-cell-mediated rejection occurred. Most importantly, we could not find any differences in (de novo) DSA. Based on our analyses at M36, class I DSA had occurred in only one patient (6%) of fast metabolizers. Due to previous transplantations, preformed Class II DSA were detectable in equal frequencies in both groups. The occurrence of de novo DSA apparently did not result in antibody-mediated rejection episodes within the three-year study period, as far as we know. However, rejections can occur later, as it is known from retrospective data that EVR-based regimens increase the risk of developing de novo DSA after RTx [37,38]. Interestingly, the prospective ELEVATE trial evaluated RTx patients with low immunological risk who were switched approximately three months after transplantation from CNI-based to EVR-based immunosuppression. One conclusion from the trial was that rejection rates in patients on the EVR-based regimen compared to patients receiving TAC had been higher; de novo DSA were not different between groups [35].

Consistent to previous data [27,35,39], after switching to EVR, we found no safety issues in either slow or fast TAC metabolizers (Table 3). However, others report high rates of adverse events and treatment discontinuation after conversion [30,40]. For example, the change in the lipid profile was as expected to occur for EVR, and showed no new safety concerns [35]. Notably, blood count and proteinuria even improved after conversion. It is known that mTOR-inhibition can be associated with a higher incidence of proteinuria compared to CNI treatment, an effect that is potentially dose-dependent [41–43]. However, it was suggested that especially late conversion promotes proteinuria. Our result is at least in line with the published results of others [44].

Of note, in this study, only one case of CMV infection occurred in fast metabolizers and no BKV infection after conversion. These data are consistent with randomized controlled trial data showing lower viral infection rates after switching to EVR [35].

The limitations of our study are the retrospective design and the limited sample size of our single-center study. However, we believe that our results are encouraging to design a prospective trial that can further evaluate our hypotheses.

In summary, we conclude from our data that selected RTx patients may benefit from a conversion from an immediate-release TAC-based immunosuppressive regimen to an EVR-based protocol to avoid further impair of kidney function associated with TAC treatment in these patients. This option could be especially interesting for patients who have already developed TAC-related adverse effects such as nephrotoxicity. Conversion to EVR is safe in selected slow and fast TAC metabolizers as the outcomes and the rate of adverse event did not noticeably differ between both TAC metabolizer types. However, these results must be confirmed in a prospective study.

Author Contributions: Conceptualization, G.T. and S.R.; Data curation, N.H.G.; Formal analysis, N.H.G. and R.K.; Methodology, G.T., S.R., and R.K.; Resources, H.P. and B.S.; Supervision, G.T.; Writing—original draft, G.T. and S.R.; and Writing—review and editing, K.S.-N., H.P., R.K., and B.S. All authors have read and agreed to the published version of the manuscript.

References

1. Kidney Disease: Improving Global Outcomes Transplant Work, G. KDIGO clinical practice guideline for the care of kidney transplant recipients. *Am. J. Transplant.* **2009**, *9* (Suppl. S3), S1–S155.
2. Schutte-Nutgen, K.; Tholking, G.; Suwelack, B.; Reuter, S. Tacrolimus—Pharmacokinetic Considerations for Clinicians. *Curr. Drug Metab.* **2018**, *19*, 342–350. [CrossRef] [PubMed]

3. Ji, E.; Choi, L.; Suh, K.S.; Cho, J.Y.; Han, N.; Oh, J.M. Combinational effect of intestinal and hepatic CYP3A5 genotypes on tacrolimus pharmacokinetics in recipients of living donor liver transplantation. *Transplantation* **2012**, *94*, 866–872. [CrossRef] [PubMed]

4. Tholking, G.; Fortmann, C.; Koch, R.; Gerth, H.U.; Pabst, D.; Pavenstadt, H.; Kabar, I.; Husing, A.; Wolters, H.; Reuter, S.; et al. The tacrolimus metabolism rate influences renal function after kidney transplantation. *PLoS ONE* **2014**, *9*, e111128. [CrossRef] [PubMed]

5. Schutte-Nutgen, K.; Tholking, G.; Steinke, J.; Pavenstadt, H.; Schmidt, R.; Suwelack, B.; Reuter, S. Fast Tac Metabolizers at Risk (-) It is Time for a C/D Ratio Calculation. *J. Clin. Med.* **2019**, *8*, 587. [CrossRef] [PubMed]

6. Tholking, G.; Siats, L.; Fortmann, C.; Koch, R.; Husing, A.; Cicinnati, V.R.; Gerth, H.U.; Wolters, H.H.; Anthoni, C.; Pavenstadt, H.; et al. Tacrolimus Concentration/Dose Ratio is Associated with Renal Function After Liver Transplantation. *Ann. Transplant.* **2016**, *21*, 167–179. [CrossRef]

7. Jouve, T.; Fonrose, X.; Noble, J.; Janbon, B.; Fiard, G.; Malvezzi, P.; Stanke-Labesque, F.; Rostaing, L. The TOMATO study (TacrOlimus MetabolizAtion in kidney TransplantatiOn): Impact of the concentration-dose ratio on death-censored graft survival. *Transplantation* **2019**. [CrossRef]

8. Egeland, E.J.; Reisaeter, A.V.; Robertsen, I.; Midtvedt, K.; Strom, E.H.; Holdaas, H.; Hartmann, A.; Asberg, A. High tacrolimus clearance—A risk factor for development of interstitial fibrosis and tubular atrophy in the transplanted kidney: A retrospective single-center cohort study. *Trans. Int.* **2019**, *32*, 257–269. [CrossRef] [PubMed]

9. Egeland, E.J.; Robertsen, I.; Hermann, M.; Midtvedt, K.; Storset, E.; Gustavsen, M.T.; Reisaeter, A.V.; Klaasen, R.; Bergan, S.; Holdaas, H.; et al. High Tacrolimus Clearance Is a Risk Factor for Acute Rejection in the Early Phase After Renal Transplantation. *Transplantation* **2017**, *101*, e273–e279. [CrossRef] [PubMed]

10. Tholking, G.; Schutte-Nutgen, K.; Schmitz, J.; Rovas, A.; Dahmen, M.; Bautz, J.; Jehn, U.; Pavenstadt, H.; Heitplatz, B.; Van Marck, V.; et al. A Low Tacrolimus Concentration/Dose Ratio Increases the Risk for the Development of Acute Calcineurin Inhibitor-Induced Nephrotoxicity. *J. Clin. Med.* **2019**, *8*, 1586. [CrossRef]

11. Budde, K.; Lehner, F.; Sommerer, C.; Reinke, P.; Arns, W.; Eisenberger, U.; Wuthrich, R.P.; Muhlfeld, A.; Heller, K.; Porstner, M.; et al. Five-year outcomes in kidney transplant patients converted from cyclosporine to everolimus: The randomized ZEUS study. *Am. J. Transplant.* **2015**, *15*, 119–128. [CrossRef] [PubMed]

12. Budde, K.; Sommerer, C.; Rath, T.; Reinke, P.; Haller, H.; Witzke, O.; Suwelack, B.; Baeumer, D.; Sieder, C.; Porstner, M.; et al. Renal function to 5 years after late conversion of kidney transplant patients to everolimus: A randomized trial. *J. Nephrol.* **2015**, *28*, 115–123. [CrossRef] [PubMed]

13. Levey, A.S.; Stevens, L.A.; Schmid, C.H.; Zhang, Y.L.; Castro, A.F.; Feldman, H.I.; Kusek, J.W.; Eggers, P.; Van Lente, F.; Greene, T.; et al. A new equation to estimate glomerular filtration rate. *Ann. Intern. Med.* **2009**, *150*, 604–612. [CrossRef] [PubMed]

14. Tholking, G.; Schmidt, C.; Koch, R.; Schuette-Nuetgen, K.; Pabst, D.; Wolters, H.; Kabar, I.; Husing, A.; Pavenstadt, H.; Reuter, S.; et al. Influence of tacrolimus metabolism rate on BKV infection after kidney transplantation. *Sci. Rep.* **2016**, *6*, 32273. [CrossRef] [PubMed]

15. Haas, M.; Loupy, A.; Lefaucheur, C.; Roufosse, C.; Glotz, D.; Seron, D.; Nankivell, B.J.; Halloran, P.F.; Colvin, R.B.; Akalin, E.; et al. The Banff 2017 Kidney Meeting Report: Revised diagnostic criteria for chronic active T cell-mediated rejection, antibody-mediated rejection, and prospects for integrative endpoints for next-generation clinical trials. *Am. J. Transplant.* **2018**, *18*, 293–307. [CrossRef]

16. Nowicka, M.; Gorska, M.; Nowicka, Z.; Edyko, K.; Edyko, P.; Wislicki, S.; Zawiasa-Bryszewska, A.; Strzelczyk, J.; Matych, J.; Kurnatowska, I. Tacrolimus: Influence of the Posttransplant Concentration/Dose Ratio on Kidney Graft Function in a Two-Year Follow-Up. *Kidney Blood Press. Res.* **2019**, *44*, 1075–1088. [CrossRef]

17. Stegall, M.D.; Cornell, L.D.; Park, W.D.; Smith, B.H.; Cosio, F.G. Renal Allograft Histology at 10 Years After Transplantation in the Tacrolimus Era: Evidence of Pervasive Chronic Injury. *Am. J. Transplant.* **2018**, *18*, 180–188. [CrossRef]

18. Einecke, G.; Reeve, J.; Halloran, P.F. Hyalinosis Lesions in Renal Transplant Biopsies: Time-Dependent Complexity of Interpretation. *Am. J. Transplant.* **2017**, *17*, 1346–1357. [CrossRef]

19. Naesens, M.; Kuypers, D.R.; Sarwal, M. Calcineurin inhibitor nephrotoxicity. *Clin. J. Am. Soc. Nephrol.* **2009**, *4*, 481–508. [CrossRef]

20. Nanmoku, K.; Shinzato, T.; Kubo, T.; Shimizu, T.; Yagisawa, T. Conversion to Everolimus in Kidney Transplant Recipients with Calcineurin Inhibitor-Induced Nephropathy: 3 Case Reports. *Trans. Proc.* **2019**, *51*, 1424–1427. [CrossRef]
21. Morales, J.; Fierro, A.; Benavente, D.; Zehnder, C.; Ferrario, M.; Contreras, L.; Herzog, C.; Buckel, E. Conversion from a calcineurin inhibitor-based immunosuppressive regimen to everolimus in renal transplant recipients: Effect on renal function and proteinuria. *Trans. Proc.* **2007**, *39*, 591–593. [CrossRef]
22. Hoskova, L.; Malek, I.; Kopkan, L.; Kautzner, J. Pathophysiological mechanisms of calcineurin inhibitor-induced nephrotoxicity and arterial hypertension. *Physiol. Res.* **2017**, *66*, 167–180. [CrossRef]
23. Gardiner, S.M.; March, J.E.; Kemp, P.A.; Fallgren, B.; Bennett, T. Regional haemodynamic effects of cyclosporine A, tacrolimus and sirolimus in conscious rats. *Br. J. Pharmacol.* **2004**, *141*, 634–643. [CrossRef]
24. Zaltzman, J.S. A comparison of short-term exposure of once-daily extended release tacrolimus and twice-daily cyclosporine on renal function in healthy volunteers. *Transplantation* **2010**, *90*, 1185–1191. [CrossRef]
25. Alperovich, G.; Maldonado, R.; Moreso, F.; Fulladosa, X.; Grinyo, J.M.; Seron, D. Glomerular enlargement assessed by paired donor and early protocol renal allograft biopsies. *Am. J. Transplant.* **2004**, *4*, 650–654. [CrossRef]
26. Ma, M.K.M.; Yung, S.; Chan, T.M. mTOR Inhibition and Kidney Diseases. *Transplantation* **2018**, *102*, S32–S40. [CrossRef]
27. Husing, A.; Schmidt, M.; Beckebaum, S.; Cicinnati, V.R.; Koch, R.; Tholking, G.; Stella, J.; Heinzow, H.; Schmidt, H.H.; Kabar, I. Long-Term Renal Function in Liver Transplant Recipients After Conversion from Calcineurin Inhibitors to mTOR Inhibitors. *Ann. Transplant.* **2015**, *20*, 707–713. [CrossRef]
28. Lui, S.L.; Chan, K.W.; Tsang, R.; Yung, S.; Lai, K.N.; Chan, T.M. Effect of rapamycin on renal ischemia-reperfusion injury in mice. *Trans. Int.* **2006**, *19*, 834–839. [CrossRef]
29. Smith, K.D.; Wrenshall, L.E.; Nicosia, R.F.; Pichler, R.; Marsh, C.L.; Alpers, C.E.; Polissar, N.; Davis, C.L. Delayed graft function and cast nephropathy associated with tacrolimus plus rapamycin use. *J. Am. Soc. Nephrol.* **2003**, *14*, 1037–1045. [CrossRef]
30. Sanchez-Escuredo, A.; Diekmann, F.; Revuelta, I.; Esforzado, N.; Ricart, M.J.; Cofan, F.; Torregrosa, J.V.; Peri, L.; Ruiz, A.; Campistol, J.M.; et al. An mTOR-inhibitor-based protocol and calcineurin inhibitor (CNI)-free treatment in kidney transplant recipients from donors after cardiac death: Good renal function, but high incidence of conversion to CNI. *Trans. Int.* **2016**, *29*, 362–368. [CrossRef]
31. Sommerer, C.; Suwelack, B.; Dragun, D.; Schenker, P.; Hauser, I.A.; Witzke, O.; Hugo, C.; Kamar, N.; Merville, P.; Junge, M.; et al. An open-label, randomized trial indicates that everolimus with tacrolimus or cyclosporine is comparable to standard immunosuppression in de novo kidney transplant patients. *Kidney Int.* **2019**, *96*, 231–244. [CrossRef]
32. Tedesco-Silva, H.; Pascual, J.; Viklicky, O.; Basic-Jukic, N.; Cassuto, E.; Kim, D.Y.; Cruzado, J.M.; Sommerer, C.; Adel Bakr, M.; Garcia, V.D.; et al. Safety of Everolimus with Reduced Calcineurin Inhibitor Exposure in De Novo Kidney Transplants: An Analysis from the Randomized TRANSFORM Study. *Transplantation* **2019**, *103*, 1953–1963. [CrossRef]
33. Manzia, T.M.; Carmellini, M.; Todeschini, P.; Secchi, A.; Sandrini, S.; Minetti, E.; Furian, L.; Spagnoletti, G.; Pisani, F.P.; Piredda, G.B.P.; et al. A 3-month, multicenter, randomized, open-label study to evaluate the impact on wound healing of the early [vs. delayed] introduction of everolimus in de novo kidney transplant recipients, with a follow-up evaluation at 12 month after transplant (NEVERWOUND study). *Transplantation* **2019**. [CrossRef]
34. Rivelli, R.F.; Goncalves, R.T.; Leite, M., Jr.; Santos, M.A.; Delgado, A.G.; Cardoso, L.R.; Takiya, C.M. Early withdrawal of calcineurin inhibitor from a sirolimus-based immunosuppression stabilizes fibrosis and the transforming growth factor-beta signalling pathway in kidney transplant. *Nephrology* **2015**, *20*, 168–176. [CrossRef] [PubMed]
35. de Fijter, J.W.; Holdaas, H.; Oyen, O.; Sanders, J.S.; Sundar, S.; Bemelman, F.J.; Sommerer, C.; Pascual, J.; Avihingsanon, Y.; Pongskul, C.; et al. Early Conversion from Calcineurin Inhibitor—To Everolimus-Based Therapy Following Kidney Transplantation: Results of the Randomized ELEVATE Trial. *Am. J. Transplant.* **2017**, *17*, 1853–1867. [CrossRef]
36. Cataneo-Davila, A.; Zuniga-Varga, J.; Correa-Rotter, R.; Alberu, J. Renal function outcomes in kidney transplant recipients after conversion to everolimus-based immunosuppression regimen with CNI reduction or elimination. *Trans. Proc.* **2009**, *41*, 4138–4146. [CrossRef]

37. Kamar, N.; Del Bello, A.; Congy-Jolivet, N.; Guilbeau-Frugier, C.; Cardeau-Desangles, I.; Fort, M.; Esposito, L.; Guitard, J.; Game, X.; Rostaing, L. Incidence of donor-specific antibodies in kidney transplant patients following conversion to an everolimus-based calcineurin inhibitor-free regimen. *Clin. Transplant.* **2013**, *27*, 455–462. [CrossRef] [PubMed]
38. Croze, L.E.; Tetaz, R.; Roustit, M.; Malvezzi, P.; Janbon, B.; Jouve, T.; Pinel, N.; Masson, D.; Quesada, J.L.; Bayle, F.; et al. Conversion to mammalian target of rapamycin inhibitors increases risk of de novo donor-specific antibodies. *Trans. Int.* **2014**, *27*, 775–783. [CrossRef]
39. Fischer, L.; Klempnauer, J.; Beckebaum, S.; Metselaar, H.J.; Neuhaus, P.; Schemmer, P.; Settmacher, U.; Heyne, N.; Clavien, P.A.; Muehlbacher, F.; et al. A randomized, controlled study to assess the conversion from calcineurin-inhibitors to everolimus after liver transplantation–PROTECT. *Am. J. Transplant.* **2012**, *12*, 1855–1865. [CrossRef]
40. Budde, K.; Lehner, F.; Sommerer, C.; Arns, W.; Reinke, P.; Eisenberger, U.; Wuthrich, R.P.; Scheidl, S.; May, C.; Paulus, E.M.; et al. Conversion from cyclosporine to everolimus at 4.5 months posttransplant: 3-year results from the randomized ZEUS study. *Am. J. Transplant.* **2012**, *12*, 1528–1540. [CrossRef]
41. Diekmann, F.; Andres, A.; Oppenheimer, F. mTOR inhibitor-associated proteinuria in kidney transplant recipients. *Transplant. Rev.* **2012**, *26*, 27–29. [CrossRef] [PubMed]
42. Wiseman, A.C.; McCague, K.; Kim, Y.; Geissler, F.; Cooper, M. The effect of everolimus versus mycophenolate upon proteinuria following kidney transplant and relationship to graft outcomes. *Am. J. Transplant.* **2013**, *13*, 442–449. [CrossRef]
43. Ponticelli, C.; Graziani, G. Proteinuria after kidney transplantation. *Trans. Int.* **2012**, *25*, 909–917. [CrossRef] [PubMed]
44. Giron, F.; Baez, Y.; Nino-Murcia, A.; Rodriguez, J.; Salcedo, S. Conversion therapy to everolimus in renal transplant recipients: Results after one year. *Transplant. Proc.* **2008**, *40*, 711–713. [CrossRef]

Intraoperative Fluid Restriction is Associated with Functional Delayed Graft Function in Living Donor Kidney Transplantation

Gertrude J Nieuwenhuijs-Moeke [1,*], Tobias M Huijink [2], Robert A Pol [2], Mostafa El Moumni [2], Johannes GM Burgerhof [3], Michel MRF Struys [1,4] and Stefan P Berger [5]

1 Department of Anesthesiology, University of Groningen, University Medical Centre Groningen, Hanzeplein 1, 9713 GZ, Groningen, The Netherlands; m.m.r.f.struys@umcg.nl

2 Department of Surgery, University of Groningen, University Medical Centre Groningen, Hanzeplein 1, 9713 GZ, Groningen, The Netherlands; t.m.huijink@umcg.nl (T.M.H.); r.pol@umcg.nl (R.A.P.); m.el.moumni@umcg.nl (M.E.M.)

3 Department of Epidemiology, University of Groningen, University Medical Centre Groningen, Hanzeplein 1, 9713 GZ, Groningen, The Netherlands; j.g.m.burgerhof@umcg.nl

4 Department of Anesthesiology and Peri-operative Medicine, Ghent University, Corneel Heymanslaan 10, 9000 Gent, Belgium

5 Department of Nephrology, University of Groningen, University Medical Centre Groningen, Groningen, The Netherlands; s.p.berger@umcg.nl

* Correspondence: g.j.nieuwenhuijs-moeke@umcg.nl

Abstract: Background: In 2016 we observed a marked increase in functional delayed graft function (fDGF) in our living donor kidney transplantation (LDKT) recipients from 8.5% in 2014 and 8.8% in 2015 to 23.0% in 2016. This increase coincided with the introduction of a goal-directed fluid therapy (GDFT) protocol in our kidney transplant recipients. Hereupon, we changed our intraoperative fluid regimen to a fixed amount of 50 mL/kg body weight (BW) and questioned whether the intraoperative fluid regimen was related to this increase in fDGF. Methods: a retrospective cohort analysis of all donors and recipients in our LDKT program between January 2014–February 2017 ($n = 275$ pairs). Results: Univariate analysis detected various risk factors for fDGF. Dialysis dependent recipients were more likely to develop fDGF compared to pre-emptively transplanted patients ($p < 0.001$). Recipients developing fDGF received less intraoperative fluid (36 (25.9–50.0) mL/kg BW vs. 47 (37.3–55.6) mL/kg BW ($p = 0.007$)). The GDFT protocol resulted in a reduction of intraoperative fluid administration on average by 850 mL in total volume and 21% in mL/kg BW compared to our old protocol ($p < 0.001$). In the unadjusted analysis, a higher intraoperative fluid volume in mL/kg BW was associated with a lower risk for the developing fDGF (OR 0.967, CI (0.941–0.993)). After adjustment for the confounders, prior dialysis and the use of intraoperative noradrenaline, the relationship of fDGF with fluid volume was still apparent (OR 0.970, CI (0.943–0.998)). Conclusion: Implementation of a GDFT protocol led to reduced intraoperative fluid administration in the LDKT recipients. This intraoperative fluid restriction was associated with the development of fDGF.

Keywords: fluid management; kidney transplantation; delayed graft function; goal-directed fluid therapy

---

1. Introduction

During the procedure of organ donation and transplantation a number of potentially harmful processes will inevitably occur, affecting the viability of the kidney graft. Both donor and recipient are subjected to anesthesia and surgery, which will produce a sequence of systemic and local changes, including a significant proinflammatory and procoagulatory response [1]. The donor organ is by definition, exposed to a number of phases of injury from the moment the donor suffers from cerebral injury (in case of brain death) until the kidney is reconnected to the circulation in the recipient. These phases include a profound systemic and local proinflammatory and procoagulatory response during donor management and retrieval, associated with hypoxia and ischemia of the kidney. In addition, prolonged warm ischemia in the deceased circulatory death (DCD) donor will affect the viability of the donor kidney. These combined effects on the graft-to-be result in a cascade of renal damage that will reveal itself at the time of transplantation, when the donor kidney is reperfused in the recipient and has been named an ischemia-reperfusion injury (IRI) [2]. Typically, IRI will clinically manifest as immediate nonfunction of the transplant with the need for dialysis treatment until the graft recovers from the insult and starts eventually to function. This 'secondary' recovery is called delayed graft function.

DGF, a form of acute kidney injury post-transplantation, is an uncommon complication after living donor kidney transplantation (LDKT), most likely due to very short ischemia times and healthy living donors. Incidences reported vary between 1%–8% [3,4]. In transplantation with kidneys from deceased brain death (DBD) donors, however, the incidence of DGF increases to 15%–25% and may rise up to 72% in transplantation with kidneys from deceased DCD donors [5,6]. DGF is a risk factor for acute rejection (AR) and the combination of DGF and AR reduces graft and patient survival [7–9]. Also in the absence of AR, DGF has been shown to be an independent risk factor for long term graft loss. Reported risk factors for DGF are: deceased donor, longer ischemia times, donor and recipient older age, female donor, male recipient, history of dialysis, higher body mass index (BMI), hypertension in the donor, diabetes in the recipient, retransplantation, higher panel-reactive antibody levels, and higher human leukocyte antigens (HLA) mismatch [3,5,7,10]. This variety of risk factors underscores the complex pathological mechanisms underlying DGF.

Regarding the intraoperative period, several studies suggest that an adequate/supranormal fluid state is associated with a reduced risk of DGF [5,7,11–14]. These studies, however, are mainly retrospective and often comprise a variety of donor types with variable incidences of DGF hampering an adequate analysis. Central venous pressure (CVP)-guided fluid therapy has been suggested until recently [11,12], but CVP does not correlate well with intravascular fluid state and its use to guide fluid therapy is currently discouraged [15]. Blood pressure and heart rate are also affected by several variables, unrelated to the circulatory state of the patient, like pain, temperature, anesthetics, and analgesics, making them less suitable as an indicator of the intravascular volume [16,17].

Recently, goal directed fluid therapy (GDFT) has been shown to improve patient outcomes after major (abdominal) surgery [18–20]. During 2015, our department implemented a GDFT approach in kidney transplant recipients to replace our standard intraoperative fluid regimen of four to five liters (L) of balanced crystalloids. In the first half year of 2016 a marked increase in DGF and functional (f)DGF in our LDKT population was noticed. During 2014 and 2015, respectively, 8.5% and 8.8% of the patients experienced fDGF. From January to June 2016 the incidence of functional delayed graft function (fDGF) rose to 23.0%, which was a significant increase compared to 2014 and 2015 ($p = 0.039$ and $p = 0.021$, respectively). Since the incidence of fDGF in this population has been stable over the past two decades and no protocol changes were implemented with the exception of the GDFT protocol, we questioned whether this increase in fDGF was due to the altered fluid regimen. To our surprise, a retrospective analysis revealed that the implementation of GDFT protocol had resulted in a reduced intraoperative fluid administration which seemed associated with the increase in fDGF. Based on these results, we promptly changed the intraoperative fluid protocol in September 2016 to a fixed amount of 50 mL/kg BW with a lower limit of 2500 mL and upper limit of 6000 mL (50 kg–120 kg), unless patients comorbidity determined otherwise. After six months the incidence of fDGF was back to baseline at 8.2%.

Since we were interested in whether the amount of fluid administered intraoperatively was indeed an independent factor predicting fDGF in this LDKT population, we performed a retrospective cohort analysis of all donors and recipients in our living donor program between January 2014–February 2017.

2. Materials and Methods

2.1. *Study Design and Population*

This retrospective cohort analysis comprised all consecutive donor and recipient pairs of the LDKT program of the University Medical Centre of Groningen (UMCG) between January 2014 and February 2017. The Institutional Review Board approved the study (METc 201600968), which was conducted in adherence to the Declaration of Helsinki. Due to the observational and retrospective character of the analysis, the requirement for informed consent was waived.

2.2. *Definition of DGF*

Twenty-two definitions of DGF were identified in literature based on dialysis, serum creatinine levels, urine output or a combination of these 3 [21], Most commonly used was dialysis requirement the first week after transplantation (also used in this analysis for DGF). This dialysis-based definition, however, is criticized for its subjectivity since there are center- or physician-specific thresholds for the use of dialysis after transplantation [22]. Furthermore, since approximately half of our LDKT population was transplanted preemptively, this dialysis-based definition was unsuitable for this analysis. Another definition, referred to as functional (f)DGF, is failure of serum creatinine level to decrease spontaneously by at least 10% daily on 3 consecutive days during the first postoperative week, discounting creatinine decreases due to dialysis. Moore and colleagues showed that fDGF is independently associated with reduced death-censored graft survival in contrast to DGF based on the dialysis definition and suggested a superiority of this definition over the dialysis-based definition [23]. To prevent misclassification in patients with excellent early graft function, failure of creatinine to decrease on postoperative day three was not classified as fDGF if optimal graft function had already been achieved by day 2. In this analysis, we compared patients undergoing LDKT with fDGF and without fDGF (nofDGF).

2.3. *Intra- and Postoperative Management and Surgical Procedure*

Anesthetic management was according to local protocol. Propofol was used for induction of anesthesia and either propofol or sevoflurane were used for maintenance of anesthesia. Sufentanil or remifentanil were used to control nociception and rocuronium or cis-atracurium for muscle relaxation. Until the implementation of the GDFT protocol, donors and recipients were given 4–5 L of balanced crystalloids throughout the procedure unless their comorbidity determined otherwise. During 2015, a GDFT protocol was gradually implemented in the recipients (not in the donors). For a detailed description of this protocol, see below. From September 2016 fluid protocol in recipients was changed to a fixed amount of 50 mL/kg BW intraoperatively. Timeline of fluid management in recipients is given in Figure 1. Fluid management in donors was not actively changed during our observation period. Regarding the type of fluid, predominantly Ringers' lactate (RL) was used. If hyponatremia occurred RL was replaced by 0.9% saline. Colloids were not given and administration of blood products was according to our local transfusion protocol with thresholds based upon patients comorbidity. Regarding hemodynamics, the goal was to keep the blood pressure within 80% range of the baseline blood pressure of the patient. As baseline, we used blood pressure measured at the preoperative visit. If hypotension occurred, the first step was to adjust depth of anesthesia or analgesia. If that was insufficient or not possible, patients received one or more doses of ephedrine or phenylephrine or a continuous infusion of noradrenaline was started. Kidney donation was performed using a hand-assisted laparoscopic approach. Thereafter the kidney was flushed and perfused with cold University of Wisconsin solution (ViaSpan®, BMS, Bruxelles, Belgium or CoStorSol®, Bridge to Life, Elkhorn, WI, USA) and stored on ice. Transplantation was performed according to local, standardized protocol. Postoperative fluid management comprised 1 L NaCl 0.45%-Glucose 2.5% per 24 h, complemented with the volume of diuresis in the former hour.

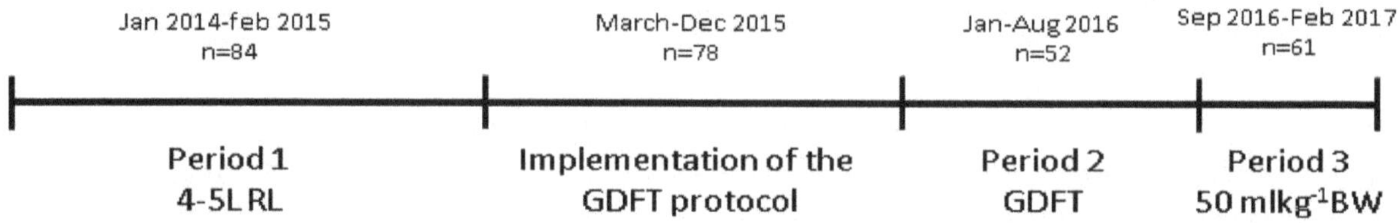

Figure 1. Timeline of various intraoperative fluid protocols in recipients. L: liters; RL: Ringers' lactate; GDFT: goal directed fluid therapy, BW: body weight.

2.4. Goal-Directed Fluid Therapy Protocol.

GDFT was performed with the use of the FloTrac®in combination with the EV1000®monitor (Edwards Lifesciences Corporation, Irvine, CA, USA). The system was used according to manufacturer's instructions. A standard institutional GDFT protocol was used with adjustment of the goal. Instead of a stroke volume variation (SVV) < 12%, commonly used in abdominal surgery, we aimed for a SVV < 10% throughout the procedure. When the SVV was >10% additional fluid was given until SVV was <10%. If SVV < 10%, fluid administration was left to the discretion of the attending anesthesiologist, however, when cardiac index (CI) was below age-adjusted normal values, a noradrenaline infusion was started. If measurement of the SVV was not possible (e.g., due to cardiac arrhythmias) a protocol based on stroke volume (SV) was used. In this case, if a fluid bolus of 250 mL resulted in an increase of the SV of 10%, additional fluid was given, if not, the trend of the SV was monitored and fluid administration was left to the discretion of the attending anesthesiologist. When SV decreased >10%, additional fluid was given. The FloTrac®was used with the EV1000 monitor, which does not communicate with our digital PDMS. Therefore SV, SVV, and CI values could not be retrieved for this analysis.

2.5. Patient Data

Demographic and postoperative data were obtained from digital patient medical records. The following variables were taken into account: age, gender, BMI, smoking, hypertension, use of antihypertensive drugs, measured glomerular filtration rate (mGFR) with use of iodine 125-iothalamate in the donor, blood pressure (measured the day of hospital admission), difference in blood pressure between donor and recipient measured by systolic/diastolic/mean of the recipient minus systolic/diastolic/mean of the donor, underlying kidney disease, number of HLA mismatches, history of dialysis, related or unrelated donor transplantation. For all recipients, the age-adjusted Charlson comorbidity index (CCI) [24] and length of hospital stay was calculated. Intraoperative data were retrieved from our digital patient data monitoring system (PDMS, CS-EZIS, Chipsoft B.V., Amsterdam, the Netherlands) and consisted of duration of surgery, intraoperative volume and type of fluid, cumulative hypotensive periods defined as a systolic blood pressure < 80 mmHg and MAP < 60 mmHg, intraoperative use of vasoactive substances, ischemia times, left/right kidney, side of implantation, number of arteries, sacrifice of an accessory artery, and urinary output the first 2 h postoperatively. Regarding the use of vasoactive substances, patients were scored on receiving one or more boluses of ephedrine and/or phenylephrine and whether or not noradrenaline was administered as a continuous infusion. Additionally, the maximum noradrenaline infusion rate during the procedure was noted. This was grouped into 3 categories: low infusion rate (0.02–0.10 mg/h), intermediate (0.10–0.20 mg/h), and high (>0.20 mg/h) infusion rate.

2.6. Statistics

For the statistical analysis SPSS version 23 (IBM Corp, Armonk, NY, USA) and GraphPad Prism version 7.02 (GraphPad Software Inc, La Jolla, CA, USA) were used. We performed univariate analyses to identify factors associated with fDGF. Categorical data were analyzed by chi-square or Fisher's exact tests. Continuous data were analyzed with an unpaired t-test in the case of normally distributed values. If variables were not normally distributed Mann–Whitney test was applied. Multivariate analysis was performed by means of binary logistic regression. We adjusted the amount of fluid administered intraoperatively in recipients for potentially relevant confounders with high significance in the univariate analysis. Additionally, we were interested in the impact of implementation of our GDFT protocol on the incidence of fDGF and on the amount of fluid administered intraoperatively. We therefore analyzed these data between the different time periods 1–3 (described above) with the use of Fisher's exact test and Kruskal–Wallis test. Post-hoc analysis with Mann–Whitney was used. Values are given as number (%), mean ± standard deviation (SD) or median with interquartile range (IQR). All reported p-values are two-sided. A p-value of 0.05 or less was considered significant.

3. Results

3.1. Univariate Analysis

3.1.1. Patient Characteristics

Between January 2014 and February 2017, 275 living donor kidney transplant procedures were performed in our center. Of the 275 recipients, 31 patients experienced fDGF and 244 recipients did not (nofDGF). Donor and recipients characteristics of fDGF and nofDGF kidneys are listed in Table 1. There were no statistically significant differences in baseline characteristics and kidney function (mGFR) in donors of kidneys with our without fDGF. Recipients developing fDGF were more likely to be dialysis-dependent at the time of transplantation (25 (81%) vs. 105 (43%), $p < 0.001$). The composition of the group of dialysis dependent patients did not differ between nofDGF and fDGF recipients. In the nofDGF group 76 (72%) patients were on hemodialysis at the time of transplantation and 29 (28%) on peritoneal dialysis. In the fDGF group, this was the case for 19 (76%) and six (24%), respectively. All patients on hemodialysis were dialyzed the day before transplantation to 1 kg above dry weight.

Table 1. Donor and recipient demographics. Data given as number (%), mean (SD), or median (IQR).

	nofDGF	fDGF	p
Donor	*N* = 244	*N* = 31	
Age year	54 (11.6)	51 (12.4)	0.104
Gender male	117 (48%)	20 (65%)	0.089
BMI	26.1 (3.0)	25.1 (2.7)	0.075
Smoking	67 (27%)	13 (42%)	0.140
Blood pressure			
S-RR mmHg	136 (15.3)	136 (11.8)	0.848
D-RR mmHg	79 (73–84)	81 (73–86)	0.548
MAP mmHg	98 (9.4)	98 (6.7)	0.897
Hypertension	38 (16%)	2 (6%)	0.277
Anti-hypertensive drugs			
Diuretics	11	1	>0.999
B-blocker	13	1	>0.999
Ca antagonist	10	0	0.610
ACE-I	4	0	>0.999
AT-II-ant.	16	1	0.703
mGFR			
Non-stimulated mL/min	109 (97–23)	107 (95–128)	0.846
Stimulated mL/min	116 (103–133)	118 (100–140)	0.764
ΔGFR	7 (2–12)	7 (−1–12)	0.810

Table 1. *Cont.*

	nofDGF	fDGF	*p*
Recipient	***N* = 244**	***N* = 31**	
Age year	54 (41–61)	55 (43–62)	0.991
Gender male	138 (57%)	21 (68%)	0.254
BMI	25.6 (22.6–28.4)	25.8 (24.0–29.8)	0.267
Smoking	45 (18%)	7 (23%)	0.626
Blood pressure			
S-RR mmHg	143 (20.4)	138 (23.7)	0.196
D-RR mmHg	79 (73–84)	81 (73–86)	0.548
MAP mmHg	97 (9.4)	98 (6.6)	0.897
Δ blood pressure with donor			
Δ S-RR mmHg	7.1 (22.8)	2.5 (29.1)	0.308
Δ D-RR mmHg	3.1 (13.9)	1.0 (15.0)	0.336
Δ MAP mmHg	4 (−6–14)	8 (−10–12)	0.756
Hypertension	175 (72%)	21 (68%)	0.675
Antihypertensive drugs			
Diuretics	84 (34%)	8 (25%)	0.421
B-blocker	124 (51%)	10 (32%)	0.058
Ca antagonist	131 (54%)	15 (48%)	0.703
ACE-I.	46 (19%)	5 (16%)	0.811
AT-II-ant	55 (23%)	7 (23%)	>0.999
CCI	3 (2–4)	3 (2–6)	0.157
Underlying kidney disease			
DM	15 (6%)	5 (16%)	0.358
PKD	57 (23%)	5 (16%)	0.495
Systemic autoimmune diseases	25 (10%)	3 (10%)	>0.999
Glomerulonephritis	47 (19%)	4 (13%)	0.4713
Other	100 (41%)	14 (45%)	0.701
HLA mm < 3	55 (23%)	8 (25%)	0.655
Dialysis dependent	105 (43%)	25 (81%)	<0.001 *
LURD	164 (67%)	19 (61%)	0.547

fDGF: functional delayed graft function; BMI: body mass index; S-RR: systolic blood pressure; D-RR: diastolic blood pressure; MAP: mean arterial pressure; ACE-I: angiotensin-converting enzyme inhibitor; AT-II-ant: angiotensin II receptor antagonist; CCI: Charlson comorbidity index; mGFR: measured glomerular filtration rate measured with use of iodine 125-iothalamate; DM: diabetes mellitus; PKD: polycystic kidney disease; HLA: human leucocyte antigen; LURD: living unrelated donation; *: statistically significant.

3.1.2. Intra- and Postoperative Data

Intraoperative data of donors of fDGF and nofDGF kidneys showed no differences with exception of the total amount of fluid, in which donors of fDGF kidneys received less fluid intraoperatively, which was the case for total volume (3545 mL (778.2) vs. 3845 mL (799.1), $p = 0.050$) and mL/kg BW (45 mL/kg BW (10.3) vs. 49 mL/kg BW (11.4), $p = 0.053$).

Recipients who developed fDGF received significantly less intraoperative fluid, which was the case for the total amount of fluid (3000 mL (2250–3680) vs. 3500 mL (2900–4075), $p = 0.023$) and mL kg-1BW (36 mL/kg BW (25.9–50.0) vs. 47 mL/kg BW (37.3–55.6), $p = 0.007$). Predominantly RL was given, but in case of hyponatremia RL was partially replaced by saline. This was the case in 48 (20%) of the recipients without fDGF and in 8 (26%) of the patients with fDGF ($p = 0.477$). Median volume replaced by saline was 1000 mL (500–2000) in the nofDGF group and 800 mL (500–1075) in the fDGF group ($p = 0.865$). Blood loss was comparable between groups and transfusion of red blood cells was applied in 10 (4.1%) of the patients in the noFDGF group and two (6.4%) of the fDGF group. Patients showed no difference in hypotensive periods, but recipients experiencing fDGF were treated more frequently with noradrenaline continuous infusion ($p = 0.034$), which was only the case for low dose infusion with a maximum of 0.1 mg/h. For noradrenaline administered at higher dosage (>0.1 mg/h), there was no difference between the two groups. fDGF was associated with a lower urine output during the first two hours after transplantation ($p = 0.005$ for the first hour and $p = 0.002$ for the second hour). Ten patients in the fDGF group were dialyzed after transplantation versus zero patients in the nofDGF group ($p < 0.001$). Eight of these kidneys gained function after a mean of 10.3 (3.1) days. Two kidneys suffered primary nonfunction due to a combination of ATN and mild antibody-mediated rejection (patient 114, transplanted June 2015) and non-HLA-mediated hyperacute rejection (patient 273, transplanted November 2016). Recipients experiencing fDGF showed a longer hospital stay (14 (10–20) vs. 9 (7–13) days $p < 0.001$) (Table 2).

Table 2. Intra- and postoperative donor and recipient data. Data given as number (%), mean (SD), or median (IQR).

	nofDGF	**fDGF**	*p*
Donor	***n* = 244**	***n* = 31**	
Duration min	227 (38.2)	216 (36.8)	0.134
Fluid			
Total mL	3845 (799.1)	3545 (778.2)	0.050*
mL/kg BW	49 (11.4)	45 (10.3)	0.053
Intraoperative blood pressure			
S-RR ≤ 80 mmHG	137 (56%)	21 (68%)	0.251
Cumulative duration (min)	10 (5–15)	10 (5–15)	0.772
Vasoactive substances			
Ephedrine	178 (73%)	25 (71%)	0.515
Phenylephrine	22 (9%)	4 (13%)	0.512
Noradrenaline	61 (25%)	11 (35%)	0.277
Recipient	***n* = 244**	***n* = 31**	
Duration min	212 (189–239)	224 (190–260)	0.390
Fluid			
Total mL	3500 (2900–4075)	3000 (2250–3680)	0.023*
mL/kg BW	47 (37.3–55.6)	36 (25.9–50.0)	0.007*
Intraoperative blood pressure			
S-RR < 80 mmHg	49 (20%)	6 (19%)	>0.999
Cumulative duration min	5 (5–10)	7.5 (4.5–11.2)	0.679
MAP < 60 mmHg	93 (38%)	11 (35%)	0.846
Cumulative duration min	10 (5–10)	5 (5–20)	0.759
Vasoactive substances			
Ephedrine	93 (38%)	16 (52%)	0.174
Phenylephrine	26 (11%)	3 (10%)	>0999
Noradrenaline	129 (53%)	23 (74%)	0.034*
0.02–0.10 mg h^{-1}	37 (15%)	10 (32%)	0.024*
0.10–0.20 mg h^{-1}	42 (17%)	7 (23%)	0.459
>0.20 mg h^{-1}	49 (20%)	6 (19%)	>0.999
Ischemia times (min)			
WIT	3 (3–4)	3 (3–4)	0.724
CIT	154 (140–173)	158 (141–178)	0.646
WIT2	39 (33–45)	38 (33–45)	0.982

Table 2. *Cont.*

	nofDGF	fDGF	*p*
Kidney left	177 (73%)	19 (61%)	0.209
Right fossa	203 (83%)	26 (84%)	>0.999
>1 artery	49 (20%)	8 (26%)	0.482
Artery sacrificed	11 (5%)	4 (13%)	0.074
Blood loss (mL)	250 (150–400)	250 (162.5–500)	0.499
Urineproduction	*n* = 230	*n* = 30	
1st h (mL)	405 (250–675)	255 (75–512)	0.005*
2nd h (mL)	350 (250–550)	183 (64–462)	0.002*
	n = 244	*n* = 31	
Dialysis after transplantation	0 (0%)	10 (32%)	<0.001*
Length of hospital stay days	9 (7–13)	14 (10–20)	<0.001*

Min: minutes; BW: bodyweight; S-RR: systolic blood pressure; MAP: mean arterial pressure; WIT: warm ischemia time; CIT: cold ischemia time: WIT2: warm ischemia time 2; *: statistically significant

3.2. *Multivariate Logistic Regression Analysis*

In the unadjusted analysis, a higher intraoperative administered fluid volume was associated with 3% lower odds for the development of fDGF per mL/kg BW (OR 0.967, CI (0.941–0.993), model 1). We adjusted for potentially relevant confounders with high significance in the univariate analysis, i.e., a history of dialysis and the use of intraoperative noradrenaline, after which the relationship was still apparent (OR 0.970, CI (0.943–0.998), model 2). Since the intraoperative amount of fluid in the donors approached significance in the univariate analysis with lower volumes given in the fDGF group, we also adjusted for amount of fluid in the donor, after which the relationship was still apparent (OR 0.969, CI (0.941–0.997), model 3) (Table 3).

Table 3. Multivariate logistic regression on risk factors of functional delayed graft function (fDGF).

Model	Odds ratio (95% CI)	*p*
1. Unadjusted analysis, model 1		
• Amount of fluid administered intraoperatively, recipient, mL/kg BW	0.967 (0.941–0.993)	0.015
2. Adjusted analysis, model 2		
• Amount of fluid administered intraoperatively, recipient, mL/kg BW	0.970 (0.943–0.998)	0.036
• No dialysis dependence at time of transplantation	0.186 (0.073–0.475)	<0.001
• Use of noradrenaline continuous infusion yes/no	2.018 (0.834–4.878)	0.119
3. Adjusted analysis, model 3		
• Amount of fluid administered intraoperatively, recipient, mL/kg BW	0.969 (0.941–0.997)	0.029
• No dialysis dependence at time of transplantation	0.181 (0.071–0.464)	<0.001
• Amount of fluid administered intraoperatively, donor, mL/kg BW	0.978 (0.942–1.014)	0.231

3.3. *Influence of the GDFT Protocol on the Intraoperative Fluid Volume.*

Additionally, we were interested in the impact of implementation of our GDFT protocol on the incidence of fDGF and on the amount of fluid administered intraoperatively. The GDFT protocol was gradually implemented during 2015 and in 2016 (up to September) all recipients were treated following this protocol (Figure 1). Data of the EV1000 monitor were not recorded in our PDMS, therefore we were unable to see which patients in 2015 were treated according the GDFT protocol and disregarded this period (March 2015–December 2015) in this specific analysis. We compared patients transplanted between January 2014–February 2015 (period 1, $n = 84$, old protocol) to patients transplanted between January 2016–June 2016 (period 2, $n = 52$, GDFT protocol) and patients transplanted between September 2016–February 2017 (period 3, $n = 61$, new protocol).

Incidence of fDGF during the different periods are shown in Figure 2. Implementation of GDFT was accompanied by an increase in fDGF from 8.3% in period 1 to 23% in period 2. The implementation of the new protocol in period 3 resulted in a reduction of the incidence of fDGF back to baseline (8.2%, $p = 0.029$).

Total amount of intraoperative administered fluid and mL/kg BW in recipients in the different time periods are shown in Figure 3A,B, respectively. Total amount of fluid and mL/kg BW were significantly different between the three time periods ($p < 0.001$, $p < 0.001$). Implementation of the GDFT (period 2) resulted in a decrease of intraoperative fluid administration compared to our old protocol (period 1), which was the case for total volume (2775 mL (2313–3500) vs. 3625 mL (3213–4000), $p < 0.001$) and mL/kg BW (38 mL/kg BW (30.3–45.3) vs. 48 mL/kg BW (40–60), $p < 0.001$). The implementation of the new protocol (period 3) resulted in an increase in intraoperative fluid administration to 4150 mL (3475–4575) mL and 54 mL/kg BW (47.4–60.1) compared to the old (total volume $p = 0.037$, mL/kg BW $p = 0.053$) and GDFT (total volume $p < 0.001$, mL/kg BW $p < 0.001$).

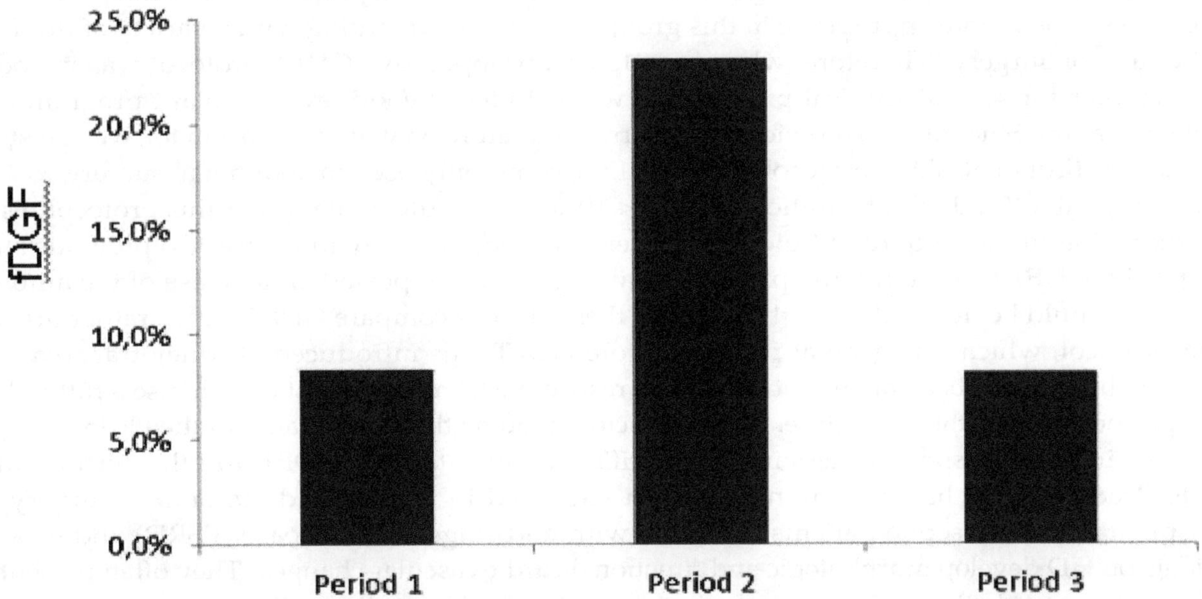

Figure 2. Incidence of fDGF in recipients during the different time periods. Period 1: January 2014–February 2015, old protocol, 4–5 L RL. Period 2: January–June 2016, GDFT protocol. Period 3: September 2016–February 2017, new protocol, 50 mL/kg BW. $p = 0.029$.

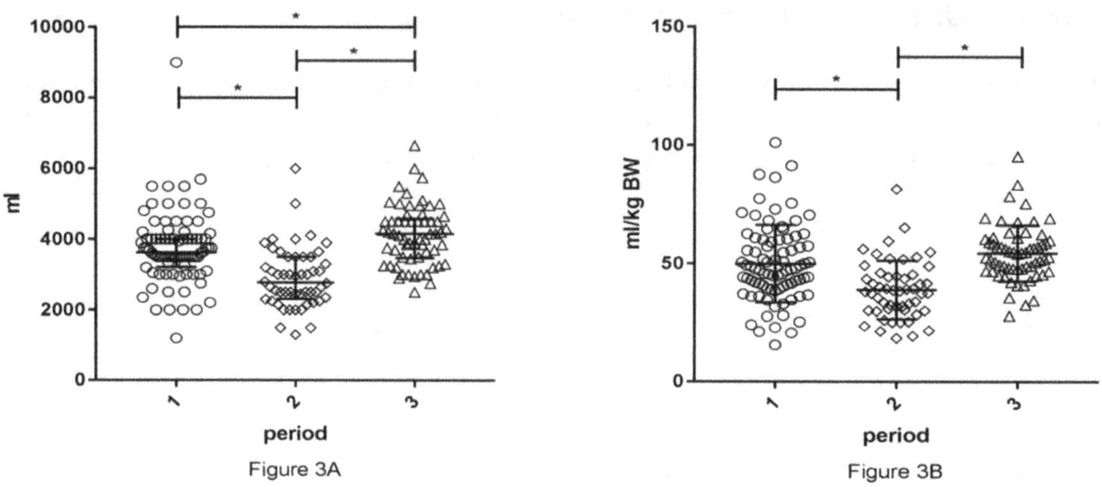

Figure 3. Volume of fluid administered intraoperatively in recipients during the different time periods. Period 1: January 2014–February 2015, old protocol, 4–5 L RL. Period 2: January–June 2016, GDFT protocol. Period 3: September 2016–February 2017, new protocol, 50 mL/kg BW. Volumes are given in mL (**A**) and mL/kg BW (**B**).

4. Discussion

This retrospective cohort analysis study shows that intraoperative fluid restriction in recipients is associated with fDGF in living donor kidney transplantation. Additionally, we showed that the implementation of a GDFT with a goal set at SVV < 10% led to a reduction of intraoperative fluid administration, on average by 850 mL in total and 21% in mL/kg BW, compared to our old protocol of 4–5 L of RL. In our opinion, this analysis provides valuable information for other centers when changes in intraoperative fluid management during kidney transplantation are considered.

Four to five liters of RL was the standard intraoperative fluid protocol in kidney transplantation in our center for over 15 years. This may seem rather liberal, but problems due to hypervolemia were rarely seen. However, following new trends on GDFT [24], a personalized intraoperative fluid approach seemed more appropriate in this group of patients presenting with a variety of fluid states at the time of surgery. Therefore, when in 2015 an intraoperative GDFT protocol was introduced in our center for several surgical procedures, we included the kidney transplant program in this implementation. Since there is no evidence in current literature on what goal to aim for, we adjusted the standard institutional GDFT protocol of SVV < 12%, commonly used in abdominal surgery, to a more generous goal in fluid administration of SVV < 10%. The implementation of this protocol resulted in a reduction in the amount of fluid administered intraoperatively in contrast to previous studies comparing GDFT to a "standard" protocol, which generally reported an increase of the amount of fluid. This could be due to the fact that most of these studies compare GDFT with a rather restrictive fluid protocol, which was general practice before GDFT was introduced. Kidney transplantation, however, has always been an exception on this restrictive trend and most centers use a rather liberal fluid protocol during this procedure. Another factor could be the performance of the FloTrac®-system in predicting fluid responsiveness in this specific patient category. GDFT and the performance of the FloTrac®-system has predominantly been validated in cardiac and abdominal surgery, liver transplantation, and septic patients. Patients with end-stage renal disease (ESRD) and especially patients on HD develop morphologic and functional cardiovascular changes. They often present with severe arterio- and atherosclerosis, inducing arterial stiffening and systolic or diastolic dysfunction. Since SVV is calculated as the percentage change of SV to the mean, derived from an arterial pulse contour analysis, it is conceivable that these cardiovascular changes influence the performance of the FloTrac®-system in predicting patients fluid state. Only one pilot study presents the effect of fluid loading on SVV measured with the use of the FloTrac®-system in patients with ESRD on HD. In this study, HD patients undergoing vascular surgery presented with a broad range of SVV (16.2 ± 6.0) after induction of anesthesia. After a fluid bolus of only 500 mL of a colloid solution almost all patients showed a SVV < 10% (6.2 ± 2.8), the threshold in our protocol [25].

The debate on perioperative fluid management is still ongoing. Controversy exists regarding assessment of the intravascular volume state, which goals to aim for, how to measure these goals, and what type of fluid should be used. Hypovolemia leads to a decreased oxygen supply to organs and tissues and may cause hypoxia, which can lead to organ dysfunction. Hypervolemia, on the other hand, can damage the endothelial glycocalyx resulting in a fluid shift from the intravascular compartment to the interstitial space and tissue edema [26]. Shin and colleagues report in their large cohort analysis of 92.094 patients undergoing noncardiac surgery that both too little and too much intraoperative fluid is associated with increased morbidity, mortality, costs, and length of hospital stay [27]. Myles and colleagues randomLy assigned 3000 patients undergoing a major abdominal procedure to a restrictive or liberal fluid regimen. In their study, a restrictive regimen was associated with increased risk of acute kidney injury with a hazard ratio of 1.71 (95% CI 1.29–2.27) [28]. These studies, however, do not take kidney transplant recipients into account. In the normal kidney, blood flow is regulated by an autoregulatory mechanism, ensuring adequate perfusion in a broad blood pressure range by afferent and efferent arterioles. In the transplanted, denervated kidney, this haemodynamic autoregulation is impaired making the renal blood flow linearly dependent on the systemic blood flow [29–31]. Furthermore, reperfusion of the ischemic kidney can be followed by vasoconstriction in the afferent arterioles. This may result in a reduced GFR due to a decrease in glomerular transcapillary hydraulic pressure difference [7,32,33]. Ensuring an adequate volume state in this specific patient category, therefore, is essential to obtain an adequate circulation both on macro- and microcirculatory level. Recently, Cavalari and colleagues reported the results of their prospective observational study, in which they compared a prospectively observed cohort of 33 deceased donor kidney transplant recipients treated with a GDFT protocol to a historical cohort of 33 kidney transplant recipients treated with their conventional fluid therapy [34]. They observed a significant reduction of cardiovascular complications, DGF. and surgical complications in the GDFT group. Surprisingly, in this study both groups received the same amount of fluid throughout the transplant procedure. Studies including deceased donor kidneys, however, comprise a variety of donor types with variable incidences of DGF hampering an adequate analysis and conclusions.

The most important predictor of fDGF in our analysis was dialysis dependency at the time of transplantation. A history of dialysis and especially hemodialysis prior to transplantation is a known risk factor of DGF [5,7,35,36]. Hypovolemia at the time of transplantation is one of the proposed underlying mechanisms [37]. Our hypothesis before implementation of the GDFT protocol was that these hypovolemic dialysis patients would present with higher SVV at time of surgery, demanding more fluid intraoperatively, compared to the relatively normovolemic or slightly hypervolemic preemptively transplanted patients. Surprisingly, comparable amounts of fluids were given to the two groups.

In our GDFT protocol, noradrenaline was used when CI was below an age-adjusted value. Therefore, an increased use of noradrenaline was seen in period 2 compared to period 1 (71% vs. 41% $p = 0.001$) due to the implementation of the GDFT. In period 3, the use of noradrenaline decreased to 50% of the patients. In the univariate analysis, the use of noradrenaline was correlated with development of fDGF, but after multivariate logistic regression this was no longer the case. However, Morita and coworkers showed that in a rat model, transplanted kidneys responded to sympaticomimetics with a reduction in renal blood flow (RBF) in contrast to the increase in RBF seen in native rat kidneys [38].

There are some limitations of this analysis that have to be addressed: A major limitation is that we were unable to evaluate outcome directly according to the fluid protocol (4–5L RL vs. GDFT) and are unable to present information or draw any conclusions regarding actual SV, SVV, CO or CI values and their relation to the observed increase of fDGF. Other limitations are those of a retrospective observational trial. There is the potential of confounding by unmeasured factors. Regarding postoperative fluid volume, the exact amount of fluid given could not be retrieved in a reliable way from our PDMS and is therefore not implemented in this analysis. Postoperative fluid management was according to a standardized protocol and comprised of 1 L NaCl 0.45%-Glucose 2.5% per 24 h, complemented with the volume of diuresis in the former hour. This means that when the kidney produces less urine the patient will be given less fluid postoperatively. Since fDGF was associated with a lower urinary output the first two hours, it is very likely that patients experiencing fDGF received less fluid postoperatively. Whether this contributed to development of fDGF or is more of a symptom remains unknown. Backpressure from congested tubules obstructed with cellular debris may contribute to a reduction in GFR [39,40]. A higher volume of urine in the first hours may have led to washout of this debris.

Finally, due to the fact that there are only 31 events there is always the possibility of overestimating the strength of associations using a multivariate analysis. A strong argument, however, is that no policy changes were implemented during the study period with the exception of the intraoperative fluid regimen. Furthermore the incidence of fDGF in our LDKT population has been stable over many years and after changing the fluid regimen back to a more liberal fixed amount of 50 mL/kg BW the incidence of fDGF instantly returned to baseline.

DGF after transplantation is a clinically relevant problem. It is associated with an increase in morbidity, patient anxiety, increased risk of acute rejection, and additional diagnostic procedures and costs. In our population the median hospital stay in patients experiencing fDGF was prolonged by five days. Furthermore, this study shows that strict protocols for perioperative fluid management are needed when studies in kidney transplantation are designed. Fluid restriction can be an important risk factor for DGF, a frequently used primary end point, even in the setting of LDKT.

5. Conclusions

Implementation of a goal-directed approach to fluid administration with a goal set at a SVV < 10% throughout the procedure led to reduced intraoperative fluid administration in the LDKT recipients in our center. This intraoperative fluid restriction was associated with the development of more fDGF. A thorough validation of GDFT protocols in patients with renal insufficiency is warranted before these are implemented in this population.

Author Contributions: G.J.N.-M.: participated in research design, data collection, data analysis, writing of the paper. T.M.H.: participated in data collection, writing of the paper; R.A.P.: participated in writing of the paper; M.E.M.: participated in data analysis, writing of the paper; J.G.B.: participated in data analysis, writing of the paper; M.M.S.: participated in research design, data analysis, writing of the paper; S.P.B.: participated in research design, data analysis, writing of the paper.

Acknowledgments: We would like to thank Cordelia Hempel and Tamar van den Berg for data retrieval and professor Anthony Absalom for his critical comments and help with language aspects.

References

1. Nijboer, W.N.; Schuurs, T.A.; van der Hoeven, J.A.; Leuvenink, H.G.; van der Heide, J.J.; van Goor, H.; Ploeg, R.J. Effects of brain death on stress and inflammatory response in the human donor kidney. *Transplant. Proc.* **2005**, *37*, 367–369. [CrossRef] [PubMed]
2. Salvadori, M.; Rosso, G.; Bertoni, E. Update on ischemia-reperfusion injury in kidney transplantation: Pathogenesis and treatment. *World J. Transplant.* **2015**, *5*, 52–67. [CrossRef] [PubMed]
3. Simpkins, C.E.; Montgomery, R.A.; Hawxby, A.M.; Locke, J.E.; Gentry, S.E.; Warren, D.S.; Segev, D.L. Cold ischemia time and allograft outcomes in live donor renal transplantation: Is live donor organ transport feasible? *Am. J. Transplant.* **2007**, *7*, 99–107. [CrossRef] [PubMed]
4. Redfield, R.R.; Scalea, J.R.; Zens, T.J.; Muth, B.; Kaufman, D.B.; Djamali, A.; Astor, B.C.; Mohamed, M. Predictors and outcomes of delayed graft function after living-donor kidney transplantation. *Transpl. Int.* **2016**, *29*, 81–87. [CrossRef] [PubMed]

5. Siedlecki, A.; Irish, W.; Brennan, D.C. Delayed graft function in the kidney transplant. *Am. J. Transplant.* **2011**, *11*, 2279–2296. [CrossRef]
6. Snoeijs, M.G.; Winkens, B.; Heemskerk, M.B.; Hoitsma, A.J.; Christiaans, M.H.; Buurman, W.A.; van Heurn, L.E. Kidney transplantation from donors after cardiac death: A 25-year experience. *Transplantation* **2010**, *90*, 1106–1112. [CrossRef]
7. Perico, N.; Cattaneo, D.; Sayegh, M.H.; Remuzzi, G. Delayed graft function in kidney transplantation. *Lancet* **2004**, *364*, 1814–1827. [CrossRef]
8. Wu, W.K.; Famure, O.; Li, Y.; Kim, S.J. Delayed graft function and the risk of acute rejection in the modern era of kidney transplantation. *Kidney Int.* **2015**, *88*, 851–858. [CrossRef]
9. Fonseca, I.; Teixeira, L.; Malheiro, J.; Martins, L.S.; Dias, L.; Castro Henriques, A.; Mendonça, D. The effect of delayed graft function on graft and patient survival in kidney transplantation: An approach using competing events analysis. *Transpl. Int.* **2015**, *28*, 738–750. [CrossRef]
10. Sharif, A.; Borrows, R. Delayed graft function after kidney transplantation: The clinical perspective. *Am. J. Kidney Dis.* **2013**, *62*, 150–158. [CrossRef]
11. Othman, M.M.; Ismael, A.Z.; Hammouda, G.E. The impact of timing of maximal crystalloid hydration on early graft function during kidney transplantation. *Anesth. Analg.* **2010**, *110*, 1440–1446. [CrossRef] [PubMed]
12. Bacchi, G.; Buscaroli, A.; Fusari, M.; Neri, L.; Cappuccilli, M.L.; Carretta, E.; Stefoni, S. The influence of intraoperative central venous pressure on delayed graft function in renal transplantation: A single-centre experience. *Transplant. Proc.* **2010**, *42*, 3387–3391. [CrossRef] [PubMed]
13. Snoeijs, M.G.; Wiermans, B.; Christiaans, M.H.; van Hooff, J.P.; Timmerman, B.E.; Schurink, G.W.H.; Buurman, W.A.; Van Heurn, L.W.E. Recipient hemodynamics during non-heart-beating donor kidney transplantation are major predictors of primary nonfunction. *Am. J. Transplant.* **2007**, *7*, 1158–1166. [CrossRef] [PubMed]
14. Aulakh, N.K.; Garg, K.; Bose, A.; Aulakh, B.S.; Chahal, H.S.; Aulakh, G.S. Influence of hemodynamics and intraoperative hydration on biochemical outcome of renal transplant recipients. *J. Anaesthesiol. Clin. Pharmacol.* **2015**, *31*, 174–179. [CrossRef] [PubMed]
15. Marik, P.E.; Cavallazzi, R. Does the central venous pressure predict fluid responsiveness? An updated meta-analysis and a plea for some common sense. *Crit. Care Med.* **2013**, *41*, 1774–1781. [CrossRef] [PubMed]
16. Ferris, R.L.; Kittur, D.S.; Wilasrusmee, C.; Shah, G.; Krause, E.; Ratner, L. Early hemodynamic changes after renal transplantation: Determinants of low central venous pressure in the recipients and correlation with acute renal dysfunction. *Med. Sci. Monit.* **2003**, *9*, 61–66.
17. Le Manach, Y.; Hofer, C.K.; Lehot, J.J.; Vallet, B.; Goarin, J.P.; Tavernier, B.; Cannesson, M. Can changes in arterial pressure be used to detect changes in Cardiac output during volume expansion in the perioperative period? *Anesthesiology* **2012**, *117*, 1165–1174. [CrossRef] [PubMed]
18. Benes, J.; Giglio, M.; Brienza, N.; Michard, F. The effects of goal-directed fluid therapy based on dynamic parameters on post-surgical outcome: A meta-analysis of randomized controlled trials. *Crit. Care* **2014**, *18*, 584. [CrossRef] [PubMed]
19. Ripollés-Melchor, J.; Espinosa, Á.; Martínez-Hurtado, E.; Abad-Gurumeta, A.; Casans-Frances, R.; Fernandez-Perez, C.; Lopez-Timoneda, F.; Calvo-Vecino, J.M. Perioperative goal-directed hemodynamic therapy in noncardiac surgery: A systematic review and meta-analysis. *J. Clin. Anesth.* **2016**, *28*, 105–115. [CrossRef] [PubMed]
20. Sun, Y.; Chai, F.; Pan, C.; Romeiser, J.L.; Gan, T.J. Effect of perioperative goal-directed hemodynamic therapy on postoperative recovery following major abdominal surgery-a systematic review and meta-analysis of randomized controlled trials. *Crit. Care* **2017**, *21*, 141. [CrossRef]
21. Decruyenaere, P.; Decruyenaere, A.; Peeters, P.; Vermassen, F. A Single-Centre Comparison of 22 Competing Definitions of Delayed Graft Function After Kidney Transplantation. *Ann. Transplant.* **2016**, *21*, 152–159. [CrossRef] [PubMed]
22. Akkina, S.K.; Connaire, J.J.; Israni, A.K.; Snyder, J.J.; Matas, A.J.; Kasiske, B.L. Similar outcomes with different rates of delayed graft function may reflect centre practice, not centre performance. *Am. J. Transplant.* **2009**, *9*, 1460–1466. [CrossRef] [PubMed]
23. Moore, J.; Shabir, S.; Chand, S.; Bentall, A.; McClean, A.; Chan, W.; Jham, S.; Benavente, D.; Sharif, A.; Ball, S.; et al. Assessing and comparing rival definitions of delayed renal allograft function for predicting subsequent graft failure. *Transplantation* **2010** *90*, 1113–1116. [CrossRef] [PubMed]

24. Pearse, R.M.; Harrison, D.A.; McDonald, N. Effect of a perioperative, cardiac output guided hemodynamic therapy algorithm on outcomes following major gastrointestinal surgery: A randomized clinical trial and updated systematic review. *JAMA* **2014**, *311*, 2181–2190. [CrossRef] [PubMed]
25. Kanda, H.; Hirasaki, Y.; Iida, T.; Kanao-Kanda, M.; Toyama, Y.; Kunisawa, T.; Iwasaki, H. Effect of fluid loading on left ventricular volume and stroke volume variability in patients with end-stage renal disease: A pilot study. *Ther. Clin. Risk Manag.* **2015**, *11*, 1619–1625. [CrossRef] [PubMed]
26. Chappell, D.; Jacob, M.; Hofmann-Kiefer, K.; Conzen, P.; Rehm, M. A rational approach to perioperative fluid management. *Anesthesiology* **2008**, *109*, 723–740. [CrossRef] [PubMed]
27. Shin, C.H.; Long, D.R.; McLean, D.; Grabitz, S.D.; Ladha, K.; Timm, F.P.; Thevathasan, T.; Pieretti, A.; Ferrone, C.; Hoeft, A.; et al. Effects of intraoperative Fluid Management on Postoperative Outcomes: A Hospital Registry Study. *Ann. Surg.* **2018**, *267*, 1084–1092. [CrossRef]
28. Myles, P.S.; Bellomo, R.; Corcoran, T.; Forbes, A.; Peyton, P.; Story, D.; Christophi, C.; Leslie, K.; McGuinness, S.; Parke, R.; et al. Restrictive versus Liberal Fluid Therapy for Major Abdominal Surgery. *N. Engl. J. Med.* **2018**, *378*, 2263–2274. [CrossRef] [PubMed]
29. Adams, P.L.; Adams, F.F.; Bell, P.D.; Navar, L.G. Impaired renal blood flow autoregulation in ischemic acute renal failure. *Kidney Int.* **1980**, *18*, 68–76. [CrossRef]
30. Shannon, J.L.; Headland, R.; MacIver, A.G.; Ferryman, S.R.; Barber, P.C.; Howie, A.J. Studies on the innervation of human renal allografts. *J. Pathol.* **1998**, *186*, 109–115. [CrossRef]
31. Thomas, M.C.; Mathew, T.H.; Russ, G.R.; Rao, M.M.; Moran, J. Perioperative blood pressure control, delayed graft function and acute rejection after renal transplantation. *Transplantation* **2003**, *75*, 1989–1995. [CrossRef] [PubMed]
32. Alejandro, V.; Scandling, J.D., Jr.; Sibley, R.K.; Dafoe, D.; Alfrey, E.; Deen, W.; Myers, B.D. Mechanisms of filtration failure during postischemic injury of the human kidney. A study of the reperfused renal allograft. *J. Clin. Investig.* **1995**, *95*, 820–831. [PubMed]
33. Wilhelm, S.M.; Simonson, M.S.; Robinson, A.V.; Stowe, N.T.; Schulak, J.A. Endothelin up-regulation and localization following renal ischemia and reperfusion. *Kidney Int.* **1999**, *55*, 1011–1018. [CrossRef] [PubMed]
34. Cavaleri, M.; Veroux, M.; Palermo, F.; Vasile, F.; Mineri, M.; Palumbo, J.; Salemi, L.; Astuto, M.; Murabito, P. Perioperative Goal-Directed Therapy during Kidney Transplantation: An Impact Evaluation on the Major Postoperative Complications. *J. Clin. Med.* **2019**, *8*, 80. [CrossRef]
35. Van Loo, A.A.; Vanholder, R.C.; Bernaert, P.R.; Vermassen, F.E.; van der Vennet, M.; Lameire, N.H. Pretransplantation hemodialysis strategy influences early renal graft function. *J. Am. Soc. Nephrol.* **1998**, *9*, 473–481.
36. Snyder, J.J.; Kasiske, B.L.; Gilbertson, D.T.; Collins, A.J. A comparison of transplant outcomes in peritoneal and hemodialysis patients. *Kidney Int.* **2002**, *62*, 1423–1430. [CrossRef]
37. Bogaard, H.J.; de Vries, J.P.; de Vries, P.M. Assessment of refill and hypovolaemia by continuous surveillance of blood volume and extracellular fluid volume. *Nephrol. Dial. Transplant.* **1994**, *9*, 1283–1287.
38. Morita, K.; Seki, T.; Nonomura, K.; Koyanagi, T.; Yoshioka, M.; Saito, H. Changes in renal blood flow in response to sympathomimetics in the rat transplanted and denervated kidney. *Int. J. Urol.* **1999**, *6*, 24–32. [CrossRef]
39. Alejandro, V.S.; Nelson, W.J.; Huie, P.; Sibley, R.K.; Dafoe, D.; Kuo, P.; Scandling, J.D., Jr.; Myers, B.D. Postischemic injury, delayed function and Na^+/K^+-ATPase distribution in the transplanted kidney. *Kidney Int.* **1995**, *48*, 1308–1315. [CrossRef]
40. Tanner, G.A.; Sloan, K.L.; Sophasan, S. Effects of renal artery occlusion on kidney function in the rat. *Kidney Int.* **1973**, *4*, 377–389. [CrossRef]

7

Lifestyle, Inflammation and Vascular Calcification in Kidney Transplant Recipients: Perspectives on Long-Term Outcomes

Camilo G. Sotomayor *, Charlotte A. te Velde-Keyzer, Martin H. de Borst, Gerjan J. Navis and Stephan J.L. Bakker

Department of Internal Medicine, University Medical Center Groningen, University of Groningen, 9700 RB Groningen, The Netherlands; c.a.keyzer@umcg.nl (C.A.t.V.-K.); m.h.de.borst@umcg.nl (M.H.d.B.); g.j.navis@umcg.nl (G.J.N.); s.j.l.bakker@umcg.nl (S.J.L.B.)

* Correspondence: c.g.sotomayor.campos@umcg.nl

Abstract: After decades of pioneering and improvement, kidney transplantation is now the renal replacement therapy of choice for most patients with end-stage kidney disease (ESKD). Where focus has traditionally been on surgical techniques and immunosuppressive treatment with prevention of rejection and infection in relation to short-term outcomes, nowadays, so many people are long-living with a transplanted kidney that lifestyle, including diet and exposure to toxic contaminants, also becomes of importance for the kidney transplantation field. Beyond hazards of immunological nature, a systematic assessment of potentially modifiable—yet rather overlooked—risk factors for late graft failure and excess cardiovascular risk may reveal novel targets for clinical intervention to optimize long-term health and downturn current rates of premature death of kidney transplant recipients (KTR). It should also be realized that while kidney transplantation aims to restore kidney function, it incompletely mitigates mechanisms of disease such as chronic low-grade inflammation with persistent redox imbalance and deregulated mineral and bone metabolism. While the vicious circle between inflammation and oxidative stress as common final pathway of a multitude of insults plays an established pathological role in native chronic kidney disease, its characterization post-kidney transplant remains less than satisfactory. Next to chronic inflammatory status, markedly accelerated vascular calcification persists after kidney transplantation and is likewise suggested a major independent mechanism, whose mitigation may counterbalance the excess risk of cardiovascular disease post-kidney transplant. Hereby, we first discuss modifiable dietary elements and toxic environmental contaminants that may explain increased risk of cardiovascular mortality and late graft failure in KTR. Next, we specify laboratory and clinical readouts, with a postulated role within persisting mechanisms of disease post-kidney transplantation (i.e., inflammation and redox imbalance and vascular calcification), as potential non-traditional risk factors for adverse long-term outcomes in KTR. Reflection on these current research opportunities is warranted among the research and clinical kidney transplantation community.

Keywords: nephrology; kidney transplant; kidney transplant recipients; long-term outcomes; graft failure; cardiovascular mortality; lifestyle; inflammation; vascular calcification; bone mineral density; dual-energy X-ray absorptiometry

---

1. Introduction

Chronic kidney disease (CKD) is a major public health problem, with a current worldwide prevalence of approximately 843 million individuals [1]. Global mean prevalence was recently reported at 13.4% for all CKD stages together (1–5) and at 10.6% if only the more severe CKD stages (3–5)

are considered [2]. Whereas the prevalence of all stages of CKD rises with age, older patients with similar levels of eGFR are less likely than their younger counterparts to progress to the need of renal replacement therapy, which has raised the question of whether all older patients who meet criteria for CKD actually have CKD [3].

The prevalence of CKD, its detection, treatment, and impact on health have been mainly studied in economically developed countries [1]. Nevertheless, even in these circumstances, it usually remains a silent, smoldering health threat, with, e.g., rates of awareness of being afflicted with kidney disease of approximately 10% among patients with CKD in an economically developed country like the United States [4]. Along the same line, in 2016, approximately 35% of patients diagnosed with incident end-stage kidney disease (ESKD) received little or no nephrology care prior to actually being diagnosed with ESKD [4]. Regrettably, prevalence of ESKD and prevalence of renal replacement therapy continue to increase (Figures 1 and 2) [4].

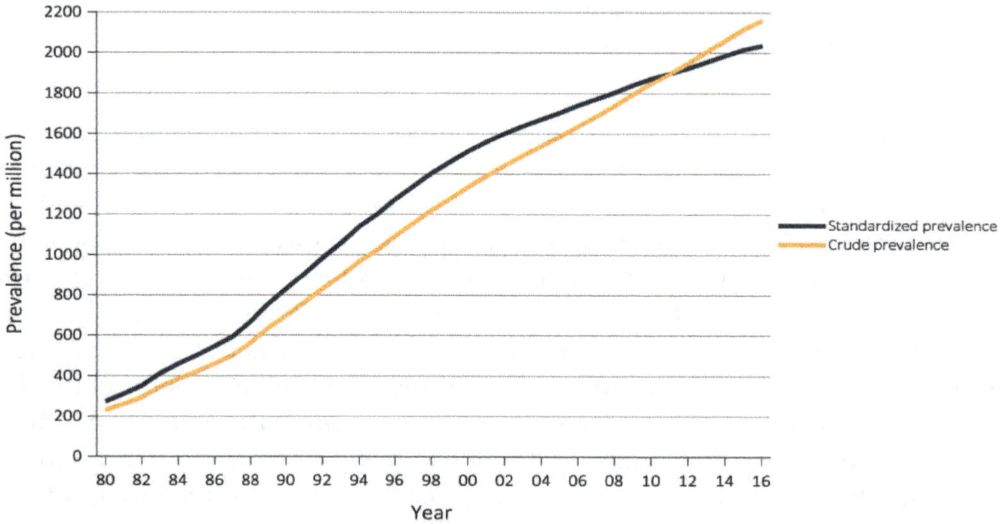

Figure 1. Prevalence of end-stage kidney disease (ESKD) in the United States (US) population, 1980–2016. This figure shows a steady increase in ESKD prevalence over recent ~35 years in the US. Standardized for age, sex, and race. Data Source: USRDS 2018 Annual Data Report [4].

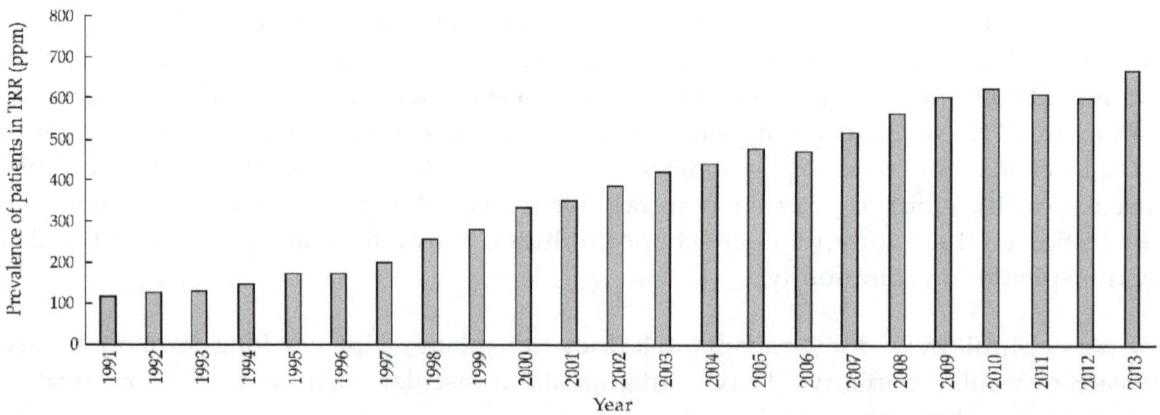

Figure 2. Prevalence of renal replacement therapy in Latin America, 1991–2013. This figure shows a steady increase in prevalence of renal replacement therapy over recent ~25 years in Latin America. Reprinted from "Latin American Dialysis and Transplant Registry: Experience and contributions to end-stage kidney disease epidemiology" [5].

Compared to chronic dialysis treatment, kidney transplantation is considered the renal replacement therapy of choice and the gold-standard treatment for most ESKD patients because it offers superior cost-effectiveness, quality of life, and life expectancy [6–10]. However, the latter has largely been due to significant improvements of short-term outcomes [11]. Advances in immunosuppression, tissue typing, treatment of infections, and surgical techniques led rates of 1-year graft survival at a pinnacle, whereas improvement of long-term outcomes post-transplant remains a major challenge in the kidney transplantation field [11].

On the one hand, the life-saving benefit of a kidney transplant remains largely hampered by cumulative injury of a multitude of hazards through immune and non-immune mechanisms of kidney damage. Over time, these mechanisms lead to chronic interstitial fibrosis and tubular atrophy as histopathological consequence and end-stage kidney allograft failure as functional repercussion, eventually requiring restart of dialysis or re-transplantation as final adverse clinical event (i.e., graft failure) [11–15].

On the other hand, kidney transplant recipients (KTR) are at particularly high risk of premature death, depicting overall mortality rates considerably higher than that of age-matched controls in the general population [16,17].

Indeed, approximately half of all kidney allograft losses are due to premature death with a functioning graft, a long-standing pattern that has remained largely unchanged over recent years [17,18].

Next, under the general understanding that cardiovascular disease is the leading cause of premature death post-kidney transplant (Figure 3) and thereby importantly challenging the improvement of longevity of KTR, great efforts have focused on the improvement of long-term cardiovascular outcomes [19–21].

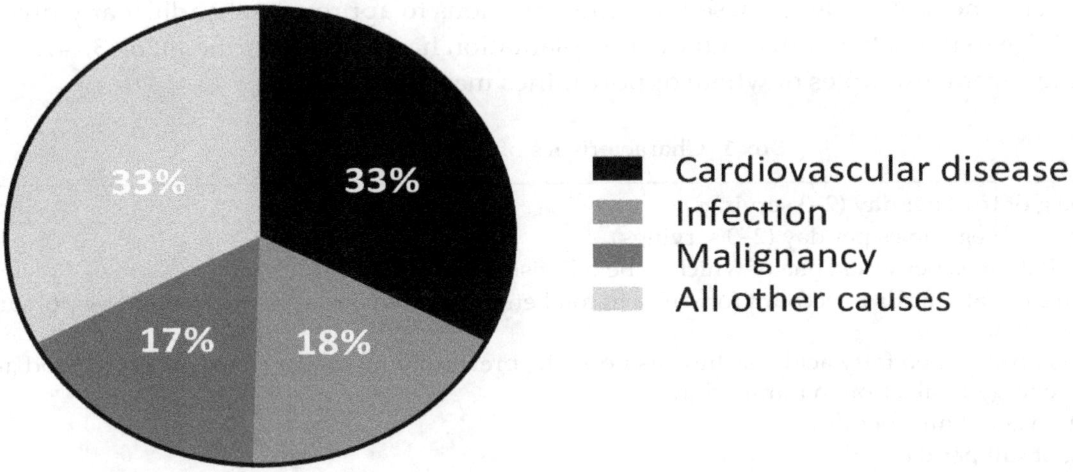

Figure 3. Mortality by causes of death with graft function in US KTR in 2015. This figure shows that cardiovascular disease was the leading cause of mortality among US KTR in 2015. Cardiovascular disease included acute myocardial infarction, atherosclerotic heart disease, congestive heart failure, cerebrovascular accident, and arrhythmia/cardiac arrest. Adapted from USRDS 2018 Annual Data Report [4].

In the clinical setting of KTR after the first-year post-transplant, beyond hazards of immunological nature, there is a pressing need to systematically study and characterize the clinical impact of potentially modifiable risk factors, such as lifestyle, diet, and exposure to toxic contaminants, which are underexplored areas in the kidney transplantation field [22–26]. This evidence is needed to guide decision making by clinicians and policy-makers in post-transplantation care. Furthermore, because kidney transplantation aims to restore kidney function but it incompletely mitigates collateral mechanisms of disease, such as chronic low-grade inflammation with persistent redox imbalance and deregulated mineral and bone metabolism, further research investigating specific clinical and laboratory readouts with a proposed involvement in such pathological pathways may point towards non-traditional risk factors and reveal novel targets for clinical intervention [27–32].

In the kidney transplantation field, future advances are expected from amelioration of adverse long-term outcomes by increasing recognition and developing novel, early, and cost-effective risk-management strategies focused on the non-immune aspects of post-kidney transplantation care and thus optimize long-term health and downturn current rates of premature death in stable KTR [11].

2. Lifestyle: Healthy Diet and Toxic Contaminants

One area with great potential for improvement is lifestyle, in particular diet and exposure to toxic contaminants. Systematic investigation of traditional and potentially modifiable risks factors in the post-kidney transplant setting may point towards otherwise overlooked early risk-management opportunities and thus provide the basis for the development of cost-effective interventional approaches to increase the lifespan of KTR. Healthy diet is a cornerstone element of cardio-metabolic health in the general population [33–38]. In general, a healthy diet is recommended as essential for cardiovascular disease prevention in all individuals. Surprisingly, however, little is known about the potential impact of a healthy diet on cardiovascular health and survival benefit in kidney patients across the continuum of CKD stages, in patients undergoing kidney replacement therapy, and remarkably limited evidence is available in the post-kidney transplantation clinical setting [39–42]. Moreover, native CKD and pre-transplant ESKD patients are generally advised to follow seemingly conflicting and challenging dietary recommendations with the aim of restricting individual nutrients such as potassium, salt, phosphorus, and protein [43]. It should be realized that there is scant evidence to support such restrictive dietary recommendations [44–46]. Finally, there is a notorious lack of studies aimed to aid on the development of evidence-based recommendations to appropriately adjust any pre-transplant dietary advice to the patient after kidney transplantation has been performed [26,43,44,47,48]. Below, we provide several examples of where opportunities may lie (Box 1).

Box 1. Characteristics of a healthy diet [49].

- ≥200 g of fruit per day (2–3 servings).
- ≥200 g of vegetables per day (2–3 servings).
- Fish 1–2 times per week, one of which to be oily fish.
- Saturated fatty acids to account for <10% of total energy intake through replacement by polyunsaturated fatty acids.
- Trans unsaturated fatty acids: as little as possible, preferably no intake from processed food and <1% of total energy intake from natural origin.
- 30 g unsalted nuts per day.
- <5 g of salt per day.
- Consumption of alcoholic beverages should be limited to 2 glasses per day (20 g/d of alcohol) for men and 1 glass per day (10 g/d of alcohol) for women.
- Sugar-sweetened soft drinks and alcoholic beverages consumption must be discouraged.

2.1. Fruit and Vegetable Consumption Post-Kidney Transplantation

With the aim of limiting potassium intake, for example, pre-transplant ESKD patients have largely been discouraged from a high consumption of fruits and vegetables, which are, however, well-known essential components of a healthy diet [50–54]. Beyond being rich in potassium, fruits and vegetables are rich in fibers, polyunsaturated and monounsaturated fatty acids, magnesium, iron, and generate less acid and contain smaller amounts of saturated fatty acids, protein, and absorbable phosphorus in comparison to meat [39,55]. At least four servings of fruit and vegetables per day are widely recommended for the prevention of major chronic diseases in the general population [49]. Indeed, increased consumption of fruits and vegetables has consistently shown to confer superior cardiovascular prognosis in the general population [52–54,56].

Recent studies show that KTR consume less fruits and vegetables than the general population, which has been associated with higher risk of cardiovascular mortality and posttransplant diabetes [57,58]. At present, however, post-kidney transplant, there is no clear incentive by transplant healthcare providers to prescribe restoration of the consumption of these basic items of a healthy diet. This attitude may respond to the fact that it remains relatively unexplored whether an increase of fruits and vegetables consumption post-kidney transplantation positively impacts outcomes of KTR, which would be hypothetically expected mainly by decreasing the excess cardiovascular burden and premature cardiovascular death. Epidemiological studies aimed to estimate a theoretical benefit of a relative increase of these specific food items are warranted as first step to, thereafter, investigate potential interventional strategies promoting novel, cost-effective, and patient-centered approaches to the nutritional management of KTR, adequately informing clinical practice and policy.

2.2. *Fish Intake Post-Kidney Transplantation and Mercury Exposure*

Similarly, fish are rich in the omega-3 polyunsaturated fatty acids (n-3 PUFA) EPA (eicosapentaenoic acid) and DHA (docosahexaenoic acid), which are suggested to yield several beneficial effects for cardiovascular health [59–62]. Circulating levels of EPA and DHA have been associated with reduced cardiovascular risk in both healthy populations and in patients with pre-existing cardiovascular disease [59–62]. Proposed beneficial health effects of marine-derived n-3 PUFA are wide-ranging, favorably impacting inflammation, fibrosis, lipid modulation, plaque stabilization, blood pressure, artery calcification processes, and endothelial function [63–66]. These properties render EPA and DHA as of encompassing therapeutic potential in the management of cardiovascular risk of KTR. Indeed, in this particular setting, recent observational studies showed that plasma levels of marine-derived n-3 PUFA are inversely associated with cardiovascular mortality risk [67,68].

It should be realized, however, that the results of randomized control trials using supplementation of these individual nutrients are not yet sufficiently powered to draw definitive conclusions and recommendations for KTR [69,70]. Moreover, no study has been devoted to evaluating the potential beneficial effect of a relatively high dietary fish intake, as mostly shown in the general population [71–75]. Indeed, fish is the main dietary source of n-3 PUFA, and its inclusion in diet seems reasonable because it is a good source of protein without potentially adverse effects of accompanying intake of high saturated fat as present in fatty meat products. Not exempt of drawbacks, however, fish is also the major source of human exposure to organic mercury (with the exception of industrial accidents or particular occupational exposures) [76–78]. Therefore, alongside the study of the potential health benefits of marine-derived n-3 PUFA, weighted investigation of a relatively higher fish intake has been performed as necessary step towards developing cautious evidence-based dietary guidelines for clinical uptake [79], suggesting that beneficial effects of a higher dietary intake of n-3 PUFA by increasing fish consumption post-kidney transplantation may not be mitigated by postulated increased cardiovascular risk due to concomitant exposure to mercury [79].

2.3. *Cadmium Exposure and Nephrotoxicity in the Post-Kidney Transplant Setting*

Cadmium is another heavy metal of environmental and lifestyle-related concern, with tobacco and diet as primary sources of exposure. Previous studies have demonstrated that cadmium may induce hypertension, which in turn is associated with accelerated kidney function decline and particularly demonstrated in KTR, by shortened allograft survival [80–84]. Most importantly, a strong body of evidence shows that the kidney is the most sensitive target organ of cadmium-induced body burden, through postulated direct mechanisms of cadmium-induced injury in this organ, wherein it accumulates with a half-life of up to 45 years [85–89]. It is important to note that, particularly in settings of long-term oxidative stress such as that of KTR, cadmium-induced nephrotoxicity may be associated with impaired kidney function at concentrations that are otherwise considered non-toxic [90–92]. Taking also into account that the most effective way to reduce cardiovascular disease in KTR may indeed be preservation of graft function, the aforementioned constellation of factors turn the investigation of cadmium-associated risk of encompassing relevance within the study of long-term outcomes of kidney allograft function [21,84]. Furthermore, bodily cadmium is susceptible to therapeutic interventions [93].

Thus, cadmium-targeted interventional strategies may offer novel opportunities to decrease the long-standing high burden of late kidney graft failure; however, whether the nephrotoxic exposure to cadmium represents an overlooked hazard for preserved graft functioning remains unknown.

3. Inflammation and Oxidative Stress and Vascular Calcification

Another area of great opportunities for further improvement may lie in a better evaluation of disease mechanisms long-term after transplantation. Traditional risk factors such as diabetes mellitus, smoking, and hypertension, among others, do not suffice to account for the excess burden of premature cardiovascular death of, otherwise, stable KTR [94–97]. Indeed, cardiovascular disease has an atypical nature in KTR when compared with the general population [20,21]. Unexplained cardiovascular risk subsidizes current efforts to provide cutting-edge evidence on the potential independent hazard of novel (non-traditional) cardiovascular risk factors post-kidney transplantation [98–102].

It should be taken into account that while kidney transplantation aims to restore kidney function, it incompletely abrogates mechanisms of disease. Moreover, an aggregate of factors specific to the transplant milieu such as a chronic low-grade immunologic response to the kidney allograft, long-term toxicity of maintenance immunosuppressive, as well as various degrees of progressive uremia, contribute to perpetuate chronic inflammation, redox imbalance, and deregulated mineral and bone metabolism, which have to be proposed as major independent and evolving pathophysiological mechanisms, whose mitigation may counterbalance—at least to a considerable extent—the excess risk of cardiovascular disease and graft failure post-kidney transplantation [30,32,101,103,104]. Below, we provide several examples of where opportunities may lie.

3.1. *Inflammation and Oxidative Stress Post-Kidney Transplantation*

Indeed, while the vicious circle between inflammation and oxidative stress as final common pathway of a multitude of insults plays an established pathological role in native chronic kidney disease (CKD), its characterization post-kidney transplant has been less than satisfactory [105–109]. This is relevant because, at a physiological level, the cornerstone role of the complex interplay between inflammation and oxidative stress (Box 2) provides a theoretical and conceptual framework upon which upcoming research may deepen the understanding of the pathophysiological status of KTR once they reach a seemingly stable clinical stage [105].

Box 2. Oxidative stress.

Oxidative stress is defined as an imbalance between the generation and removal of oxidant species. The most representative biological oxidant agents are reactive oxygen species (ROS) and reactive nitrogen species (RNS). The former group includes hydrogen peroxide, superoxide anion, and hydroxyl radical, whereas within the latter group relevant species are peroxynitrite anion, nitric oxide, and nitrogen dioxide radicals. Oxidative stress occurs when ROS and/or RNS production overwhelms the endogenous antioxidant defense system, either by excess production and/or inadequate removal. The antioxidant defense system is constituted by enzymatic antioxidant agents, including catalase, glutathione peroxidase, and superoxide dismutase. Non-enzymatic antioxidant components include a diversity of biological molecules, such as ascorbic acid (vitamin C), α-tocopherol (vitamin E), reduced glutathione, carotenoids, flavonoids, polyphenols, and several other exogenous antioxidants [110].

3.1.1. Vitamin C as Anti-Inflammatory and Antioxidant Agent and Its Depletion Post-Kidney Transplant

Inflammation, specifically the established inflammatory biomarker high-sensitivity C-reactive protein (hs-CRP)—which is also an indirect marker of increased oxidant production—has been previously shown to be independently associated with increased mortality risk in KTR [98,100]. Supported by data consistently showing an inverse correlation with hs-CRP in different settings, vitamin C is well-known by its anti-inflammatory effects [111–114]. Moreover, vitamin C is a physiological antioxidant agent, with radical-scavenger and reducing activities, of paramount importance for protection against diseases and degenerative processes caused by oxidant stress [115]. This particular composite of biochemical properties renders vitamin C as compelling research candidate to broaden the understanding of the interaction of inflammation and oxidative stress in the mechanisms leading to excess risk of premature death post-kidney transplantation. It should be realized, moreover, that pre-transplant ESKD patients often have an imbalance of several critical trace elements and vitamins [39]. Vitamin C, particularly, has been shown to be removed by conventional hemodialysis membranes, leading to drastic vitamin C depletion and oxidative stress [116–118]. Through an inverse mediating effect on inflammatory signaling biomarkers, sub-physiological levels of vitamin C (depletion) may be hypothesized to be implicated in mechanisms that associate with increased risk of adverse long-term outcomes [119–123]. To date, however, relatively little is known regarding the prevalence of abnormal vitamin C status post-kidney transplantation, yet recent studies have shown that low plasma vitamin C contributes to excess risk for premature death post-kidney transplantation [124,125].

3.1.2. Advanced Glycation End products as Amplifiers of Oxidative Stress and Inflammatory Responses

Inflammation is referred to as a redox-sensitive mechanism on the basis that reactive oxygen species may activate transcription factors such as nuclear factor kappa B (NF-kB), which regulates inflammatory mediator genes expression [126]. In this regard, advanced glycation end products (AGE) are particularly interesting oxidative stress biomarkers because it has been demonstrated that, upon binding to AGE-specific receptors, AGE activate intracellular pathways that amplify inflammatory and oxidative stress responses and regulate the transcription of adhesion molecules through NF-kB activation [127]. In agreement, data derived from clinical studies in pre-transplant ESKD patients support the implication of AGE in the complex feedback loop between oxidative stress and inflammation leading to endothelial dysfunction and adverse cardiovascular effects [128–130].

Several studies have observed accumulation of AGE in native and transplant CKD patients, and a strong body of evidence on the general theory of AGE pathophysiology supports its pivotal role in the initiation and progression of mechanisms underlying cardiovascular disease. However, few attempts have been made to investigate the association of AGE with cardiovascular risk post-kidney transplantation [99,131]. Through a mediating effect on up-regulation of inflammatory, oxidative stress and endothelial dysfunction biomarkers, a relative increase of AGE may be hypothesized to actively contribute to the intracellular signaling pathways that ultimately yield excess risk of premature cardiovascular death in KTR. It remains unknown whether a hypothetical association with risk of cardiovascular mortality is independent of estimates of kidney function and traditional cardiovascular risk factors such as body mass index, diabetes, blood pressure, and smoking status.

3.1.3. Inflammation, Galectin-3, and Fibrosis

Inflammation is also referred to as a unifying mechanism of injury because—through a cornerstone signaling link with interstitial fibrosis and tubular atrophy—it may hold observations that connect hazards of several natures with structural damage and detrimental function of the kidney [12–15,132,133]. Of note, the concept that chronic rejection is responsible for all progressive long-term kidney graft failure has long ago been reformulated to a hypothesis of cumulative damage [12–15]. Thus, repeated insults of both immune and non-immune nature damage the graft by leading to interstitial fibrosis and tubular atrophy, which represents a final common pathway of injury with adverse functional consequences [13]. Galectin-3 is a β-galactoside-binding lectin with a postulated key mediating role on kidney tissue fibrosis [134–138]. In different models, it has been shown that whether a variety of insults incur on irreversible kidney fibrosis or not depends on the expression and secretion of galectin-3 [135–138]. In the general population, moreover, an increasing body of prospective evidence has related plasma galectin-3 with incident CKD [139–141]. Because galectin-3 is both a biomarker of systemic inflammation and kidney fibrosis, it may broaden our understanding and provide data to further support a unifying link between repeated inflammatory and pro-oxidant insults and increased risk of graft failure beyond the first-year post-kidney transplantation. Finally, it should be realized that the dependent role of galectin-3 on kidney fibrosis has been specifically shown in the particular post-kidney transplant setting in a murine model [138]. Within the clinical kidney transplantation field, however, a number of crucial questions remain unanswered. Especially with galectin-3, targeted pharmacological therapies are increasingly becoming available, and evidence of a hypothetical association between galectin-3 levels and risk of long-term graft survival may point towards novel interventional avenues to potentially decrease the long-standing burden of late graft failure.

3.2. Bone Disease and Vascular Calcification

Chronic kidney disease-mineral and bone disorders (CKD-MBD) is the clinical entity or syndrome that KDIGO (Kidney Disease: Improving Global Outcomes) more than a decade ago has coined to embody the disruption of the complex systems biology enclosed by the kidney, skeleton, and cardiovascular system [142]. In line with previous evidence, the results of a recent elegant study by Yilmaz et al. support the hypothesis that decline in cardiovascular risk post-kidney transplantation depends on partial resolution of inflammation but also on resolution of the CKD-MBD [143,144]. The findings of the aforementioned research group support the notion that beyond restoration of organ function post-kidney transplant, amelioration of inflammation and correction of CKD-MBD may attenuate excess cardiovascular disease through separate biological pathways. In agreement, Cozzolino et al. recently depicted inflammation and oxidative stress, on one hand, and CKD-MBD, on the other hand, as major mechanisms underlying a feedback loop that exacerbates cardiovascular disease in CKD patients (Figure 4) [145].

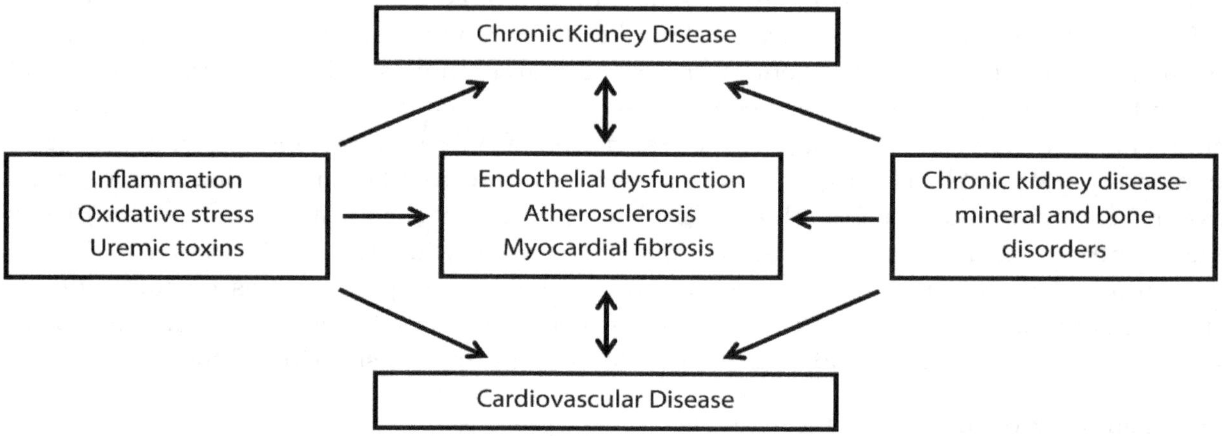

Figure 4. Cardiovascular disease in chronic kidney disease. This figure shows inflammation, oxidative stress, and uremic toxins on one side and chronic kidney disease-mineral and bone disorders on the other side of independent mechanisms linking chronic kidney and cardiovascular disease. Adapted from: "Cardiovascular disease in dialysis patients" by M. Cozzolino et al., 2019, Nephrol Dial Transplant, 33: iii28–34 [145].

Within the context of CKD-MBD, vascular calcification—a currently established cardiovascular risk factor in KTR, as shown by previous studies of our group and others [146–151]—is linked with bone disease through inter-related pathophysiological mechanisms that comprise the bone-vascular axis hypothesis, which contributes to the exceedingly high cardiovascular risk in native CKD [152–156]. Post-kidney transplant bone disease is certainly a topic of epidemiological relevance due to its high prevalence and its association with fragility fractures and reduced mobility [157–162]. Previous studies remarked that existing research had failed to explore a hypothetical contributing role of post-kidney transplant bone disease to increased risk of vascular calcification in KTR [154,158,163]. Recent evidence, however, has come to support the existence of a bone-vascular axis post-kidney transplantation, providing data to evaluate its epidemiological relevance post-kidney transplant and pointing towards an otherwise overlooked therapeutic opportunity to at least partially decrease the markedly high cardiovascular burden post-kidney transplant [164].

It has also been proposed that mediators of inflammation (e.g., interleukin 6 and tumor necrosis factor) contribute to fibroblast growth factor (FGF)-23 elevation and that, in turn, FGF-23 increases cytokine production, thus linking systemic inflammation with dysregulated phosphate metabolism in a vicious cycle [165,166]. It has been proposed that inflammatory mediators function as drug targets to decrease the burden of FGF23-associated injury in various tissues, thus offering a novel therapeutic opportunity to decrease the burden of cardiovascular diseases including vascular calcification in kidney disease patients [165,167]. Nevertheless, even in CKD patients within normal range of serum phosphate levels, vascular calcification is often observed. Calciprotein particles are calcium-phosphate nanoparticles that increase with CKD progression, which have been associated with inflammatory responses, endothelial damage, vascular stiffness, and calcification [168]. Calciprotein particles may play a pathophysiological role in the link between chronic inflammation and vascular calcification. Further research is warranted to evaluate its contribution to overall cardiovascular burden in KTR and to develop novel pharmacological strategies targeting calciprotein particles to encourage protection against the risk of vascular calcification post-kidney transplantation [169].

3.3. Immunosuppressive Therapy and Traditional Risk Factors of Vascular Calcification

The contribution of several traditional risk factors of vascular calcification may be particularly relevant in the post-kidney transplantation setting due to the effect of maintenance immunosuppressive therapy on diabetes, dyslipidemia, and vitamin D metabolism [170]. Previous studies have shown that low vitamin D along with low vitamin K may synergistically associate with higher risk of hypertension [171] and thereby contribute to higher risk of vascular calcification [172]. In KTR, particularly, we have recently shown that combined vitamin D and K deficiency is highly prevalent and is associated with increased mortality and graft failure [173]. Further research is needed to investigate both the direct and indirect role of immunosuppressive drugs in the progression of vascular calcification. There may, however, be opposing effects, because it has been described that steroids and calcineurin inhibitors inhibit inducible nitric oxide and may thereby lead to progression of vascular calcification through endothelial dysfunction [170], while mycophenolate mofetil inhibits vascular smooth muscle cell proliferation and may be protective against vascular calcification [174,175]. Similarly, we recently reported that use of cyclosporine rather than tacrolimus correlated with prevalence of osteopenia, while osteopenia was associated with higher risk of vascular calcification after kidney transplantation [164]. Future studies are warranted to assess the association between immunosuppressive agents and risk of vascular calcification, which may provide new cardiovascular risk management opportunities post-kidney transplantation.

4. Conclusions

Further research on lifestyle-related factors including diet and exposure to toxic contaminants, as well as persisting mechanisms of disease post-kidney transplantation (i.e., inflammation and redox imbalance and vascular calcification) is needed as it may bring about powerful opportunities to improve long-term outcomes post-kidney transplantation. Reflection on these current research opportunities is warranted among the research and clinical kidney transplantation community. Forthcoming analyses of the data to be generated by the long-lasting Transplant Lines Prospective Cohort Study and Biobank of Solid Organ Transplant Recipients [176] may shed light on these questions.

Author Contributions: Conceptualization, C.G.S. and S.J.L.B.; methodology, C.G.S., M.H.d.B., G.J.N., and S.J.L.B.; investigation, C.G.S. and S.J.L.B.; resources, C.G.S., M.H.d.B., and S.J.L.B.; writing—original draft preparation, C.G.S.; writing—review and editing, C.G.S., M.H.d.B., C.A.t.V.-K., G.J.N., and S.J.L.B.; supervision, M.H.d.B., G.J.N., and S.J.L.B.; project administration, C.G.S. and S.J.L.B.; funding acquisition, C.G.S. and S.J.L.B. All authors have read and agreed to the published version of the manuscript.

Disclaimer: The data reported in Figure 1 have been supplied by the United States Renal Data System. The interpretation and reporting of these data are the responsibility of the author(s) of this manuscript and in no way should be seen as an official policy or interpretation of the U.S. government.

References

1. Jager, K.J.; Kovesdy, C.; Langham, R.; Rosenberg, M.; Jha, V.; Zoccali, C. A single number for advocacy and communication-worldwide more than 850 million individuals have kidney diseases. *Nephrol. Dial. Transpl.* **2019**, *34*, 1803–1805. [CrossRef] [PubMed]
2. Hill, N.R.; Fatoba, S.T.; Oke, J.L.; Hirst, J.A.; O'callaghan, C.A.; Lasserson, D.S.; Hobbs, F.D.R. Global Prevalence of Chronic Kidney Disease-A Systematic Review and Meta-Analysis. *PLoS ONE* **2016**, *11*, e0158765. [CrossRef] [PubMed]
3. Eriksen, B.O.; Ingebretsen, O.C. The progression of chronic kidney disease: A 10-year population-based study of the effects of gender and age. *Kidney Int.* **2006**, *69*, 375–382. [CrossRef] [PubMed]
4. United States Renal Data System. *USRDS 2018 Annual Data Report: Atlas of Chronic Kidney Disease and End-Stage Renal Disease in the United States*; Bethesda, M., Ed.; National Institutes of Health; National Institute of Diabetes and Digestive and Kidney Diseases: Bethesda, MD, USA, 2018. Available online: https://www.usrds.org/Default.aspx (accessed on 8 September 2019).
5. Cusumano, A.M.; Rosa-Diez, G.J.; Gonzalez-Bedat, M.C. Latin American Dialysis and Transplant Registry: Experience and contributions to end-stage renal disease epidemiology. *World J. Nephrol.* **2016**, *5*, 389. [CrossRef] [PubMed]
6. Mohnen, S.M.; Van Oosten, M.J.M.; Los, J.; Leegte, M.J.H.; Jager, K.J.; Hemmelder, M.H.; Logtenberg, S.J.J.; Stel, V.S.; Hakkaart-Van Roijen, L.; De Wit, G.A. Healthcare costs of patients on different renal replacement modalities – Analysis of Dutch health insurance claims data. *PLoS ONE* **2019**, *14*, e0220800. [CrossRef]
7. Suthanthiran, M.; Strom, T.B. Renal Transplantation. *N. Engl. J. Med.* **1994**, *331*, 365–376. [CrossRef]
8. Wolfe, R.A.; Ashby, V.B.; Milford, E.L.; Ojo, A.O.; Ettenger, R.E.; Agodoa, L.Y.C.; Held, P.J.; Port, F.K. Comparison of Mortality in All Patients on Dialysis, Patients on Dialysis Awaiting Transplantation, and Recipients of a First Cadaveric Transplant. *N. Engl. J. Med.* **1999**, *341*, 1725–1730. [CrossRef]
9. Oniscu, G.C.; Brown, H.; Forsythe, J.L.R. Impact of Cadaveric Renal Transplantation on Survival in Patients Listed for Transplantation. *J. Am. Soc. Nephrol.* **2005**, *16*, 1859–1865. [CrossRef] [PubMed]
10. Tonelli, M.; Wiebe, N.; Knoll, G.; Bello, A.; Browne, S.; Jadhav, D.; Klarenbach, S.; Gill, J. Systematic Review: Kidney Transplantation Compared With Dialysis in Clinically Relevant Outcomes. *Am. J. Transpl.* **2011**, *11*, 2093–2109. [CrossRef]
11. Lamb, K.E.; Lodhi, S.; Meier-Kriesche, H.U. Long-term renal allograft survival in the United States: A critical reappraisal. *Am. J. Transpl.* **2011**, *11*, 450–462. [CrossRef]
12. Nankivell, B.J.; Borrows, R.J.; Fung, C.L.-S.; O'Connell, P.J.; Allen, R.D.M.; Chapman, J.R. The natural history of chronic allograft nephropathy. *N. Engl. J. Med.* **2003**, *349*, 2326–2333. [CrossRef] [PubMed]
13. Nankivell, B.J.; Chapman, J.R. Chronic allograft nephropathy: Current concepts and future directions. *Transplantation* **2006**, *81*, 643–654. [CrossRef] [PubMed]
14. Nankivell, B.J.; Kuypers, D.R.J. Diagnosis and prevention of chronic kidney allograft loss. *Lancet* **2011**, *378*, 1428–1437. [CrossRef]
15. Nankivell, B.J.; Borrows, R.J.; Fung, C.L.-S.; O'Connell, P.J.; Allen, R.D.M.; Chapman, J.R. Natural history, risk factors, and impact of subclinical rejection in kidney transplantation. *Transplantation* **2004**, *78*, 242–249. [CrossRef]

16. Arend, S.M.; Mallat, M.J.K.; Westendorp, R.J.W.; Van Der Woude, F.J.; Van Es, L.A. Patient survival after renal transplantation; more than 25 years follow-up. *Nephrol. Dial. Transpl.* **1997**, *12*, 1672–1679.
17. Oterdoom, L.H.; de Vries, A.P.J.; van Ree, R.M.; Gansevoort, R.T.; van Son, W.J.; van der Heide, J.J.H.; Navis, G.; de Jong, P.E.; Gans, R.O.B.; Bakker, S.J.L. N-Terminal Pro-B-Type Natriuretic Peptide and Mortality in Renal Transplant Recipients Versus the General Population. *Transplantation* **2009**, *87*, 1562–1570. [CrossRef]
18. U.S. Renal Data System. *USRDS 2010 Annual Data Report: Atlas of Chronic Kidney Disease and End-Stage Renal Disease in the United States, National Institutes of Health*; National Institute of Diabetes and Digestive and Kidney Diseases: Bethesda, MD, USA, 2010.
19. Ojo, A.O.; Hanson, J.A.; Wolfe, R.A.; Leichtman, A.B.; Agodoa, L.Y.; Port, F.K. Long-term survival in renal transplant recipients with graft function. *Kidney Int.* **2000**, *57*, 307–313. [CrossRef]
20. Shirali, A.C.; Bia, M.J. Management of cardiovascular disease in renal transplant recipients. *Clin. J. Am. Soc. Nephrol.* **2008**, *3*, 491–504. [CrossRef]
21. Jardine, A.G.; Gaston, R.S.; Fellstrom, B.C.; Holdaas, H. Prevention of cardiovascular disease in adult recipients of kidney transplants. *Lancet* **2011**, *378*, 1419–1427. [CrossRef]
22. Fry, K.; Patwardhan, A.; Ryan, C.; Trevillian, P.; Chadban, S.; Westgarth, F.; Chan, M. Development of Evidence-Based Guidelines for the Nutritional Management of Adult Kidney Transplant Recipients. *J. Ren. Nutr.* **2009**, *19*, 101–104. [CrossRef]
23. Zelle, D.M.; Kok, T.; Dontje, M.L.; Danchell, E.I.; Navis, G.; van Son, W.J.; Bakker, S.J.L.; Corpeleijn, E. The role of diet and physical activity in post-transplant weight gain after renal transplantation. *Clin. Transpl.* **2013**, *27*, E484–E490. [CrossRef] [PubMed]
24. Nolte Fong, J.V.; Moore, L.W. Nutrition Trends in Kidney Transplant Recipients: The Importance of Dietary Monitoring and Need for Evidence-Based Recommendations. *Front. Med.* **2018**, *5*, 302. [CrossRef] [PubMed]
25. Klaassen, G.; Zelle, D.M.; Navis, G.J.; Dijkema, D.; Bemelman, F.J.; Bakker, S.J.L.; Corpeleijn, E. Lifestyle intervention to improve quality of life and prevent weight gain after renal transplantation: Design of the Active Care after Transplantation (ACT) randomized controlled trial. *BMC Nephrol.* **2017**, *18*, 296. [CrossRef] [PubMed]
26. Sabbatini, M.; Ferreri, L.; Pisani, A.; Capuano, I.; Morgillo, M.; Memoli, A.; Riccio, E.; Guida, B. Nutritional management in renal transplant recipients: A transplant team opportunity to improve graft survival. *Nutr. Metab. Cardiovasc. Dis.* **2019**, *29*, 319–324. [CrossRef] [PubMed]
27. Monier-Faugere, M.-C.; Mawad, H.; Qi, Q.; Friedler, R.M.; Malluche, H.H. High Prevalence of Low Bone Turnover and Occurrence of Osteomalacia after Kidney Transplantation. *J. Am. Soc. Nephrol.* **2000**, *11*, 1093–1099. [PubMed]
28. Sprague, S.M.; Belozeroff, V.; Danese, M.D.; Martin, L.P.; Olgaard, K. Abnormal bone and mineral metabolism in kidney transplant patients—A review. *Am. J. Nephrol.* **2008**, *28*, 246–253. [CrossRef]
29. Evenepoel, P.; Lerut, E.; Naesens, M.; Bammens, B.; Claes, K.; Kuypers, D.; Vermeersch, P.; Meijers, B.; Van Damme, B.; Vanrenterghem, Y. Localization, etiology and impact of calcium phosphate deposits in renal allografts. *Am. J. Transpl.* **2009**, *9*, 2470–2478. [CrossRef]
30. Kalantar-Zadeh, K.; Molnar, M.Z.; Kovesdy, C.P.; Mucsi, I.; Bunnapradist, S. Management of mineral and bone disorder after kidney transplantation. *Curr. Opin. Nephrol. Hypertens.* **2012**, *21*, 389–403. [CrossRef]
31. Lou, I.; Foley, D.; Odorico, S.K.; Leverson, G.; Schneider, D.F.; Sippel, R.; Chen, H. How Well Does Renal Transplantation Cure Hyperparathyroidism? *Ann. Surg.* **2015**, *262*, 653–659. [CrossRef]
32. Wolf, M.; Weir, M.R.; Kopyt, N.; Mannon, R.B.; Von Visger, J.; Deng, H.; Yue, S.; Vincenti, F. A Prospective Cohort Study of Mineral Metabolism After Kidney Transplantation. *Transplantation* **2016**, *100*, 184–193. [CrossRef]
33. Willett, W. Diet and health: What should we eat? *Science* **1994**, *264*, 532–537. [CrossRef] [PubMed]
34. Stampfer, M.J.; Hu, F.B.; Manson, J.E.; Rimm, E.B.; Willett, W.C. Primary Prevention of Coronary Heart Disease in Women through Diet and Lifestyle. *N. Engl. J. Med.* **2000**, *343*, 16–22. [CrossRef] [PubMed]
35. Hu, F.B.; Manson, J.E.; Stampfer, M.J.; Colditz, G.; Liu, S.; Solomon, C.G.; Willett, W.C. Diet, lifestyle, and the risk of type 2 diabetes mellitus in women. *N. Engl. J. Med.* **2001**, *345*, 790–797. [CrossRef]
36. Chiuve, S.E.; McCullough, M.L.; Sacks, F.M.; Rimm, E.B. Healthy Lifestyle Factors in the Primary Prevention of Coronary Heart Disease Among Men. *Circulation* **2006**, *114*, 160–167. [CrossRef]
37. Chiuve, S.E.; Rexrode, K.M.; Spiegelman, D.; Logroscino, G.; Manson, J.E.; Rimm, E.B. Primary prevention of stroke by healthy lifestyle. *Circulation* **2008**, *118*, 947–954. [CrossRef] [PubMed]

38. Chiuve, S.E.; Fung, T.T.; Rexrode, K.M.; Spiegelman, D.; Manson, J.E.; Stampfer, M.J.; Albert, C.M. Adherence to a low-risk, healthy lifestyle and risk of sudden cardiac death among women. *JAMA* **2011**, *306*, 62–69. [CrossRef]

39. Kalantar-Zadeh, K.; Fouque, D. Nutritional Management of Chronic Kidney Disease. *N. Engl. J. Med.* **2017**, *377*, 1765–1776. [CrossRef]

40. Kelly, J.T.; Palmer, S.C.; Wai, S.N.; Ruospo, M.; Carrero, J.-J.; Campbell, K.L.; Strippoli, G.F.M. Healthy Dietary Patterns and Risk of Mortality and ESRD in CKD: A Meta-Analysis of Cohort Studies. *Clin. J. Am. Soc. Nephrol.* **2017**, *12*, 272–279. [CrossRef]

41. Chauveau, P. Nutrition in chronic kidney disease: Nephrology dialysis transplantation notable advances in 2018. *Nephrol. Dial. Transpl.* **2019**, *34*, 893–896. [CrossRef]

42. Saglimbene, V.M.; Wong, G.; Ruospo, M.; Palmer, S.C.; Garcia-Larsen, V.; Natale, P.; Teixeira-Pinto, A.; Campbell, K.L.; Carrero, J.-J.; Stenvinkel, P.; et al. Article Fruit and Vegetable Intake and Mortality in Adults undergoing Maintenance Hemodialysis. *Clin. J. Am. Soc. Nephrol.* **2019**, *14*, 250–260. [CrossRef]

43. Levin, A.; Stevens, P.E.; Bilous, R.W.; Coresh, J.; De Francisco, A.L.M.; De Jong, P.E.; Griffith, K.E.; Hemmelgarn, B.R.; Iseki, K.; Lamb, E.J.; et al. Notice. *Kidney Int. Suppl.* **2013**, *3*, 1. [CrossRef]

44. Palmer, S.C.; Hanson, C.S.; Craig, J.C.; Strippoli, G.F.M.; Ruospo, M.; Campbell, K.; Johnson, D.W.; Tong, A. Dietary and fluid restrictions in CKD: A thematic synthesis of patient views from qualitative studies. *Am. J. Kidney Dis.* **2015**, *65*, 559–573. [CrossRef] [PubMed]

45. Mcmahon, E.J.; Campbell, K.L.; Bauer, J.D.; Mudge, D.W. Altered dietary salt intake for people with chronic kidney disease. *Cochrane Database Syst. Rev.* **2015**, *18*, CD010070. [CrossRef]

46. Liu, Z.; Su, G.; Guo, X.; Wu, Y.; Liu, X.; Zou, C.; Zhang, L.; Yang, Q.; Xu, Y.; Ma, W. Dietary interventions for mineral and bone disorder in people with chronic kidney disease. *Cochrane Database Syst. Rev.* **2015**, *16*, CD010350. [CrossRef] [PubMed]

47. Gordon, E.J.; Prohaska, T.R.; Gallant, M.; Siminoff, L.A. Self-care strategies and barriers among kidney transplant recipients: A qualitative study. *Chronic Illn.* **2009**, *5*, 75–91. [CrossRef]

48. Stanfill, A.; Bloodworth, R.; Cashion, A. Lessons learned: Experiences of gaining weight by kidney transplant recipients. *Prog. Transpl.* **2012**, *22*, 71–78. [CrossRef]

49. Piepoli, M.F.; Hoes, A.W.; Agewall, S.; Albus, C.; Brotons, C.; Catapano, A.L.; Cooney, M.-T.; Corrà, U.; Cosyns, B.; Deaton, C.; et al. European Guidelines on cardiovascular disease prevention in clinical practice. *Eur. Heart J.* **2016**, *37*, 2315–2381. [CrossRef]

50. Lloyd-Jones, D.M.; Hong, Y.; Labarthe, D.; Mozaffarian, D.; Appel, L.J.; Van Horn, L.; Greenlund, K.; Daniels, S.; Nichol, G.; Tomaselli, G.F.; et al. Defining and setting national goals for cardiovascular health promotion and disease reduction: The american heart association's strategic impact goal through 2020 and beyond. *Circulation* **2010**, *121*, 586–613. [CrossRef]

51. Crowe, F.L.; Roddam, A.W.; Key, T.J.; Appleby, P.N.; Overvad, K.; Jakobsen, M.U.; Tjonneland, A.; Hansen, L.; Boeing, H.; Weikert, C.; et al. Fruit and vegetable intake and mortality from ischaemic heart disease: Results from the European Prospective Investigation into Cancer and Nutrition (EPIC)-Heart study. *Eur. Heart J.* **2011**, *32*, 1235–1243. [CrossRef]

52. Lim, S.S.; Vos, T.; Flaxman, A.D.; Danaei, G.; Shibuya, K.; Adair-Rohani, H.; AlMazroa, M.A.; Amann, M.; Anderson, H.R.; Andrews, K.G.; et al. A comparative risk assessment of burden of disease and injury attributable to 67 risk factors and risk factor clusters in 21 regions, 1990–2010: A systematic analysis for the Global Burden of Disease Study 2010. *Lancet* **2012**, *380*, 2224–2260. [CrossRef]

53. Larsson, S.C.; Virtamo, J.; Wolk, A. Total and specific fruit and vegetable consumption and risk of stroke: A prospective study. *Atherosclerosis* **2013**, *227*, 147–152. [CrossRef] [PubMed]

54. Zhang, X.; Shu, X.-O.; Xiang, Y.-B.; Yang, G.; Li, H.; Gao, J.; Cai, H.; Gao, Y.-T.; Zheng, W. Cruciferous vegetable consumption is associated with a reduced risk of total and cardiovascular disease mortality. *Am. J. Clin. Nutr.* **2011**, *94*, 240–246. [CrossRef] [PubMed]

55. Cases, A.; Cigarrán-Guldrís, S.; Mas, S.; Gonzalez-Parra, E. Vegetable-Based Diets for Chronic Kidney Disease? It Is Time to Reconsider. *Nutrients* **2019**, *11*, 1263. [CrossRef] [PubMed]

56. Forouzanfar, M.H.; Alexander, L.; Anderson, H.R.; Bachman, V.F.; Biryukov, S.; Brauer, M.; Burnett, R.; Casey, D.; Coates, M.M.; Cohen, A.; et al. Global, regional, and national comparative risk assessment of 79 behavioural, environmental and occupational, and metabolic risks or clusters of risks in 188 countries, 1990–2013: A systematic analysis for the Global Burden of Disease Study 2013. *Lancet* **2015**, *386*, 2287–2323. [CrossRef]
57. Sotomayor, C.G.; Gomes-Neto, A.W.; Eisenga, M.F.; Nolte, I.M.; Anderson, J.L.; de Borst, M.H.; Osté, M.C.; Rodrigo, R.; Gans, R.O.; Berger, S.P.; et al. Consumption of fruits and vegetables and cardiovascular mortality in renal transplant recipients: A prospective cohort study. *Nephrol. Dial. Transpl.* **2020**, *35*, 357–365. [CrossRef] [PubMed]
58. Gomes-Neto, A.W.; Osté, M.C.; Sotomayor, C.; Berg, E.V.D.; Geleijnse, J.M.; Gans, R.O.; Navis, G.J.; Bakker, S.J. Fruit and Vegetable Intake and Risk of Posttransplantation Diabetes in Renal Transplant Recipients. *Diabetes Care* **2019**, *42*, 1644–1652. [CrossRef]
59. Mozaffarian, D.; Gottdiener, J.S.; Siscovick, D.S. Intake of tuna or other broiled or baked fish versus fried fish and cardiac structure, function, and hemodynamics. *Am. J. Cardiol.* **2006**, *97*, 216–222. [CrossRef]
60. Chin, J.P.; Gust, A.P.; Nestel, P.J.; Dart, A.M. Marine oils dose-dependently inhibit vasoconstriction of forearm resistance vessels in humans. *Hypertension* **1993**, *21*, 22–28. [CrossRef]
61. Nestel, P.J. Fish oil and cardiovascular disease: Lipids and arterial function. *Am. J. Clin. Nutr.* **2000**, *71*, 228S–231S. [CrossRef]
62. Kristensen, S.D.; Bach Iversen, A.M.; Schmidt, E.B. n−3 polyunsaturated fatty acids and coronary thrombosis. *Lipids* **2001**, *36*, S79–S82. [CrossRef]
63. Bar-Or, A.; Bashinskaya, V.V.; Kulakova, O.G.; Boyko, A.N.; Favorov, A.V.; Favorova, O.O.; Medicina, F.D.E.; Bos, S.D.; Berge, T.; Celius, E.G.; et al. The genetics of multiple sclerosis: SNPs to pathways to pathogenesis. *PLoS ONE* **2012**, *7*, 457. [CrossRef]
64. Christensen, J.H. Omega-3 polyunsaturated Fatty acids and heart rate variability. *Front. Med.* **2011**, *2*, 84. [CrossRef] [PubMed]
65. Masson, S.; Marchioli, R.; Mozaffarian, D.; Bernasconi, R.; Milani, V.; Dragani, L.; Tacconi, M.; Marfisi, R.M.; Borgese, L.; Cirrincione, V.; et al. Plasma n-3 polyunsaturated fatty acids in chronic heart failure in the GISSI-heart failure trial: Relation with fish intake, circulating biomarkers, and mortality. *Am. Heart J.* **2013**, *165*, 208–215. [CrossRef] [PubMed]
66. Calder, P.C. Omega-3 fatty acids and inflammatory processes. *Nutrients* **2010**, *2*, 355–374. [CrossRef] [PubMed]
67. Eide, I.A.; Jenssen, T.; Hartmann, A.; Diep, L.M.; Dahle, D.O.; Reisæter, A.V.; Bjerve, K.S.; Christensen, J.H.; Schmidt, E.B.; Svensson, M. The association between marine n-3 polyunsaturated fatty acid levels and survival after renal transplantation. *Clin. J. Am. Soc. Nephrol.* **2015**, *10*, 1246–1256. [CrossRef] [PubMed]
68. Gomes-Neto, A.W.; Sotomayor, C.G.; Pranger, I.; van den Berg, E.; Gans, R.O.; Soedamah-Muthu, S.; Navis, G.J.; Bakker, S.J. Intake of Marine-Derived Omega-3 Polyunsaturated Fatty Acids and Mortality in Renal Transplant Recipients. *Nutrients* **2017**, *9*, 363. [CrossRef]
69. Tatsioni, A.; Chung, M.; Sun, Y.; Kupelnick, B.; Lichtenstein, A.H.; Perrone, R.; Chew, P.; Lau, J.; Bonis, P.A. Effects of fish oil supplementation on kidney transplantation: A systematic review and meta-analysis of randomized, controlled trials. *J. Am. Soc. Nephrol.* **2005**, *16*, 2462–2670. [CrossRef]
70. Lim, A.K.; Manley, K.J.; Roberts, M.A.; Fraenkel, M.B. Fish oil for kidney transplant recipients. *Cochrane Database Syst. Rev.* **2016**, *8*, CD005282. [CrossRef]
71. Kromhout, D.; Feskens, E.J.; Bowles, C.H. The protective effect of a small amount of fish on coronary heart disease mortality in an elderly population. *Int. J. Epidemiol.* **1995**, *24*, 340–345. [CrossRef]
72. Stone, N.J. Fish consumption, fish oil, lipids, and coronary heart disease. *Circulation* **1996**, *94*, 2337–2340. [CrossRef]
73. Krauss, R.M.; Eckel, R.H.; Howard, B.; Appel, L.J.; Daniels, S.R.; Deckelbaum, R.J.; Erdman, J.W.; Kris-Etherton, P.; Goldberg, I.J.; Kotchen, T.A.; et al. AHA Dietary Guidelines: revision 2000: A statement for healthcare professionals from the Nutrition Committee of the American Heart Association. *Circulation* **2000**, *102*, 2284–2299. [CrossRef] [PubMed]
74. Psota, T.L.; Gebauer, S.K.; Kris-Etherton, P. Dietary Omega-3 Fatty Acid Intake and Cardiovascular Risk. *Am. J. Cardiol.* **2006**, *98*, 3–18. [CrossRef] [PubMed]

75. Wang, C.; Harris, W.S.; Chung, M.; Lichtenstein, A.H.; Balk, E.M.; Kupelnick, B.; Jordan, H.S.; Lau, J. n-3 Fatty acids from fish or fish-oil supplements, but not α-linolenic acid, benefit cardiovascular disease outcomes in primary- and secondary-prevention studies: A systematic review. *Am. J. Clin. Nutr.* **2006**, *84*, 5–17. [CrossRef] [PubMed]
76. World Health Organization. *Preventing Disease through Healthy Environment—Exposure to Mercury: A Major Public Health Concern*; WHO: Geneva, Switzerland, 2010.
77. Hightower, J.M.; Moore, D. Mercury levels in high-end consumers of fish. *Environ. Health Perspect.* **2003**, *111*, 604–608. [CrossRef] [PubMed]
78. Joshi, A.; Douglass, C.W.; Kim, H.D.; Joshipura, K.J.; Park, M.C.; Rimm, E.B.; Carino, M.J.; Garcia, R.I.; Morris, J.S.; Willett, W.C. The relationship between amalgam restorations and mercury levels in male dentists and nondental health professionals. *J. Public Health Dent.* **2003**, *63*, 52–60. [CrossRef]
79. Sotomayor, C.G.; Gomes-Neto, A.W.; Gans, R.O.; de Borst, M.; Berger, S.P.; Rodrigo, R.; Navis, G.J.; Touw, D.J.; Bakker, S.J.; Sotomayor, C.G.; et al. Fish Intake, Circulating Mercury and Mortality in Renal Transplant Recipients. *Nutrients* **2018**, *10*, 1419. [CrossRef]
80. Schroeder, J.C.; DiNatale, B.C.; Murray, I.A.; Flaveny, C.A.; Liu, Q.; Laurenzana, E.M.; Lin, J.M.; Strom, S.C.; Omiecinski, C.J.; Amin, S.; et al. The uremic toxin 3-indoxyl sulfate is a potent endogenous agonist for the human aryl hydrocarbon receptor. *Biochemistry* **2010**, *49*, 393–400. [CrossRef]
81. Tellez-Plaza, M.; Navas-Acien, A.; Crainiceanu, C.M.; Guallar, E. Cadmium exposure and hypertension in the 1999–2004 National Health and Nutrition Examination Survey (NHANES). *Environ. Health Perspect.* **2008**, *116*, 51–56. [CrossRef]
82. Mange, K.C.; Cizman, B.; Joffe, M.; Feldman, H.I. Arterial hypertension and renal allograft survival. *JAMA* **2000**, *283*, 633–638. [CrossRef]
83. Mange, K.C.; Feldman, H.I.; Joffe, M.M.; Fa, K.; Bloom, R.D. Blood Pressure and the Survival of Renal Allografts from Living Donors. *J. Am. Soc. Nephrol.* **2004**, *15*, 187–193. [CrossRef]
84. Weir, M.R.; Burgess, E.D.; Cooper, J.E.; Fenves, A.Z.; Goldsmith, D.; McKay, D.; Mehrotra, A.; Mitsnefes, M.M.; Sica, D.A.; Taler, S.J. Assessment and management of hypertension in transplant patients. *J. Am. Soc. Nephrol.* **2015**, *26*, 1248–1260. [CrossRef] [PubMed]
85. Akesson, A.; Lundh, T.; Vahter, M.; Bjellerup, P.; Lidfeldt, J.; Nerbrand, C.; Samsioe, G.; Strömberg, U.; Skerfving, S. Tubular and glomerular kidney effects in Swedish women with low environmental cadmium exposure. *Environ. Health Perspect.* **2005**, *113*, 1627–1631. [CrossRef] [PubMed]
86. Buser, M.C.; Ingber, S.Z.; Raines, N.; Fowler, D.A.; Scinicariello, F. Urinary and blood cadmium and lead and kidney function: NHANES 2007–2012. *Int. J. Hyg. Environ. Health* **2016**, *219*, 261–267. [CrossRef] [PubMed]
87. Huang, M.; Choi, S.J.; Kim, D.W.; Kim, N.Y.; Park, C.H.; Do Yu, S.; Kim, D.S.; Park, K.S.; Song, J.S.; Kim, H.; et al. Risk assessment of low-level cadmium and arsenic on the kidney. *J. Toxicol. Environ. Health A* **2009**, *72*, 1493–1498. [CrossRef] [PubMed]
88. Geeth Gunawardana, C.; Martinez, R.E.; Xiao, W.; Templeton, D.M.; Geeth, C. Cadmium inhibits both intrinsic and extrinsic apoptotic pathways in renal mesangial cells. *Am. J. Physiol. Ren. Physiol.* **2006**, *290*, 1074–1082. [CrossRef] [PubMed]
89. Prozialeck, W.C.; Edwards, J.R. Mechanisms of cadmium-induced proximal tubule injury: New insights with implications for biomonitoring and therapeutic interventions. *J. Pharm. Exp.* **2012**, *343*, 2–12. [CrossRef]
90. Shaikh, Z.A.; Vu, T.T.; Zaman, K. Oxidative stress as a mechanism of chronic cadmium-induced hepatotoxicity and renal toxicity and protection by antioxidants. *Toxicol. Appl. Pharm.* **1999**, *154*, 256–263. [CrossRef]
91. Johri, N.; Jacquillet, G.; Unwin, R. Heavy metal poisoning: The effects of cadmium on the kidney. *BioMetals* **2010**, *23*, 783–792. [CrossRef]
92. Liu, J.; Qu, W.; Kadiiska, M.B. Role of oxidative stress in cadmium toxicity and carcinogenesis. *Toxicol. Appl. Pharm.* **2009**, *238*, 209–214. [CrossRef]
93. Andersen, O. Chelation of cadmium. *Environ. Health Perspect.* **1984**, *54*, 249–266. [CrossRef]
94. Kasiske, B.L.; Guijarro, C.; Massy, Z.A.; Wiederkehr, M.R.; Ma, J.Z. Cardiovascular disease after renal transplantation. *J. Am. Coll. Cardiol.* **1996**, *7*, 158–165.
95. Kasiske, B.L.; Vazquez, M.A.; Harmon, W.E.; Brown, R.S.; Danovitch, G.M.; Gaston, R.S.; Roth, D.; Scandling, J.D.; Singer, G.G.; The American Society of Transplantation. Recommendations for the outpatient surveillance of renal transplant recipients. American Society of Transplantation. *J. Am. Soc. Nephrol.* **2000**, *11*, S1–S86. [PubMed]

96. Ducloux, D.; Kazory, A.; Chalopin, J.M. Predicting coronary heart disease in renal transplant recipients: A prospective study. *Kidney Int.* **2004**, *66*, 441–447. [CrossRef] [PubMed]
97. Kiberd, B.; Panek, R. Cardiovascular outcomes in the outpatient kidney transplant clinic: The Framingham risk score revisited. *Clin. J. Am. Soc. Nephrol.* **2008**, *3*, 822–828. [CrossRef]
98. Winkelmayer, W.C.; Lorenz, M.; Kramar, R.; Födinger, M.; Hörl, W.H.; Sunder-Plassmann, G. C-reactive protein and body mass index independently predict mortality in kidney transplant recipients. *Am. J. Transpl.* **2004**, *4*, 1148–1154. [CrossRef]
99. Hartog, J.W.L. Risk factors for chronic transplant dysfunction and cardiovascular disease are related to accumulation of advanced glycation end-products in renal transplant recipients. *Nephrol. Dial. Transpl.* **2006**, *21*, 2263–2269. [CrossRef]
100. Abedini, S.; Holme, I.; März, W.; Weihrauch, G.; Fellström, B.; Jardine, A.; Cole, E.; Maes, B.; Neumayer, H.H.; Grønhagen-Riska, C.; et al. Inflammation in renal transplantation. *Clin. J. Am. Soc. Nephrol.* **2009**, *4*, 1246–1254. [CrossRef]
101. Turkmen, K.; Tonbul, H.Z.; Toker, A.; Gaipov, A.; Erdur, F.M.; Cicekler, H.; Anil, M.; Ozbek, O.; Selcuk, N.Y.; Yeksan, M.; et al. The relationship between oxidative stress, inflammation, and atherosclerosis in renal transplant and end-stage renal disease patients. *Ren. Fail.* **2012**, *34*, 1229–1237. [CrossRef]
102. Ocak, N.; Dirican, M.; Ersoy, A.; Sarandol, E. Adiponectin, leptin, nitric oxide, and C-reactive protein levels in kidney transplant recipients: Comparison with the hemodialysis and chronic renal failure. *Ren. Fail.* **2016**, *38*, 1639–1646. [CrossRef]
103. van Gennip, A.C.E.; Broers, N.J.H.; ter Meulen, K.J.; Canaud, B.; Christiaans, M.H.L.; Cornelis, T.; Gelens, M.A.C.J.; Hermans, M.M.H.; Konings, C.J.A.M.; van der Net, J.B.; et al. Endothelial dysfunction and low-grade inflammation in the transition to renal replacement therapy. *PLoS ONE* **2019**, *14*, e0222547. [CrossRef]
104. Mazzaferro, S.; Pasquali, M.; Taggi, F.; Baldinelli, M.; Conte, C.; Muci, M.L.; Pirozzi, N.; Carbone, I.; Francone, M.; Pugliese, F. Progression of coronary artery calcification in renal transplantation and the role of secondary hyperparathyroidism and inflammation. *Clin. J. Am. Soc. Nephrol.* **2009**, *4*, 685–690. [CrossRef] [PubMed]
105. Himmelfarb, J.; Stenvinkel, P.; Ikizler, T.A.; Hakim, R.M. The elephant in uremia: Oxidant stress as a unifying concept of cardiovascular disease in uremia. *Kidney Int.* **2002**, *62*, 1524–1538. [CrossRef] [PubMed]
106. Cachofeiro, V.; Goicochea, M.; de Vinuesa, S.G.; Oubiña, P.; Lahera, V.; Luño, J. Oxidative stress and inflammation, a link between chronic kidney disease and cardiovascular disease. *Kidney Int.* **2008**, *74*, S4–S9. [CrossRef] [PubMed]
107. Liu, J.; Tian, J.; Chaudhry, M.; Maxwell, K.; Yan, Y.; Wang, X.; Shah, P.T.; Khawaja, A.A.; Martin, R.; Robinette, T.J.; et al. Attenuation of Na/K-ATPase Mediated Oxidant Amplification with pNaKtide Ameliorates Experimental Uremic Cardiomyopathy. *Sci. Rep.* **2016**, *6*, 34592. [CrossRef]
108. Jerotic, D.; Matic, M.; Suvakov, S.; Vucicevic, K.; Damjanovic, T.; Savic-Radojevic, A.; Pljesa-Ercegovac, M.; Coric, V.; Stefanovic, A.; Ivanisevic, J.; et al. Association of Nrf2, SOD2 and GPX1 Polymorphisms with Biomarkers of Oxidative Distress and Survival in End-Stage Renal Disease Patients. *Toxins* **2019**, *11*, 431. [CrossRef]
109. La Russa, D.; Pellegrino, D.; Montesanto, A.; Gigliotti, P.; Perri, A.; La Russa, A.; Bonofiglio, R. Oxidative Balance and Inflammation in Hemodialysis Patients: Biomarkers of Cardiovascular Risk? *Oxid. Med. Cell Longev.* **2019**, *2019*, 1–7. [CrossRef]
110. Sies, H. (Ed.) *Oxidative Stress II: Oxidants and Antioxidants*; Academic Press: New York, NY, USA, 1991.
111. Langlois, M.; Duprez, D.; Delanghe, J.; De Buyzere, M.; Clement, D.L. Serum vitamin C concentration is low in peripheral arterial disease and is associated with inflammation and severity of atherosclerosis. *Circulation* **2001**, *103*, 1863–1868. [CrossRef]
112. Korantzopoulos, P.; Kolettis, T.M.; Kountouris, E.; Dimitroula, V.; Karanikis, P.; Pappa, E.; Siogas, K.; Goudevenos, J.A. Oral vitamin C administration reduces early recurrence rates after electrical cardioversion of persistent atrial fibrillation and attenuates associated inflammation. *Int. J. Cardiol.* **2005**, *102*, 321–326. [CrossRef]
113. Mikirova, N.; Casciari, J.; Rogers, A.; Taylor, P. Effect of high-dose intravenous vitamin C on inflammation in cancer patients. *J. Transl. Med.* **2012**, *10*. [CrossRef]

114. Mikirova, N.; Casciari, J.; Riordan, N.; Hunninghake, R. Clinical experience with intravenous administration of ascorbic acid: Achievable levels in blood for different states of inflammation and disease in cancer patients. *J. Transl. Med.* **2013**, *11*, 191. [CrossRef]
115. Frei, B.; England, L.; Ames, B.N. Ascorbate is an outstanding antioxidant in human blood plasma. *Proc. Natl. Acad. Sci. USA* **1989**, *86*, 6377–6381. [CrossRef] [PubMed]
116. Wang, S.; Eide, T.C.; Sogn, E.M.; Berg, K.J.; Sund, R.B. Plasma ascorbic acid in patients undergoing chronic haemodialysis. *Eur. J. Clin. Pharm.* **1999**, *55*, 527–532. [CrossRef]
117. Morena, M.; Cristol, J.P.; Bosc, J.Y.; Tetta, C.; Forret, G.; Leger, C.L.; Delcourt, C.; Papoz, L.; Descomps, B.; Canaud, B. Convective and diffusive losses of vitamin C during haemodiafiltration session: A contributive factor to oxidative stress in haemodialysis patients. *Nephrol. Dial. Transpl.* **2002**, *17*, 422–427. [CrossRef] [PubMed]
118. Sullivan, J.F.; Eisenstein, A.B. Ascorbic acid depletion during hemodialysis. *JAMA* **1972**, *220*, 1697–1699. [CrossRef] [PubMed]
119. Jacob, R.A. Assessment of Human Vitamin C Status. *J. Nutr.* **1990**, *120*, 1480–1485. [CrossRef]
120. Johnston, C.S.; Solomon, R.E.; Corte, C. Vitamin C depletion is associated with alterations in blood histamine and plasma free carnitine in adults. *J. Am. Coll. Nutr.* **1996**, *15*, 586–591. [CrossRef]
121. Zhang, K.; Li, Y.; Cheng, X.; Liu, L.; Bai, W.; Guo, W.; Wu, L.; Zuo, L. Cross-over study of influence of oral vitamin C supplementation on inflammatory status in maintenance hemodialysis patients. *BMC Nephrol.* **2013**, *14*, 252. [CrossRef]
122. Attallah, N.; Osman-Malik, Y.; Frinak, S.; Besarab, A. Effect of intravenous ascorbic acid in hemodialysis patients with EPO-hyporesponsive anemia and hyperferritinemia. *Am. J. Kidney Dis.* **2006**, *47*, 644–654. [CrossRef]
123. May, J.M.; Harrison, F.E. Role of vitamin C in the function of the vascular endothelium. *Antioxid. Redox Signal.* **2013**, *19*, 2068–2083. [CrossRef]
124. Sotomayor, C.G.; Eisenga, M.F.; Gomes Neto, A.W.; Ozyilmaz, A.; Gans, R.O.B.; de Jong, W.H.A.; Zelle, D.M.; Berger, S.P.; Gaillard, C.A.J.M.; Navis, G.J.; et al. Vitamin C Depletion and All-Cause Mortality in Renal Transplant Recipients. *Nutrients* **2017**, *9*, 568. [CrossRef]
125. Gacitúa, T.A.; Sotomayor, C.G.; Groothof, D.; Eisenga, M.F.; Pol, R.A.; de Borst, M.H.; Gans, R.O.B.; Berger, S.P.; Rodrigo, R.; Navis, G.J.; et al. Plasma Vitamin C and Cancer Mortality in Kidney Transplant Recipients. *J. Clin. Med.* **2019**, *8*, 2064. [CrossRef] [PubMed]
126. Schreck, R.; Rieber, P.; Baeuerle, P.A. Reactive oxygen intermediates as apparently widely used messengers in the activation of the NF-kappa B transcription factor and HIV-1. *EMBO J.* **1991**, *10*, 2247–2258. [CrossRef]
127. Yan, S.D.; Schmidt, A.M.; Anderson, G.M.; Zhang, J.; Brett, J.; Zou, Y.S.; Pinsky, D.; Stern, D. Enhanced cellular oxidant stress by the interaction of advanced glycation end products with their receptors/binding proteins. *J. Biol. Chem.* **1994**, *269*, 9889–9897. [PubMed]
128. Linden, E.; Cai, W.; He, J.C.; Xue, C.; Li, Z.; Winston, J.; Vlassara, H.; Uribarri, J. Endothelial dysfunction in patients with chronic kidney disease results from advanced glycation end products (AGE)-mediated inhibition of endothelial nitric oxide synthase through RAGE activation. *Clin. J. Am. Soc. Nephrol.* **2008**, *3*, 691–698. [CrossRef]
129. Stinghen, A.E.M.; Massy, Z.A.; Vlassara, H.; Striker, G.E.; Boullier, A. Uremic Toxicity of Advanced Glycation End Products in CKD. *J. Am. Soc. Nephrol.* **2016**, *27*, 354–370. [CrossRef] [PubMed]
130. Stam, F.; van Guldener, C.; Becker, A.; Dekker, J.M.; Heine, R.J.; Bouter, L.M.; Stehouwer, C. DA Endothelial Dysfunction Contributes to Renal Function-Associated Cardiovascular Mortality in a Population with Mild Renal Insufficiency: The Hoorn Study. *J. Am. Soc. Nephrol.* **2006**, *17*, 537–545. [CrossRef]
131. Calviño, J.; Cigarran, S.; Gonzalez-Tabares, L.; Menendez, N.; Latorre, J.; Cillero, S.; Millan, B.; Cobelo, C.; Sanjurjo-Amado, A.; Quispe, J.; et al. Advanced glycation end products (AGEs) estimated by skin autofluorescence are related with cardiovascular risk in renal transplant. *PLoS ONE* **2018**, *13*, e0201118. [CrossRef]
132. Choi, B.S.; Shin, M.J.; Shin, S.J.; Kim, Y.S.; Choi, Y.J.; Kim, Y.-S.; Moon, I.S.; Kim, S.Y.; Koh, Y.B.; Bang, B.K.; et al. Clinical significance of an early protocol biopsy in living-donor renal transplantation: Ten-year experience at a single center. *Am. J. Transpl.* **2005**, *5*, 1354–1360. [CrossRef]

133. Heilman, R.L.; Devarapalli, Y.; Chakkera, H.A.; Mekeel, K.L.; Moss, A.A.; Mulligan, D.C.; Mazur, M.J.; Hamawi, K.; Williams, J.W.; Reddy, K.S. Impact of Subclinical Inflammation on the Development of Interstitial Fibrosis and Tubular Atrophy in Kidney Transplant Recipients. *Am. J. Transpl.* **2010**, *10*, 563–570. [CrossRef]
134. Henderson, N.C.; Mackinnon, A.C.; Farnworth, S.L.; Kipari, T.; Haslett, C.; Iredale, J.P.; Liu, F.T.; Hughes, J.; Sethi, T. Galectin-3 expression and secretion links macrophages to the promotion of renal fibrosis. *Am. J. Pathol.* **2008**, *172*, 288–298. [CrossRef]
135. Kolatsi-Joannou, M.; Price, K.L.; Winyard, P.J.; Long, D.A. Modified citrus pectin reduces galectin-3 expression and disease severity in experimental acute kidney injury. *PLoS ONE* **2011**, *6*, 18683. [CrossRef]
136. Frenay, A.-R.S.; Yu, L.; van der Velde, A.R.; Vreeswijk-Baudoin, I.; López-Andrés, N.; van Goor, H.; Silljé, H.H.; Ruifrok, W.P.; de Boer, R.A. Pharmacological inhibition of galectin-3 protects against hypertensive nephropathy. *Am. J. Physiol. Ren. Physiol.* **2015**, *308*, F500–F509. [CrossRef]
137. Martinez-Martinez, E.; Ibarrola, J.; Calvier, L.; Fernandez-Celis, A.; Leroy, C.; Cachofeiro, V.; Rossignol, P.; Lopez-Andres, N. Galectin-3 blockade reduces renal fibrosis in two normotensive experimental models of renal damage. *PLoS ONE* **2016**, *11*, e0166272. [CrossRef]
138. Dang, Z.; Mackinnon, A.; Marson, L.P.; Sethi, T. Tubular Atrophy and Interstitial Fibrosis After Renal Transplantation Is Dependent on Galectin-3. *Transplantation* **2012**, *93*, 477–484. [CrossRef]
139. O'Seaghdha, C.; Hwang, S.; Ho, J.; Vasan, R.; Levy, D.; Fox, C. Elevated Galectin-3 Precedes the Development of CKD. *J. Am. Soc. Nephrol.* **2013**, *24*, 1470–1477. [CrossRef]
140. Rebholz, C.M.; Selvin, E.; Liang, M.; Ballantyne, C.M.; Hoogeveen, R.C.; Aguilar, D.; McEvoy, J.W.; Grams, M.E.; Coresh, J. Plasma galectin-3 levels are associated with the risk of incident chronic kidney disease. *Kidney Int.* **2018**, *93*, 252–259. [CrossRef]
141. Alam, M.L.; Katz, R.; Bellovich, K.A.; Bhat, Z.Y.; Brosius, F.C.; de Boer, I.H.; Gadegbeku, C.A.; Gipson, D.S.; Hawkins, J.J.; Himmelfarb, J.; et al. Soluble ST2 and Galectin-3 and Progression of CKD. *Kidney Int. Rep.* **2018**, *4*, 103–111. [CrossRef]
142. Moe, S.M.; Drüeke, T.; Lameire, N.; Eknoyan, G. Chronic Kidney Disease-Mineral-Bone Disorder: A New Paradigm. *Adv. Chronic. Kidney Dis.* **2007**, *14*, 3–12. [CrossRef]
143. Simmons, E.M.; Langone, A.; Sezer, M.T.; Vella, J.P.; Recupero, P.; Morrow, J.D.; Ikizler, T.A.; Himmelfarb, J. Effect of renal transplantation on biomarkers of inflammation and oxidative stress in end-stage renal disease patients. *Transplantation* **2005**, *79*, 914–919. [CrossRef]
144. Yilmaz, M.I.; Sonmez, A.; Saglam, M.; Cayci, T.; Kilic, S.; Unal, H.U.; Karaman, M.; Cetinkaya, H.; Eyileten, T.; Gok, M.; et al. A longitudinal study of inflammation, CKD-mineral bone disorder, and carotid atherosclerosis after renal transplantation. *Clin. J. Am. Soc. Nephrol.* **2015**, *10*, 471–479. [CrossRef]
145. Cozzolino, M.; Mangano, M.; Stucchi, A.; Ciceri, P.; Conte, F.; Galassi, A. Cardiovascular disease in dialysis patients. *Nephrol. Dial. Transpl.* **2018**, *33*, iii28–iii34. [CrossRef] [PubMed]
146. DeLoach, S.S.; Joffe, M.M.; Mai, X.; Goral, S.; Rosas, S.E. Aortic calcification predicts cardiovascular events and all-cause mortality in renal transplantation. *Nephrol. Dial. Transpl.* **2009**, *24*, 1314–1319. [CrossRef] [PubMed]
147. Nguyen, P.T.; Henrard, S.; Coche, E.; Goffin, E.; Devuyst, O.; Jadoul, M. Coronary artery calcification: A strong predictor of cardiovascular events in renal transplant recipients. *Nephrol. Dial. Transpl.* **2010**, *25*, 3773–3778. [CrossRef] [PubMed]
148. Roe, P.; Wolfe, M.; Joffe, M.; Rosas, S.E. Inflammation, coronary artery calcification and cardiovascular events in incident renal transplant recipients. *Atherosclerosis* **2010**, *212*, 589–594. [CrossRef]
149. Claes, K.J.; Heye, S.; Bammens, B.; Kuypers, D.R.; Meijers, B.; Naesens, M.; Vanrenterghem, Y.; Evenepoel, P. Aortic calcifications and arterial stiffness as predictors of cardiovascular events in incident renal transplant recipients. *Transpl. Int.* **2013**, *26*, 973–981. [CrossRef]
150. Davis, B.; Marin, D.; Hurwitz, L.M.; Ronald, J.; Ellis, M.J.; Ravindra, K.V.; Collins, B.H.; Kim, C.Y. Application of a Novel CT-Based Iliac Artery Calcification Scoring System for Predicting Renal Transplant Outcomes. *Am. J. Roent* **2016**, *206*, 436–441. [CrossRef]
151. Benjamens, S.; Pol, R.A.; Glaudemans, A.W.J.M.; Wieringa, I.; Berger, S.P.; Bakker, S.J.L.; Slart, R.H.J.A. A high abdominal aortic calcification score by dual X-ray absorptiometry is associated with cardiovascular events after kidney transplantation. *Nephrol. Dial. Transpl.* **2018**, *33*, 2253–2259. [CrossRef]

152. Braun, J.; Oldendorf, M.; Moshage, W.; Heidler, R.; Zeitler, E.; Luft, F.C. Electron beam computed tomography in the evaluation of cardiac calcifications in chronic dialysis patients. *Am. J. Kidney Dis.* **1996**, *27*, 394–401. [CrossRef]
153. London, G.; Marty, C.; Marchais, S.J.; Guerin, A.P.; Metivier, F.; de Vernejoul, M. Arterial Calcifications and Bone Histomorphometry in End-Stage Renal Disease. *J. Am. Soc. Nephrol.* **2004**, *15*, 1943–1951. [CrossRef]
154. Seifert, M.E.; Hruska, K.A. The Kidney-Vascular-Bone Axis in the Chronic Kidney Disease-Mineral Bone Disorder. *Transplantation* **2016**, *100*, 497–505. [CrossRef]
155. Adragao, T.; Herberth, J.; Monier-Faugere, M.-C.; Branscum, A.J.; Ferreira, A.; Frazao, J.M.; Dias Curto, J.; Malluche, H.H. Low Bone Volume-A Risk Factor for Coronary Calcifications in Hemodialysis Patients. *Clin. J. Am. Soc. Nephrol.* **2009**, *4*, 450–455. [CrossRef] [PubMed]
156. Asci, G.; Ok, E.; Savas, R.; Ozkahya, M.; Duman, S.; Toz, H.; Kayikcioglu, M.; Branscum, A.J.; Monier-Faugere, M.C.; Herberth, J.; et al. The link between bone and coronary calcifications in CKD-5 patients on haemodialysis. *Nephrol. Dial. Transpl.* **2011**, *26*, 1010–1015. [CrossRef]
157. Bouquegneau, A.; Salam, S.; Delanaye, P.; Eastell, R.; Khwaja, A. Mini-Review Bone Disease after Kidney Transplantation. *Clin. J. Am. Soc. Nephrol.* **2016**, *11*, 1282–1296. [CrossRef] [PubMed]
158. Malluche, H.H.; Monier-Faugere, M.-C.; Herberth, J. Bone disease after renal transplantation. *Nat. Rev. Neprhol.* **2010**, *6*, 32–40. [CrossRef] [PubMed]
159. Drüeke, T.B.; Evenepoel, P. The Bone after Kidney Transplantation. *Clin. J. Am. Soc. Nephrol.* **2019**, *14*, 795–797. [CrossRef] [PubMed]
160. Neves, C.L.; Dos Reis, L.M.; Batista, D.G.; Custodio, M.R.; Graciolli, F.G.; Martin, R.D.C.T.; Neves, K.R.; Dominguez, W.V.; Moyses, R.M.; Jorgetti, V. Persistence of bone and mineral disorders 2 years after successful kidney transplantation. *Transplantation* **2013**, *96*, 290–296. [CrossRef]
161. Iyer, S.P.; Nikkel, L.E.; Nishiyama, K.K.; Dworakowski, E.; Cremers, S.; Zhang, C.; Mcmahon, D.J.; Boutroy, S.; Liu, X.S.; Ratner, L.E.; et al. Kidney Transplantation with Early Corticosteroid Withdrawal: Paradoxical Effects at the Central and Peripheral Skeleton. *J. Am. Soc. Nephrol.* **2014**, *25*, 1331–1341. [CrossRef]
162. Keronen, S.; Martola, L.; Finne, P.; Burton, I.S.; Kröger, H.; Honkanen, E. Changes in Bone Histomorphometry after Kidney Transplantation. *Clin. J. Am. Soc. Nephrol.* **2019**, *14*, 894–903. [CrossRef]
163. Moe, S.M. Vascular calcification and renal osteodystrophy relationship in chronic kidney disease. *Eur. J. Clin. Investig.* **2006**, *36*, 51–62. [CrossRef]
164. Sotomayor, C.G.; Benjamens, S.; Gomes-Neto, A.W.; Pol, R.A.; Groothof, D.; te Velde-Keyzer, C.A.; Chong, G.; Glaudemans, A.W.J.M.; Berger, S.P.; Bakker, S.J.L.; et al. Bone Mineral Density and Aortic Calcification. *Transplantation* **2020**. [CrossRef]
165. Czaya, B.; Faul, C. FGF23 and inflammation—a vicious coalition in CKD. *Kidney Int.* **2019**, *96*, 813–815. [CrossRef] [PubMed]
166. Singh, S.; Grabner, A.; Yanucil, C.; Schramm, K.; Czaya, B.; Krick, S.; Czaja, M.J.; Bartz, R.; Abraham, R.; Di Marco, G.S.; et al. Fibroblast growth factor 23 directly targets hepatocytes to promote inflammation in chronic kidney disease. *Kidney Int.* **2016**, *90*, 985–996. [CrossRef] [PubMed]
167. Egli-Spichtig, D.; Imenez Silva, P.H.; Glaudemans, B.; Gehring, N.; Bettoni, C.; Zhang, M.Y.H.; Pastor-Arroyo, E.M.; Schönenberger, D.; Rajski, M.; Hoogewijs, D.; et al. Tumor necrosis factor stimulates fibroblast growth factor 23 levels in chronic kidney disease and non-renal inflammation. *Kidney Int.* **2019**, *96*, 890–905. [CrossRef] [PubMed]
168. Hamano, T.; Matsui, I.; Mikami, S.; Tomida, K.; Fujii, N.; Imai, E.; Rakugi, H.; Isaka, Y. Fetuin-mineral complex reflects extraosseous calcification stress in CKD. *J. Am. Soc. Nephrol.* **2010**, *21*, 1998–2007. [CrossRef] [PubMed]
169. Kuro-O, M. Klotho and endocrine fibroblast growth factors: markers of chronic kidney disease progression and cardiovascular complications? *Nephrol. Dial. Transpl.* **2019**, *34*, 15–21. [CrossRef]
170. Cianciolo, G.; Capelli, I.; Angelini, M.L.; Valentini, C.; Baraldi, O.; Scolari, M.P.; Stefoni, S. Importance of vascular calcification in kidney transplant recipients. *Am. J. Nephrol.* **2014**, *39*, 418–426. [CrossRef]
171. Van Ballegooijen, A.J.; Cepelis, A.; Visser, M.; Brouwer, I.A.; Van Schoor, N.M.; Beulens, J.W. Joint Association of Low Vitamin D and Vitamin K Status with Blood Pressure and Hypertension. *Hypertension* **2017**, *69*, 1165–1172. [CrossRef] [PubMed]

172. Hou, Y.-C.; Lu, C.-L.; Zheng, C.-M.; Chen, R.-M.; Lin, Y.-F.; Liu, W.-C.; Yen, T.-H.; Chen, R.; Lu, K.-C. Correction: Hou et al. Emerging Role of Vitamins D and K in Modulating Uremic Vascular Calcification: The Aspect of Passive Calcification. *Nutrients* **2019**, *11*, 152. [CrossRef] [PubMed]
173. van Ballegooijen, A.J.; Beulens, J.W.J.; Keyzer, C.A.; Navis, G.J.; Berger, S.P.; de Borst, M.H.; Vervloet, M.G.; Bakker, S.J.L. Joint association of vitamins D and K status with long-term outcomes in stable kidney transplant recipients. *Nephrol. Dial. Transpl.* **2020**, *35*, 706–714. [CrossRef] [PubMed]
174. Nguyen, P.T.H.; Coche, E.; Goffin, E.; Beguin, C.; Vlassenbroek, A.; Devuyst, O.; Robert, A.; Jadoul, M. Prevalence and determinants of coronary and aortic calcifications assessed by chest CT in renal transplant recipients. *Am. J. Nephrol.* **2007**, *27*, 329–335. [CrossRef] [PubMed]
175. Shimizu, H.; Takahashi, M.; Takeda, S.I.; Inoue, S.; Fujishiro, J.; Hakamata, Y.; Kaneko, T.; Murakami, T.; Takeuchi, K.; Takeyoshi, I.; et al. Mycophenolate mofetil prevents transplant arteriosclerosis by direct inhibition of vascular smooth muscle cell proliferation. *Transplantation* **2004**, *77*, 1661–1667. [CrossRef] [PubMed]
176. Eisenga, M.F.; Gomes-Neto, A.W.; Van Londen, M.; Ziengs, A.L.; Douwes, R.M.; Stam, S.P.; Osté, M.C.J.; Knobbe, T.J.; Hessels, N.R.; Buunk, A.M.; et al. Rationale and design of TransplantLines: A prospective cohort study and biobank of solid organ transplant recipients. *BMJ Open* **2018**, *8*, 24502. [CrossRef] [PubMed]

8

Clusterin as a New Marker of Kidney Injury in Children Undergoing Allogeneic Hematopoietic Stem Cell Transplantation

Kinga Musiał [1,*], Monika Augustynowicz [1], Izabella Miśkiewicz-Migoń [2], Krzysztof Kałwak [2], Marek Ussowicz [2] and Danuta Zwolińska [1]

1 Department of Pediatric Nephrology, Wrocław Medical University, 50-556 Wrocław, Poland; monika.augustynowicz@umed.wroc.pl (M.A.); danuta.zwolinska@umed.wroc.pl (D.Z.)

2 Department of Bone Marrow Transplantation, Oncology and Pediatric Hematology, Wrocław Medical University, 50-556 Wrocław, Poland; imiskiewicz@usk.wroc.pl (I.M.-M.); krzysztof.kalwak@umed.wroc.pl (K.K.); marek.ussowicz@umed.wroc.pl (M.U.)

* Correspondence: kinga.musial@umed.wroc.pl

† Short title: Clusterin in children after alloHSCT.

Abstract: Background and aims: The markers of renal damage defining subclinical AKI are not widely used in children undergoing allogeneic hematopoietic stem cell transplantation (alloHSCT). The aim of the study was to evaluate serum and urinary clusterin as indices of kidney injury after alloHSCT in relation to damage (kidney injury molecule (KIM)-1) and functional (cystatin C) markers. Material and methods: Serum and urinary clusterin, KIM-1 and cystatin C concentrations were assessed by ELISA in 27 children before alloHSCT, 24 h, 1, 2, 3 and 4 weeks after alloHSCT and in controls. Results: All parameters were significantly higher in HSCT patients compared to controls even before the transplantation. The serum concentrations increased after HSCT and this rising trend was kept until the third (clusterin) or 4th (KIM-1, cystatin C) week. Urinary clusterin and KIM-1 were elevated until the third week and then decreased yet remained higher than before HSCT. Urinary cystatin C has risen from the second week after HSCT and decreased after the third week but was still higher than before alloHSCT. Conclusions: The features of kidney injury are present even before alloHSCT. Clusterin seems useful in the assessment of subclinical AKI and may become a new early marker of sublethal kidney injury in children.

Keywords: acute kidney injury; cystatin C; hyperfiltration; kidney injury molecule (KIM)-1; tubular damage

---

1. Introduction

Renal tubular epithelial cells are prone to hypoxia and metabolic stress, thus they become first target cells in the course of kidney injury. Contrast-induced nephropathy is a classic example of reversible acute kidney injury (AKI) with tubular involvement [1]. Animal and human studies showed that contrast administration triggers both systemic and renal cytotoxic effects [2,3]. However, if the conditions are unfavorable, further irreversible changes may lead to progression to chronic kidney disease [4].

Acute kidney injury is a well-documented phenomenon characteristic for HSCT [5–8]. However, most studies on AKI take into account the KDIGO classifications, focusing on the serum creatinine values and diuresis [9]. Such criteria do not ease the AKI diagnosis. In order to secure the patient with positive fluid balance and prevent oliguria, additional hydration and forced diuresis are implemented. These conditions may bias the values of estimated glomerular filtration rate (eGFR) and urine output.

Recent classifications have expanded the definition of AKI beyond the functional criteria. They distinguish four options, based on the combined evaluation of function and damage markers [10]. This new approach defines normal renal function as an absence of any index alteration, subclinical AKI as an isolated increase of any damage marker, functional AKI when solely function markers are modified and combined AKI with both function and damage markers altered [10,11].

The search for new markers was conditioned by the failure of serum creatinine as an early marker of renal function decrement. The indices of cellular damage—especially of tubular injury—are of particular interest as new markers of the so-called "subclinical AKI" [10]. The preliminary studies concerning children after cardiosurgery or hematopoietic stem cell transplantation (HSCT) proved that combination of the biomarkers of renal function and tubular damage may be of added value in the early diagnosis of AKI [12,13].

Indeed, the risk of AKI is increased in children undergoing hematopoietic stem cell transplantation (HSCT), mainly due to the nephrotoxicity of drugs. Additionally, renal hypoperfusion, infections and immune complications (including graft versus host disease) count. Moreover, patients with allogeneic HSCT suffer from AKI more often than those undergoing the autologous transplantation [14,15]. The assessment of renal function in the early (up to 28 days) post-transplantation period seems of paramount importance, because it may reveal the potential direction of future changes into either full renal recovery or acute kidney disease or chronic kidney disease [16,17]. First promising results in the population of children undergoing HSCT should urge further search for reliable early markers of kidney injury [13].

2. Aim of Study

Therefore, the objective of the study was to assess the usefulness of serum and urinary clusterin as new indices of kidney injury in the early post-HSCT period in relation to other renal damage (KIM-1) and functional (cystatin C) markers and to estimate their potential value as factors differentiating between children transplanted because of oncological and non-oncological reasons.

3. Material and Methods

3.1. Study Design and Settings

This observational pilot study concerned 27 children (15 girls, 12 boys) undergoing first alloHSCT in the Department of Bone Marrow Transplantation, Pediatric Oncology and Hematology, in 2019 (patient flow is shown in Figure 1). The observation period started before introducing conditioning therapy, then parameter examinations were performed 24 h, 1, 2, 3 and 4 weeks after HSCT.

The exclusion criteria for the patients were the age below 2 years and over 18 years, autologous HSCT and retransplantation. The whole alloHSCT group contained 27 patients (median age 4.5 years, interquartile range 3.1–8.0 years). The subdivision into two groups was carried out depending on the indications for allotransplantation. Seventeen patients (median age 6.6 years, interquartile range 4.0–9.8 years) were qualified for transplantation due to oncological reasons, 10 (median age 4.5 years, interquartile range 3.1–7.0 years) underwent HSCT due to non-oncological indications (mainly severe aplastic anemia). In 79% of cases the donor was unrelated, in 18%-related and in 3%-haploidentical.

The conditioning therapy concerned myeloablative (busulfan, cyclophosphamide and fludarabine or fludarabine, treosulfan, thiotepa) or non-myeloablative (cyclophosphamide, fludarabine) regimens. In most patients graft versus host disease (GvHD) protocol contained pre-HSCT ATG, cyclosporine A since 1 day before HSCT and methotrexate given in the 1st, 3rd and 6th day after transplantation. Nineteen out of 27 patients developed GvHD. None of the patients died in the observation period.

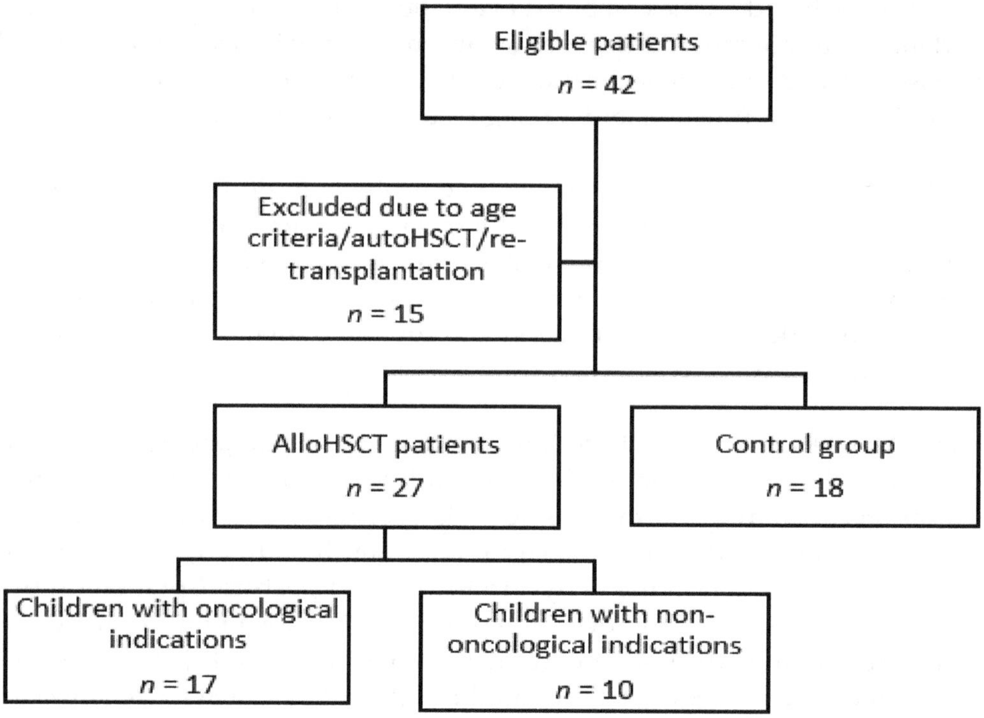

Figure 1. Patient flow.

The control group contained 18 age-matched children (9 girls, 9 boys; median age 7.8 years, interquartile range 7.0–9.8 years) with monosymptomatic nocturnal enuresis and normal kidney function.

Informed consent was obtained from the patients over 16 and their parents, if necessary.

3.2. Methods

Blood samples were drawn from peripheral veins after an overnight fast. Samples were clotted for 30 min, centrifuged at room temperature, 1000 g for 15 min, then serum was stored at −80 °C until assayed. Urine was collected aseptically from the first morning sample, centrifuged at room temperature, 1000 g for 15 min and then stored at −80 °C until assayed.

The serum and urine concentrations of clusterin, cystatin C and KIM-1 were evaluated by commercially available ELISA kits (clusterin EIAab, reagent kit E1180h; cystatin C R & D Systems, reagent kit DSCTC0; KIM-1 EIAab, reagent kit E0785 h). Standards, serum and urine samples were transferred to 96-well microplates precoated with recombinant antibodies to human clusterin, cystatin C, KIM-1 and creatinine. Captured proteins were then detected using monoclonal antibodies against clusterin, cystatin C and KIM-1 conjugated to horseradish peroxidase. Next, the assay was developed with tetramethylbenzidine substrate and blue color was developed proportionately to the amount of captured protein. The addition of acid stop solution ended the color development and converted it to the endpoint yellow. The intensity of the latter was measured in a microplate reader at 450 nm, with the correction wavelength at 550/650 nm. Each sample was tested in duplicate and the arithmetical mean was considered a final result. Measurements were performed according to the manufacturer's instructions; results were calculated by reference to standard curves. Detection limits were as follows: clusterin 1.56 ng/mL; cystatin C 3.13 ng/mL; KIM-1 0.15 ng/mL. The intra-assay and inter-assay coefficients of variation (% CV) for examined parameters did not exceed 8.5% and 9.4%, respectively.

The assessment of kidney function relied on hematological protocols assessing serum creatinine in fixed time points. Serum and urine chemistry parameters were measured using automated routine diagnostic tests on the Beckman Coulter AU2700 analyzer. The serum creatinine was assessed with the use of enzymatic method (creatinine OSR61204 reagent, creatininase–sarcosine oxidase reactions). Serum and urine concentrations of all parameters was measured before conditioning, 24 h after allotransplantation and then 1 week, 2, 3, 4 weeks after alloHSCT. eGFR was calculated in all time points, based on the Schwarz formula [18]. The eGFR changes were confronted with the pre-transplantation values.

All urinary concentrations of evaluated parameters were normalized to urinary creatinine values.

AKI was diagnosed based on the pRIFLE criteria [9]. Hyperfiltration was defined as eGFR ≥ 140 mL/min/1.73 m^2, according to recent meta-analysis and pediatric experience [19,20].

3.3. Statistical Analysis

Results were expressed as median values and interquartile ranges. The null hypothesis of normality of distribution of analyzed variables was rejected by Shapiro–Wilk test. Thus, the comparisons between paired and unpaired data were evaluated by using nonparametric tests (Friedman, Wilcoxon, Kruskal–Wallis, Mann–Whitney U). The correlations between parameters were assessed with the use of Spearman's correlation coefficient R. Statistical analysis was performed using the package Statistica ver. 13.3 (StatSoft). A p-value < 0.05 was considered significant.

4. Results

None of the patients presented with eGFR < 60 mL/min/1.73 m^2 and median eGFR values in both groups were above 90 mL/min/1.73 m^2 at any time point (Table 1) Most oncological patients demonstrated hyperfiltration until the 3rd week after transplantation (with peak incidence in the first week after HSCT). Non-oncological children with eGFR > 140 mL/min/1.73 m^2 were in minority. The median eGFR values in non-oncological children were comparable to those of the controls during the whole study except for the early (24 h after HSCT) measurement, when they became significantly higher (Table 1). Contrarily, the eGFR records in oncological patients remained significantly elevated compared to controls from point zero until the 3rd week after alloHSCT. They were increased throughout the whole study period compared to the non-oncological patients (Table 1).

Table 1. eGFR values in examined groups.

eGFR (mL/min/1.73 m^2) Median Value (Interquartile Range)	Before alloHSCT	24 h after alloHSCT	1 Week after alloHSCT	2 Weeks after alloHSCT	3 Weeks after alloHSCT	4 Weeks after alloHSCT
Oncological patients	142 (112–149) ^{a}	183 (153–216) ^{a,b}	172 (155–205) ^{a,b}	188 (166–195) ^{a,b}	149 (140–174) ^{a,b,c}	134 (123–149) ^{a,c}
Non-oncological patients	107 (96–129)	140 (126–176) ^{b}	131 (118–149) ^{b}	130 (114–136) ^{b}	129 (100–145) ^{b}	126 (92–134)

^{a} $p < 0.05$ oncological pts vs. non-oncological pts; ^{b} $p < 0.05$ any time point vs. before alloHSCT; ^{c} $p < 0.05$ 2 weeks after vs. 3 weeks after; eGFR estimated glomerular filtration rate; alloHSCT allogeneic hematopoietic stem cell transplantation.

The urinary clusterin, KIM-1 and cystatin C concentrations were significantly elevated in all patients compared to controls, irrespective of the indication for transplantation (oncological or non-oncological), even before alloHSCT. Normalization of the urinary concentrations of clusterin, KIM-1 and cystatin C for urinary creatinine maintained these differences (Figures 2–4). In the case of clusterin, the urinary values have increased nearly 3-fold 24 h after transplantation, then kept the plateau phase until the second week and rose again in the 3rd week. Finally, they decreased in the 4th week after HSCT, yet remained higher than before HSCT (Figure 2). The urinary KIM-1 values rose by 50% 24 h after HSCT, then kept growing until the 3rd week and finally decreased (Figure 3). Urinary cystatin C demonstrated the delayed elevation from the 2nd week after transplantation, lasting only until the 3rd week and followed by a significant decrease 1 week later (Figure 4). After 4 weeks of observation, all urinary biomarkers were still significantly elevated compared to the pre-transplantation values.

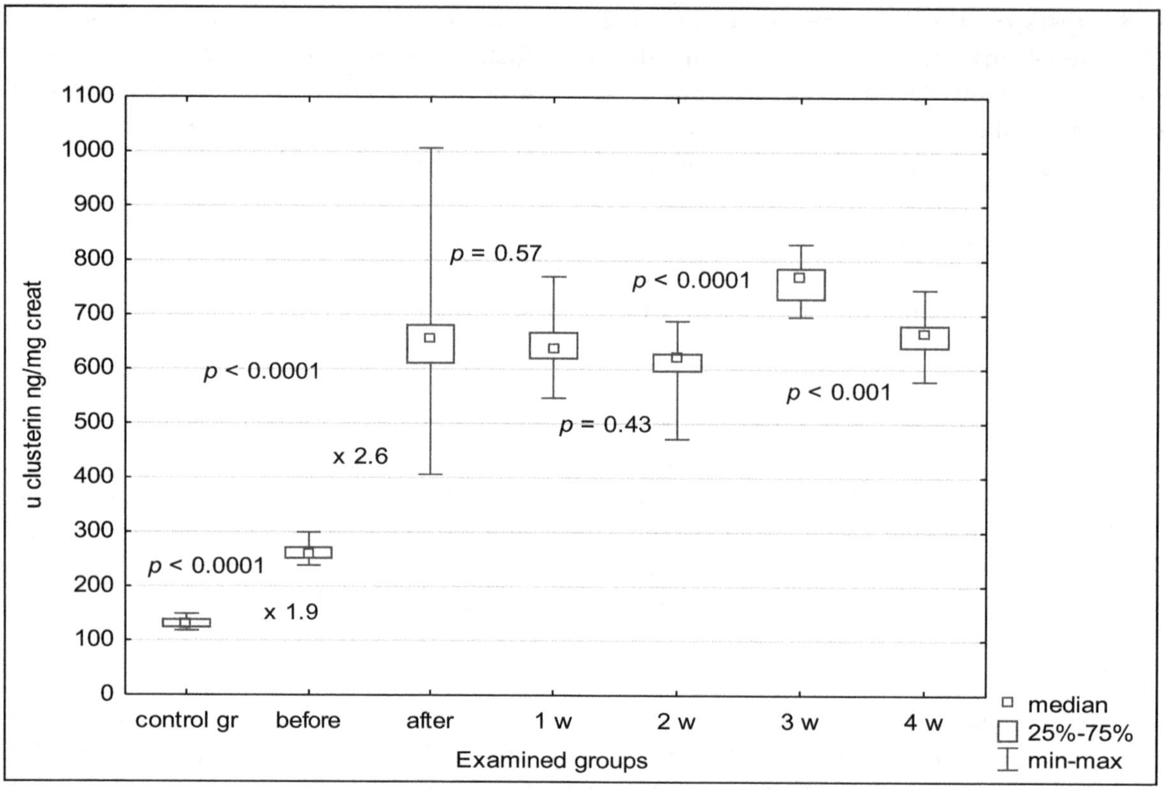

Figure 2. Urinary clusterin values in examined groups. before—before alloHSCT; after—24 h after alloHSCT; 1 w (2 w, 3 w, 4 w)—1 week (2, 3, 4 weeks) after alloHSCT.

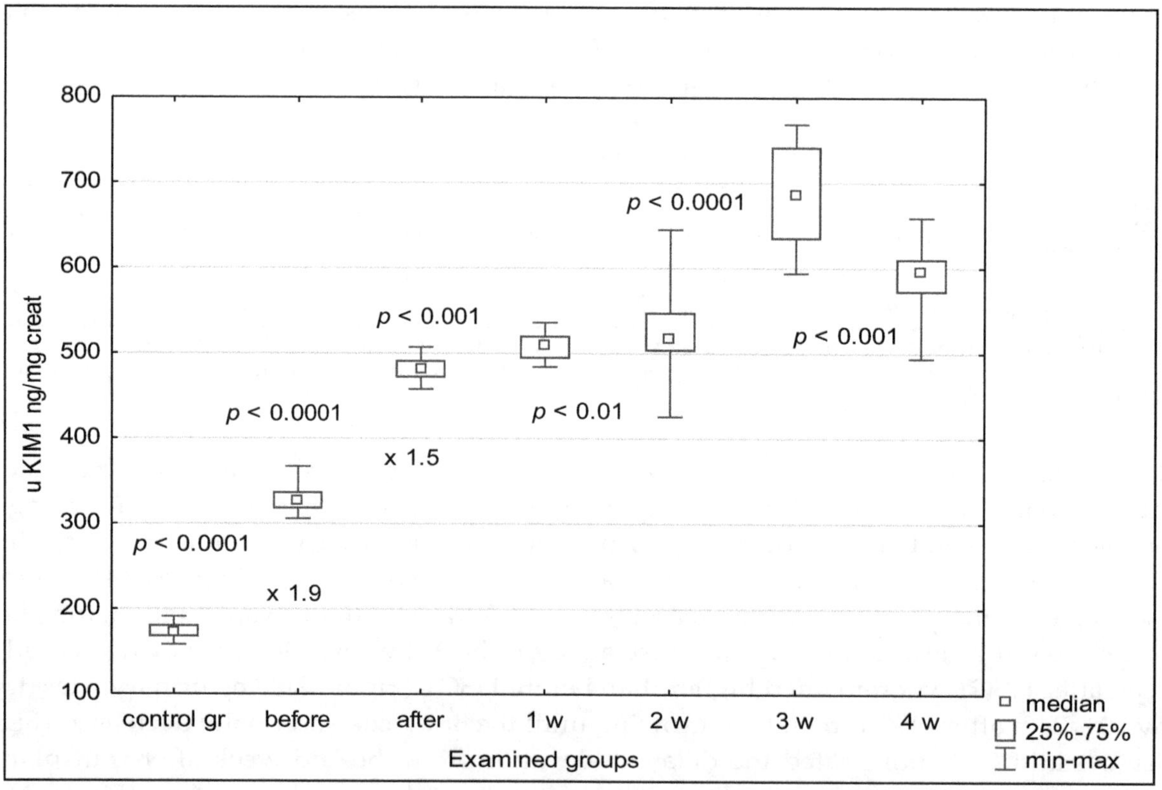

Figure 3. Urinary KIM-1 values in examined groups. before—before alloHSCT; after—24 h after alloHSCT; 1 w (2 w, 3 w, 4 w)—1 week (2, 3, 4 weeks) after alloHSCT.

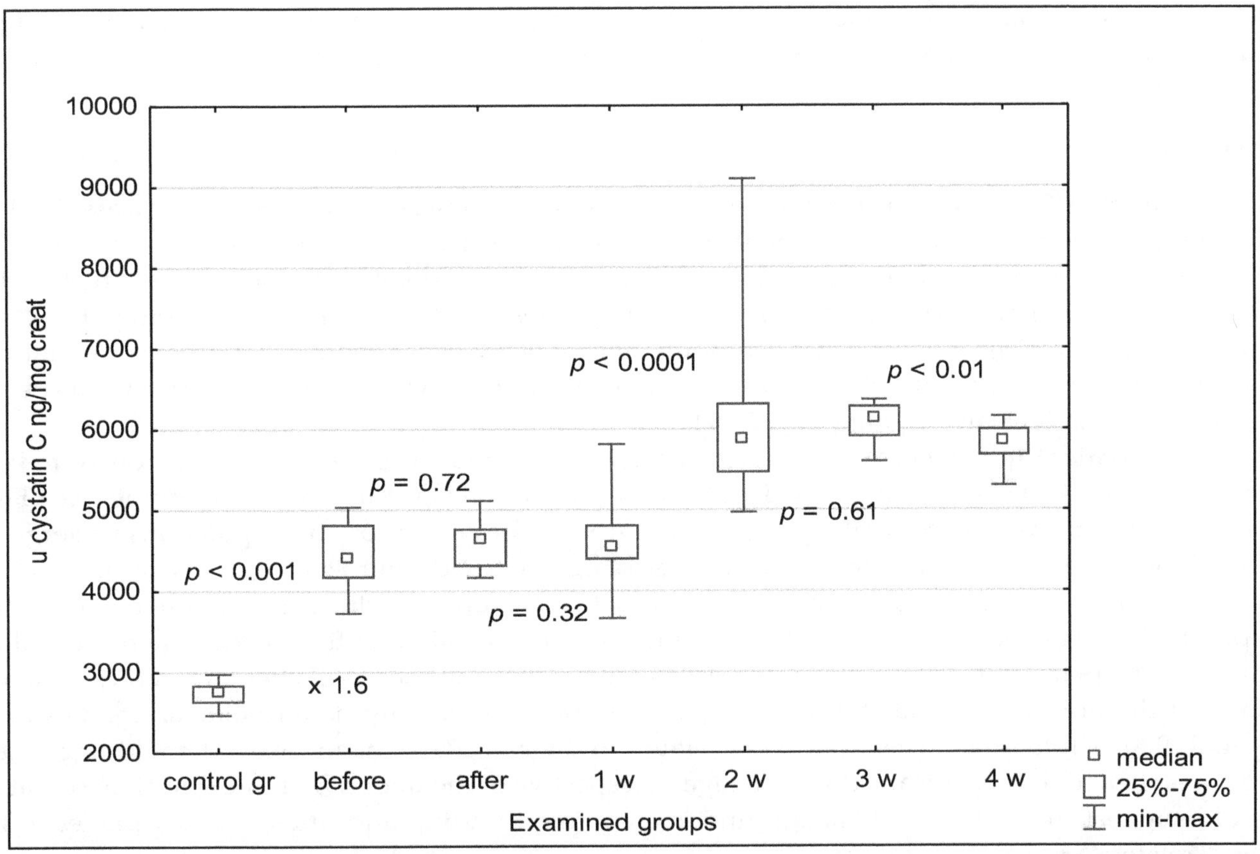

Figure 4. Urinary cystatin C values in examined groups. before—before alloHSCT; after—24 h after alloHSCT; 1 w (2 w, 3 w, 4 w)—1 week (2, 3, 4 weeks) after alloHSCT.

The serum concentrations of clusterin, KIM-1 and cystatin C in children before transplantation were significantly higher than in controls (Table 2). The serum values further increased 24 h after HSCT and the rise was most spectacular in the case of clusterin (over 2-fold) compared to 50%–60% elevation of other markers. Then the concentrations rose systematically until the 3rd week (clusterin) or 4th week (KIM-1, cystatin C) after alloHSCT. There was no significant difference in the urinary or serum marker values between oncological and non-oncological patients at any time point (Table 2).

Table 2. Serum parameter values in examined groups.

Serum Parameter Median Value (Interquartile Range)	s Clusterin (ng/mL)	s KIM1 (ng/mL)	s Cystatin C (ng/mL)
Control group	1.3 (1.2–1.4)	2.3 (2.2–2.4)	148 (141.7–164.3)
Before alloHSCT	3.1 (3.0–3.1) [a]	4.2 (4.1–4.3) [a]	408 (387.6–433) [a]
24 hafter alloHSCT	7.9 (7.2–8.4) [a,b]	6.7 (6.3–6.8) [a,b]	634.8 (604.6–689.1) [a,b]
1 week after alloHSCT	8.9 (8.8–9.1) [a,c]	6.7 (6.0–6.8) [a]	905.6 (879–961.6) [a,c]
2 weeks after alloHSCT	9.5 (9.3–10) [a,d]	8 (7.8–8.2) [a,d]	898 (878.7–926.3) [a]
3 weeks after alloHSCT	13.3 (12.8–13.6) [a,e]	8.9 (8.8–8.9) [a,e]	1106 (1053–1157) [a,e]
4 weeks after alloHSCT	13.3 (12.8–13.6) [a]	9.2 (9.1–9.2) [a,f]	1262 (1222–1288) [a,f]

[a] $p < 0.05$ any time point vs. control group; [b] $p < 0.05$ 24 h after alloHSCT vs. before alloHSCT; [c] $p < 0.05$ 1 week after alloHSCT vs. 24 h after alloHSCT; [d] $p < 0.05$ 2 weeks after alloHSCT vs. 1 week after alloHSCT; [e] $p < 0.05$ 3 weeks after alloHSCT vs. 2 weeks after alloHSCT; [f] $p < 0.05$ 4 weeks after alloHSCT vs. 3 weeks after alloHSCT. No significant correlations were detected between the analyzed parameters.

AKI was diagnosed in 4 patients (3 oncological and 1 non-oncological), according to the pRIFLE criteria. Risk stage was diagnosed in 3 of them, 1 developed Injury stage. None of the patients required renal replacement therapy.

5. Discussion

Although AKI is a common finding in the patients undergoing alloHSCT, most of the classifications assessing the degree of renal impairment concentrate on the functional indices. However, damage markers seem a promising and objective alternative in the assessment of kidney injury. The fact that the number of potential AKI markers is increasing proves that the problem is emerging. Thus, our aim was to confront the known indices of tubular injury (KIM-1) and glomerular function (cystatin C, eGFR) with a new marker of cellular stress and damage. Clusterin has not been analyzed in a specific population of patients undergoing HSCT so far.

Every patient in this study group, irrespective of the indication for HSCT, demonstrated the features of cellular damage seen even before the procedure of transplantation. The interpretation of this unexpected result was quite challenging, because up-to-date studies on the populations undergoing HSCT have never compared their records to those of age-matched controls with normal renal function and no history of kidney injury. The pre-transplantation therapies, including chemotherapeutics and nephrotoxic drugs, seem of paramount importance as an explanation for this phenomenon. Indeed, all patients transplanted due to oncological reasons have undergone series of chemotherapies, whereas many of the non-oncological children were treated with potentially nephrotoxic antibiotics prior to alloHSCT. All these interventions were related to their primary diagnoses and could trigger the pre-transplantation subclinical kidney damage. Irrespective of the underlying cause, such observation would suggest that subclinical background is a common finding and, thus, the key player in the HSCT-related AKI.

The post-transplantation aggravation of cellular damage was rather predictable, taking into account the nephrotoxic and cytotoxic potentials of conditioning regimens, anti-GvHD prophylaxis and treatment of infections. The essential finding was that these signs of injury concerned both serum and urine, depicting not only renal, but also systemic cell damage after HSCT.

Among all analyzed parameters, the serum and urinary clusterin values have shown the most spectacular changes in children before HSCT compared to controls and before HSCT compared to 24 h after HSCT. The serum and urinary values before transplantation were at least two times higher than in controls and rose over 2.5-fold after transplantation. In the meantime, the other serum markers increased by no more than 60%, whereas the urinary values became 14% higher (KIM-1) or remained unchanged (cystatin C). Only in the case of clusterin the post-HSCT response was more spectacular than the difference between control group and pre-HSCT values.

Clusterin is a 75–80 kDa heat shock protein secreted by both epithelial and secretory cells in response to stress. Its protective and anti-apoptotic roles against renal ischemia-reperfusion injury have been demonstrated in murine kidneys [21]. Interestingly, clusterin was detected in both renal tubular epithelial and mesangial cells. Its decreased expression aggravated postischemic renal injury, as well as proteinuria in the course of glomerulopathy. Clusterin knockout mice suffered from the progression of renal inflammation and fibrosis after ischemia–reperfusion injury [22]. Investigation concerning humans is restricted to single reports on the urinary clusterin in patients with diabetes mellitus and promising results of a diagnostic multi-biomarker kit including urine clusterin in the scope of indices of chronic kidney injury [23,24].

Taking into account the experimental data, the above mentioned reports and our results, we could put forward the hypothesis about the protective role of clusterin in the kidney injury due to HSCT. Such presumption would provide the explanation for increasing levels in both serum and urine as a response to systemic and kidney stress conditions. Moreover, clusterin has turned out the most accurate marker predicting drug-induced AKI in adults, better than cystatin C or KIM-1 [25]. Interestingly, all three markers became higher compared to non-AKI controls already 1–3 days before the onset of AKI.

This may suggest the reason for the early pre-transplant elevation of all indices compared to healthy controls. It also shows the added value of all tested markers in diagnosing nephrotoxicity. Moreover, yet, testing big cohorts may give unequivocal results in the pediatric population, questioning for example the accuracy of KIM-1 as a predictor of AKI in children [26].

In our study group, urinary KIM-1 behaved similarly to urinary clusterin, although the elevation after HSCT did not reach 50%. However, the rising trend persisted until the third week and then a significant decrease was noticed. Yet, the values remained higher than before transplantation. Such scheme would talk into the tubular damage aggravating since the HSCT procedure. The serum KIM-1 concentrations kept the systematic growth throughout the whole observation period, except for the plateau phase between 24 h and one week after HSCT. These results have suggested the ongoing tubular damage in the course of HSCT procedure, triggered most probably by nephrotoxic drugs. Increased serum KIM-1 could point at its release by the cells damaged in the course of conditioning therapy, anti-GvHD prophylaxis or current infection treatment, as well as the accumulation of a molecule that cannot be filtered freely through glomeruli due to its molecular mass of 90–110 kDa. The possible long-term consequence has been discovered in experimental studies, when chronic KIM-1 elevation in mice promoted fibrosis, thus linking AKI to CKD [27].

However, both abovementioned markers seemed similar in the mode of early reaction to kidney injury. The usefulness of clusterin and KIM-1 could be strengthened by the fact that their elevated serum and urine values were noticed even before transplantation, both in oncological and non-oncological patients, whereas pre-transplantation eGFR changes concerned only oncological children. In detail, their eGFR values were significantly higher compared to controls and most of the patients demonstrated hyperfiltration. This finding was confirmed by other authors, who put the main stress on hypermetabolic states and previous chemotherapy as causative factors of hyperfiltration [28]. The eGFR discrepancies could also be the consequence of many transplant-related covariates like catabolism, inflammation or weight loss, directly influencing serum creatinine [29].

Whether this hyperfiltration could be the early sign of progression into chronic kidney injury, remains unexplained, because the longer time of observation would be needed. However, the elevation of both damage parameters and eGFR could be the proof for the pre-transplantation kidney injury in oncological patients. This finding justifies the current attempts to prevent renal injury or at least to minimize the impact of potential nephrotoxins on the kidney. The reduction of nephrotoxic exposure is one of the effective tools already used in oncological patients [30]. The animal models suggest the possibility to prevent AKI with the use of phosphodiesterase-5 inhibitors prior to potentially nephrotoxic treatment [31,32]. Independent of the chosen strategy, the threat of renal injury should urge careful follow-up of the patient in order to avoid additional insults triggering irreversible damage to the kidney.

Cystatin Cis an established marker of glomerular function and a good predictor of AKI in children, so it seemed a good candidate to verify the abovementioned discrepant eGFR results. However, it did not confirm differences between oncological and non-oncological patients [33]. Out of the three examined markers, cystatin C was the only one with low molecular weight (13 kDa) freely filtered through glomeruli. Therefore, the fact that the elevation of cystatin C in serum has outrun the increase of the urinary value was the direct proof of the serum origin of cystatin C found in the urine. Having said that, the increased values of urinary clusterin and KIM-1, both of higher molecular weight than cystatin C, must have been of tubular cell origin. Therefore, their elevation was probably proportionate to the degree of cell damage and, in case of clusterin, to the intensity of protective mechanisms against kidney injury.

Summarizing, in our study clusterin has outperformed the targeted glomerular (cystatin C) and tubular (KIM-1) indices of kidney function. Therefore, it seems a promising early marker of the sublethal kidney injury, covering both tubular and glomerular spectrum of renal damage. Whether clusterin may become a duplex renal functional and damage marker, is yet to be established in the studies performed on a larger group of patients.

We also must acknowledge the limitations of our study. First, the clinical data were collected according to the hematological protocols, not taking into account all nephrological aspects. Thus, the full information about urine output is missing. This is the first report on the clusterin serum and urinary values in children, so it is impossible to confront them with the age-related reference values. We are also aware of the low number of patients and the heterogeneity of examined groups, which limits the power of conclusions and urges the continuation of the study throughout a longer period on a larger group of patients.

6. Conclusions

All children demonstrated the features of cell damage already before alloHSCT; thus, the subclinical AKI is a common finding in this population. Clusterin seems more useful in the assessment of subclinical AKI than the classical indices of tubular (KIM-1) and glomerular (cystatin C) damage analyzed separately. It may become a new early marker of sublethal kidney injury in this group of patients.

Author Contributions: Conceptualization: K.M., M.A., D.Z.; investigation: K.M., M.A., I.M.-M., M.U.; resources: I.M.-M., K.K., M.U.; formal analysis: K.M.; writing—original draft: K.M. writing—review and editing: K.M., D.Z.; visualization: K.M.; funding acquisition: K.K., D.Z. All authors have read and agreed to the published version of the manuscript.

References

1. Mamoulakis, C.; Tsarouhas, K.; Fragkiadoulaki, I.; Heretis, I.; Wilks, M.; Spandidos, D.; Tsitsimpikou, C.; Tsatsakis, A. Contrast-induced nephropathy: Basic concepts, pathophysiological implications and prevention strategies. *Pharmacol. Ther.* **2017**, *180*, 99–112. [CrossRef] [PubMed]
2. Mamoulakis, C.; Fragkiadoulaki, I.; Karkala, P.; Georgiadis, G.; Zisis, I.E.; Stivaktakis, P.; Kalogeraki, A.; Tsiaoussis, T.; Burykina, T.; Lazopoulos, G.; et al. Contrast-indiced nephropathy in an animal model: Evaluation of novel biomarkers in blood and tissue samples. *Toxicol. Rep.* **2019**, *6*, 395–400. [CrossRef [PubMed]
3. Tsarouhas, K.; Tsitsimpikou, C.; Papantoni, X.; Lazaridou, D.; Koutouzis, M.; Mazzaris, S.; Rezaee, R.; Mamoulakis, C.; Georgoulias, P.; Nepka, C.; et al. Oxidative stress and kidney injury in trans-radial catheterization. *Biomed. Rep.* **2018**, *8*, 417–425. [CrossRef] [PubMed]
4. Chevalier, R.L. The proximal tubule is the primary target of injury and progression of kidney disease: Role of the glomerulotubular junction. *Am. J. Physiol. Renal Physiol.* **2016**, *311*, F145–F161. [CrossRef]
5. Koh, K.N.; Sunkara, A.; Kang, G. Acute Kidney Injury in Pediatric Patients Receiving Allogeneic Hematopoietic Cell Transplantation: Incidence, Risk Factors, and Outcomes. *Biol. Blood Marrow Transplant.* **2018**, *24*, 758–764. [CrossRef]
6. Raina, R.; Herrera, N.; Krishnappa, V.; Sethi, S.K.; Deep, A.; Kao, W.; Bunchman, T.; Abu-Arja, R. Hematopoietic stem cell transplantation and acute kidney injury in children: A comprehensive review. *Pediatr. Transplant.* **2017**, *21*, e12935. [CrossRef]
7. Didsbury, M.S.; Mackie, F.E.; Kennedy, S.E. A systematic review of acute kidney injury in pediatric allogeneic hematopoietic stem cell recipients. *Pediatr. Transplant.* **2015**, *19*, 460–470. [CrossRef]
8. Kizilbash, S.J.; Kashtan, C.E.; Chavers, B.M.; Cao, Q.; Smith, A.R. Acute kidney injury and the risk of mortality in children undergoing hematopoietic stem cell transplantation. *Biol. Blood Marrow Transplant.* **2016**, *22*, 1264–1270. [CrossRef]
9. Sutherland, S.M.; Byrnes, J.J.; Kothari, M.; Longhurst, C.A.; Dutta, S.; Garcia, P.; Goldstein, S.L. AKI in hospitalized children: Comparing the pRIFLE, AKIN, and KDIGO definitions. *Clin. J. Am. Soc. Nephrol.* **2015**, *10*, 554–561. [CrossRef]
10. Haase, M.; Kellum, J.A.; Ronco, C. Subclinical AKI—An emerging syndrome with important consequences. *Nat. Rev. Nephrol.* **2012**, *8*, 735–739. [CrossRef]

11. Ronco, C.; Kellum, J.A.; Haase, M. Subclinical AKI is still AKI. *Crit. Care* **2012**, *16*, 313. [CrossRef] [PubMed]
12. Basu, R.K.; Wong, H.R.; Krawczeski, C.D.; Wheeler, D.S.; Manning, P.B.; Chawla, L.S.; Devarajan, P.; Goldstein, S.L. Combining functional and tubular damage biomarkers improves diagnostic precision for acute kidney injury after cardiac surgery. *J. Am. Coll. Cardiol.* **2014**, *64*, 2753–2762. [CrossRef] [PubMed]
13. Benoit, S.W.; Dixon, B.P.; Goldstein, S.L.; Bennett, M.R.; Lane, A.; Lounder, D.T.; Rotz, S.J.; Gloude, N.J.; Lake, K.E.; Litts, B.; et al. A novel strategy for identifying early acute kidney injury in pediatric hematopoietic stem cell transplantation. *Bone Marrow Transplant.* **2019**, *54*, 1453–1461. [CrossRef] [PubMed]
14. Kanduri, S.R.; Cheungpasitporn, W.; Thongprayoon, C.; Bathini, T.; Kovvuru, K.; Garla, V.; Medaura, J.; Vaitla, P.; Kashani, K.B. Incidence and mortality of acute kidney injury in patients undergoing hematopoietic stem cell transplantation: A systematic review and meta-analysis. *QJM* **2020**. [CrossRef] [PubMed]
15. Caliskan, Y.; Besisik, S.K.; Sargin, D.; Ecder, T. Early renal injury after myeloablative allogeneic and autologous hematopoietic cell transplantation. *Bone Marrow Transplant.* **2006**, *38*, 141–147. [CrossRef]
16. Basu, R.K. Targeting acute kidney injury: Can an innovative approach to existing and novel biomarkers shift the paradigm? *Nephron* **2019**, *143*, 207–210. [CrossRef]
17. Chawla, L.S.; Bellomo, R.; Bihorac, A.; Goldstein, S.L.; Siew, E.D.; Bagshaw, S.M.; Bittleman, D.; Cruz, D.; Endre, Z.H.; Fitzgerald, R.L.; et al. Acute kidney disease and renal recovery: Consensus report of the Acute Disease Quality Initiative (ADQI) 16 workgroup. *Nat. Rev. Nephrol.* **2017**, *13*, 241–257. [CrossRef]
18. Schwartz, G.J.; Muñoz, A.; Schneider, M.F.; Mak, R.H.; Kaskel, F.; Warady, B.A.; Furth, S.L. New equations to estimate GFR in children with CKD. *J. Am. Soc. Nephrol.* **2009**, *20*, 629–637. [CrossRef]
19. Cachat, F.; Combescure, C.; Cauderay, M.; Girardin, E.; Chehade, H. A systematic review of glomerular hyperfiltration assessment and definition in the medical literature. *Clin. J. Am. Soc. Nephrol.* **2015**, *10*, 382–389. [CrossRef]
20. Iduoriyekemwen, N.J.; Ibadin, M.O.; Aikhionbare, H.A.; Idogun, S.E.; Abiodun, M.T. Glomerular hyperfiltration in excess weight adolescents. *Niger. J. Clin. Pract.* **2019**, *22*, 842–848. [CrossRef]
21. Zhou, W.; Guan, Q.; Kwan, C.C.H.; Chen, H.; Gleave, M.E.; Nguan, C.Y.C.; Du, C. Loss of clusterin expression worsens renal ischemia-reperfusion injury. *Am. J. Physiol. Renal Physiol.* **2010**, *298*, F568–F578. [CrossRef] [PubMed]
22. Guo, J.; Guan, Q.; Liu, X.; Wang, H.; Gleave, M.E.; Nguan, C.Y.C.; Du, C. Relationship of clusterin with renal inflammation and fibrosis after the recovery phase of ischemia-reperfusion injury. *BMC Nephrol.* **2016**, *17*, 133. [CrossRef] [PubMed]
23. Kim, S.S.; Song, S.H.; Kim, J.H.; Jeon, Y.K.; Kim, B.H.; Kang, M.-C.; Chun, S.W.; Hong, S.H.; Chung, M.; Kim, Y.K.; et al. Urine clusterin/apolipoprotein J is linked to tubular damage and renal outcomes in patients with type 2 diabetes mellitus. *Clin. Endocrinol.* **2017**, *87*, 156–164. [CrossRef] [PubMed]
24. Watson, D.; Yang, J.; Sarwal, R.D.; Sigdel, T.K.; Liberto, J.; Damm, I.; Louie, V.; Sigdel, S.; Livingstone, D.; Soh, K.; et al. A novel multi-biomarker assay for non-invasive quantitative monitoring of kidney injury. *J. Clin. Med.* **2019**, *8*, 499. [CrossRef] [PubMed]
25. Da, Y.; Akalya, K.; Murali, T.; Vathsala, A.; Tan, C.-S.; Low, S.; Lim, H.-N.; Teo, B.-W.; Lau, T.; Ong, L.; et al. Serial quantification of urinary protein biomarkers to predict drug-induced acute kidney injury. *Curr. Drug Metab.* **2019**, *20*, 656–664. [CrossRef] [PubMed]
26. Fazel, M.; Sarveazad, A.; Ali, K.M.; Yousefifard, M.; Hosseini, M. Accuracy of urine kidney injury molecule-1 in predicting acute kidney injury in children; a systematic review and meta-analysis. *Arch. Acad. Emerg. Med.* **2020**, *8*, e44. [PubMed]
27. Humphreys, B.D.; Xu, F.; Sabbisetti, V.; Grgic, I.; Naini, S.M.; Wang, N.; Chen, G.; Xiao, S.; Patel, D.; Henderson, J.M.; et al. Chronic epithelial kidney injury molecule-1 expression causes murine kidney fibrosis. *J. Clin. Investig.* **2013**, *123*, 4023–4035. [CrossRef]
28. Kwatra, N.S.; Meany, H.J.; Ghelani, S.J.; Zahavi, D.; Pandya, N.; Majd, M. Glomerular hyperfiltration in children with cancer: Prevalence and a hypothesis. *Pediatr. Radiol.* **2017**, *47*, 221–226. [CrossRef]
29. Filler, G.; Lee, M. Educational review: Measurement of GFR in special populations. *Pediatr. Nephrol.* **2018**, *33*, 2037–2046. [CrossRef]
30. Young, J.; Dahale, D.; Demmel, K.; O'Brien, M.; Geller, J.I.; Courter, J.; Haslam, D.B.; Danziger-Isakov, L.; Goldstein, S.L. Reducing acute kidney injury in pediatric oncology patients: An improvement project targeting nephrotoxic medications. *Pediatr. Blood Cancer* **2020**, *67*, e28396. [CrossRef]

31. Georgiadis, G.; Zisis, I.-E.; Docea, A.O.; Tsarouhas, K.; Fragkiadoulaki, I.; Mavridis, C.; Karavitakis, M.; Stratakis, S.; Stylianou, K.; Tsitsimpikou, C.; et al. Current concepts on the reno-protective effects of phosphodiesterase 5 inhibitors in acute kidney injury: Systematic search and review. *J. Clin. Med.* **2020**, *9*, 1284. [CrossRef] [PubMed]
32. Iordache, A.M.; Buga, A.M.; Albulescu, D.; Vasile, R.C.; Mitrut, R.; Georgiadis, G.; Zisis, I.-E.; Mamoulakis, C.; Tsatsakis, A.; Docea, A.O.; et al. Phosphodiesterase-5 inhibitors ameliorate structural kidney damage in a rat model of contrast-induced nephropathy. *Food Chem. Toxicol.* **2020**, *143*, 111535. [CrossRef] [PubMed]
33. Nakhjavan-Shahraki, B.; Yousefifard, M.; Ataei, N.; Baikpour, M.; Ataei, F.; Bazargani, B.; Abbasi, A.; Ghelichkhani, P.; Javidilarijani, F.; Hosseini, M. Accuracy of cystatin C in prediction of acute kidney injury in children; serum or urine levels: Which one works better? A systematic review and meta-analysis. *BMC Nephrol.* **2017**, *18*, 120. [CrossRef] [PubMed]

9

Beliefs of UK Transplant Recipients about Living Kidney Donation and Transplantation: Findings from a Multicentre Questionnaire-Based Case–Control Study

Pippa K. Bailey [1,2,*], Fergus J. Caskey [1,2], Stephanie MacNeill [1], Charles Tomson [3], Frank J. M. F. Dor [4] and Yoav Ben-Shlomo [1]

[1] Population Health Sciences, Bristol Medical School, University of Bristol, Bristol BS8 2PS, UK; fergus.caskey@bristol.ac.uk (F.J.C.); stephanie.macneill@bristol.ac.uk (S.M.); y.ben-shlomo@bristol.ac.uk (Y.B.-S.)
[2] Southmead Hospital, North Bristol NHS Trust, Bristol BS10 5NB, UK
[3] The Newcastle upon Tyne Hospitals NHS Foundation Trust, Newcastle upon Tyne NE7 7DN, UK; ctomson@doctors.org.uk
[4] Imperial College Healthcare NHS Trust, London W12 0HS, UK; frank.dor@nhs.net
* Correspondence: pippa.bailey@bristol.ac.uk

Abstract: Differing beliefs about the acceptability of living-donor kidney transplants (LDKTs) have been proposed as explaining age, ethnic and socioeconomic disparities in their uptake. We investigated whether certain patient groups hold beliefs incompatible with LDKTs. This questionnaire-based case–control study was based at 14 hospitals in the United Kingdom. Participants were adults transplanted between 1 April 2013 and 31 March 2017. LDKT recipients were compared to deceased-donor kidney transplant (DDKT) recipients. Beliefs were determined by the direction and strength of agreement with ten statements. Multivariable logistic regression was used to investigate the association between beliefs and LDKT versus DDKT. Sex, age, ethnicity, religion, and education were investigated as predictors of beliefs. A total of 1240 questionnaires were returned (40% response). DDKT and LDKT recipients responded in the same direction for 9/10 statements. A greater strength of agreement with statements concerning the 'positive psychosocial effects' of living kidney donation predicted having an LDKT over a DDKT. Older age, Black, Asian and Minority Ethnic (BAME) group ethnicity, and having a religion other than Christianity were associated with greater degree of uncertainty regarding a number of statements, but there was no evidence that individuals in these groups hold strong beliefs against living kidney donation and transplantation. Interventions should address uncertainty, to increase LDKT activity in these groups.

Keywords: living kidney donation; living-donor kidney transplantation; beliefs; inequity

---

1. Introduction

Living-donor kidney transplantation offers the best treatment in terms of life-expectancy and quality of life [1–6] for most people with kidney failure. The healthcare costs associated with living-donor kidney transplants (LDKTs) are less than for dialysis or deceased-donor kidney transplants (DDKTs) [7,8]. The medium-term risks of donating a kidney are small [9–12] and the quality of life of donors returns to pre-donation levels after donation [13,14].

Only 20% of those listed on the UK national transplant waiting list receive an LDKT each year [15]. Certain individuals with renal disease appear to be disadvantaged: people from Black and Asian ethnic groups in the UK are less likely to receive an LDKT when compared to White people with kidney disease [16,17]. Socioeconomic deprivation is also associated with reduced access to living-donor kidney transplantation [16,17]. Older people with kidney disease are less likely to receive an LDKT when compared to younger patients [17], and women are less likely to receive an LDKT when compared to men [18,19]. Ensuring equity in living-donor kidney transplantation has been highlighted as a UK and international research priority by patients and clinicians [20–22]. Differing beliefs in the acceptability of living kidney donation and transplantation have been proposed as a possible explanation for the observed differences in access [17,23,24].

In this questionnaire-based case–control study, we compared the beliefs of LDKT and DDKT recipients about the acceptability of living kidney donation and transplantation. We investigated whether beliefs about living-donor kidney transplantation were associated with an individual's sex, age, ethnicity, religion and education. We aimed to identify groups with beliefs against living-donor kidney transplantation, that may explain the observed disparities in the uptake of LDKTs.

2. Experimental Section

2.1. Participants

The study was based at 14 UK hospitals (listed in Supplementary Methods). We wanted to investigate beliefs about living-donor kidney transplantation specifically, and not kidney transplantation in general. Therefore, we did not invite people with Chronic Kidney Disease or those on dialysis to participate, as some of these individuals may have held beliefs against transplantation in general, as opposed to living-donor kidney transplantation specifically. We obtained from each site an anonymised list of all individuals who received kidney transplants between 1 April 2013 and 31 March 2017, stratified by LDKT and DDKT status. Individuals aged <18 years at the time of transplantation, and individuals lacking mental capacity according to the Mental Capacity Act 2005, were excluded. We performed stratified random sampling using Stata 15 [25] to select, on average, 110 LDKTs and 110 DDKTs from each site, weighted by the number of transplants performed annually at each study site. Sex and 5-year age group strata-matched sampling was used to ensure a similar sample distribution by age and sex. The case–control study was designed to detect a 7-point difference in a continuous measure of patient activation (analysis of this variable not presented here) between LDKT cases and DDKT controls with 90% power, assuming a 5% significance level. The calculation indicated that 170 patients would be needed, and that, therefore, a total of 944 would be needed to allow analyses stratified by Index of Multiple Deprivation rank quintile and allow for 10% missing data. This sample size allows for the detection of a far smaller difference (0.16 Standard Deviation) for a dichotomous exposure or between 6–8% for a categorical outcome [26].

2.2. Questionnaire Content and Survey Tools

Paper questionnaires were mailed by post to participants by research collaborators at the study sites. Questionnaires were accompanied by a patient information sheet, an invitation letter and a return postage paid envelope. A website-address was provided so that participants could complete the questionnaire online if preferred. Non-responders were sent a second questionnaire after 4–6 weeks. Anonymised data were extracted from returned paper questionnaires at the University of Bristol and uploaded onto a secure REDCap database [27].

Transplant beliefs were assessed using questions developed by Stothers et al. [28,29]. In development, the questions were reviewed by three expert focus groups, then evaluated in a pilot study to test content reliability and validity [28]. Test–retest analysis was reported as demonstrating excellent internal consistency, and there was no evidence of 'skew' or 'halo' effects (an overall perception/feeling of satisfaction that influences all responses rather than allowing a thoughtful consideration of each individual question) [28]. Participants were asked to read ten statements describing a belief regarding living-donor kidney transplantation (Box 1). These included statements regarding the acceptability of receiving a donated kidney, coercion or pressure on family to donate, rewards for the donor, required closeness of relationship, the subsequent effect on relationship, beliefs about recipients asking family to donate, donation from offspring to parents, and the risks of donation. Participants were asked to tick one of the following options: (i) Strongly disagree, (ii) Disagree, (iii) Agree, (iv) Strongly agree, (v) Don't know.

Box 1. Belief statements.

1. It is morally acceptable to take a kidney from a healthy person.
2. Donors often agree to donate due to feelings of guilt or family pressure.
3. Donating a kidney is a rewarding experience for the live donors.
4. Donating a kidney to someone requires an extremely close personal relationship.
5. A living-donor kidney transplant may strengthen the relationship between the donor and recipient.
6. Approaching a potential donor who then says no will change the relationship between the two people.
7. Asking someone to donate makes the recipient seem selfish.
8. It is acceptable for a parent to receive a kidney from his/her child (over 18 years old).
9. Decisions about donation should be made by the donor alone. The recipient should not ask for a kidney.
10. Since the donor operation is not risk free, someone who needs a kidney transplant should wait for a kidney from someone who has died.

Questionnaires assessed participant demographics as indicated in Box 2.

Box 2. Participant demographic data collected.

- Sex
  - Male; Female
- 10-year age group
  - 10–19 years; 20–29 years; 30–39 years; 40–49 years; 50–59 years; 60–69 years; 70–79 years; 80–89 years
- Religion
  - No religion; Christian; Muslim; Jewish; Hindu; Sikh; Buddhism
- Socioeconomic position
  - No formal education; Primary school; Secondary school; Vocational/Technical; University—undergraduate; University—postgraduate; Other
- Ethnicity coded using the UK's Office for National Statistics 2011 census categories [30]
  - White;
  - Asian/Asian British;
  - Black/African/Caribbean/Black British;
  - Mixed/Multiple (White and Black Caribbean, White and Black African, Any other Mixed/Multiple ethnic background);
  - Other (Arab, Any other ethnic group)

2.3. *Statistical Analysis*

We compared demographic characteristics between DDKT and LDKT recipients using chi^2 tests. The proportion of DDKT and LDKT recipients selecting each level of agreement with a belief statement was calculated and initially compared using chi^2 tests. We used multivariable logistic regression to look at the association of transplant type (LDKT versus DDKT) with a recipient's agreement with a belief statement. For the multivariable logistic regression, the response options were coded 1–4 (1 = strongly disagree, 2 = disagree, 3 = agree, 4 = strongly agree) with 'Don't know' coded as missing.

For each belief statement we ran an unadjusted model and one adjusted for potential confounders. We specified, a priori, potential confounders including sex, age, education level, ethnicity and religion. We used robust standard errors to account for clustering within renal centres. Statistical analyses were performed in Stata 15 [25].

Basic descriptive statistical tests (chi^2 tests) then were performed to look for differences in response (agreement = strongly agreed and agreed; disagreement = strongly disagreed and disagreed; and don't know) across different patient demographic groups. For these analyses, age was dichotomised into age <60 years and age ≥60 years, ethnicity into White, Black, Asian and Minority Ethnic (BAME) groups, education into university education or no university education, and religion divided into three categories: no religion, Christianity, or other religion. Small numbers of respondents from certain ethnic groups and from religions other than Christianity or none limited subgroup analysis. Small numbers and single participant responders in some groups risked identification: we were therefore required to combine Islam, Hinduism, Judaism, Buddhism, and Sikhism as 'religions other than Christianity' for analysis.

2.4. Ethical Approval and Consent

We received NHS Research Ethics Committee (REC) (REC reference 17/LO/1602) and Health Research Authority (HRA) approval. A consent form formed the first page of the questionnaire. The study was funded by a Kidney Research UK Project Grant (RP_028_20170302). The clinical and research activities being reported are consistent with the Principles of the Declaration of Istanbul as outlined in the 'Declaration of Istanbul on Organ Trafficking and Transplant Tourism'.

3. Results

A total of 1240 questionnaires were returned from 3103 patients (40% response). Participant characteristics are reported in Table 1.

LDKT recipients were more likely to respond than DDKT recipients (46% vs. 34%) and women were more likely to respond than men (43% vs. 37%) (Table S1). However, the study participants were a population representative sample (Table S2). Overall, the proportion of missing data was small (<3% for belief questions and <10% for all demographic variables) (Supplementary Missing data).

3.1. Comparison of LDKT and DDKT Recipients

DDKT recipients expressed greater uncertainty than LDKT recipients regarding all belief statements, with a greater proportion of DDKT than LDKT recipients selecting 'Don't know' for every question (Table 2).

The direction of belief for DDKT and LDKT recipients was the same for nine statements (Table 2). The majority of both DDKT and LDKT recipients agreed with the statements: (1) It is morally acceptable to take a kidney from a healthy person; (3) Donating a kidney is a rewarding experience for live donors; (5) A living-donor kidney transplant may strengthen the relationship between the donor and recipient; (8) It is acceptable for a parent to receive a kidney from his/her child (over 18 years old); (9) Decisions about donation should be made by the donor alone. The recipient should not ask for a kidney. The majority of both DDKT and LDKT recipients disagreed that: (4) Donating a kidney to someone requires an extremely close personal relationship; (10) Since the donor operation is not risk free, someone who needs a kidney transplant should wait for a kidney from someone who has died. For these seven statements, DDKT and LDKT recipients who indicated that they had a belief (rather than did not know) reported the same direction of belief but for all questions a greater proportion of LDKT recipients indicated a stronger belief than DDKTs.

No difference between DDKT and LDKT recipients was found with either direction or strength of belief with respect to Statement (3)—'Asking someone to donate makes the recipient seem selfish'.

Statement (6)—'Approaching a potential donor who then says no will change the relationship between the two people'—was associated with the greatest uncertainty for all participants; 36% of DDKT recipients and 34% of LDKT recipients selecting 'Don't know' for this question.

DDKT and LDKT recipients differed in the direction of their belief with respect to only one statement. For statement (2)—'Donors often agree to donate due to feelings of guilt or family pressure'—the majority of LDKT recipients disagreed whilst DDKT recipients were split between disagreement, agreement and not knowing (Table 2).

3.2. *Predictors of Case–Control Status*

The strength of agreement with seven belief statements predicted case–control status, even after adjustment for potential confounders (Table 3). A greater level of agreement with statements 1, 3, 5, and 8 predicted being an LDKT over a DDKT recipient. These statements concern the 'acceptability' of living donation and transplantation, and its 'positive effects' ('rewarding experience' and 'strengthening relationship'). A greater level of disagreement with statements 2, 6 and 10 predicted being an LDKT over a DDKT recipient. These statements relate to beliefs about individuals experiencing 'pressure to donate' and the 'risks/negative impacts of living donation'.

3.3. *Participant Characteristics and Beliefs (Table S3a–e)*

3.3.1. Sex

For only one of the ten statements, responses from women and men differed. The majority of women and men agreed with Statement 8—'It is acceptable for a parent to receive a kidney from his/her child (over 18 years old)'—but a greater proportion of women disagreed compared to men (14% versus 8%, chi^2 p-value < 0.001 across all categories of agreement).

3.3.2. Age

For four of the ten statements, older respondents indicated greater uncertainty by selecting 'Don't know' rather than indicating a direction of belief. Individuals aged ≥60 years were more likely than individuals aged <60 years to answer 'Don't know' for statement (2)—'Donors often agree to donate due to feelings of guilt or family pressure' (36% versus 24%, chi^2 p-value < 0.001 across all categories of agreement), statement (5)—'A living-donor kidney transplant may strengthen the relationship between the donor and recipient' (23% versus 16%, chi^2 p-value 0.02 across all categories of agreement), statement (6)—'Approaching a potential donor who then says no will change the relationships between the two people' (41% versus 31%, chi^2 p-value < 0.001 across all categories of agreement), and statement (7)—'Asking someone to donate makes the recipient seem selfish' (32% versus 18%, chi^2 p-value < 0.001 across all categories of agreement).

For one statement, statement (9)—'Decisions about donation should be made by the donor alone. The recipient should not ask for a kidney'—the direction of belief differed with age. People aged ≥60 years were much more likely to agree compared to people aged <60 years (73% versus 57%, chi^2 p-value < 0.001 across all categories of agreement).

Table 1. Participant characteristics by case–control status [a].

Characteristics		Cases [b] (LDKTs) $n = 672$	Controls [b] (DDKTs) $n = 565$	Chi^2 Comparing Cases and Controls
Sex	Male	382 (57)	322 (57)	$p = 0.95$
	Female	279 (42)	235 (42)	
	Missing	11 (2)	8 (1)	
Age (years)	20–29	47 (7)	27 (5)	$p = 0.39$
	30–39	80 (12)	57 (10)	
	40–49	106 (16)	102 (18)	
	50–59	178 (27)	153 (27)	
	60–69	167 (25)	132 (23)	
	>70	77 (12)	79 (14)	
	Missing	17 (3)	15 (3)	
Ethnicity	White	581 (87)	445 (79)	$p = 0.005$
	Asian	38 (6)	41 (7)	
	Black/African/Caribbean	19 (3)	39 (7)	
	Mixed/Multiple	5 (0.7)	5 (0.9)	
	Other	10 (2)	14 (3)	
	Missing	19 (3)	21 (4)	
Religion	No religion	191 (28)	144 (26)	$p = 0.01$
	Christian	402 (60)	315 (56)	
	Muslim	10 (2)	11 (2)	
	Other religions [c]	37 (6)	56 (10)	
	Missing	22 (3)	39 (7)	
Highest level of education	No formal education/Primary school	10 (2)	20 (4)	$p = 0.03$
	Secondary school	202 (30)	191 (34)	
	Vocational/Technical	171 (26)	143 (25)	
	University-undergraduate	145 (22)	98 (17)	
	University-postgraduate	73 (11)	46 (8)	
	Other	33 (5)	24 (4)	
	Missing	38 (6)	43 (8)	

[a] The three participants for whom transplant type/case–control status was missing are excluded from this table. [b] Percentages may not total 100% due to figures being presented to the nearest whole number. [c] Hindu, Jewish, Sikh, Buddhist and Other combined due to single participant responders in some groups risking identification.

Table 2. Beliefs about living donation and living-donor kidney transplantation.

Belief Statement	Transplant Type	Strongly Disagree *n* (%)	Disagreen *n* (%)	Agreen *n* (%)	Strongly Agree *n* (%)	Don't Know *n* (%)	Chi[2] *p*-Value
1. It is morally acceptable to take a kidney from a healthy person.	DDKT [a]	8 (2)	22 (4)	293 (53)	172 (31)	52 (10)	<0.001
	LDKT [a]	24 (4)	11 (2)	252 (39)	340 (52)	28 (4)	
2. Donors often agree to donate due to feelings of guilt or family pressure.	DDKT	63 (11)	172 (31)	117 (21)	22 (4)	177 (32)	<0.001
	LDKT	134 (20)	262 (40)	81 (12)	9 (1)	170 (26)	
3. Donating a kidney is a rewarding experience for the live donors.	DDKT	6 (1)	5 (0.9)	260 (47)	158 (29)	123 (22)	<0.001
	LDKT	11 (2)	4 (0.6)	269 (41)	314 (48)	60 (9)	
4. Donating a kidney to someone requires an extremely close personal relationship.	DDKT	78 (14)	286 (52)	79 (14)	47 (9)	62 (11)	0.004
	LDKT	121 (18)	331 (50)	110 (17)	59 (9)	38 (6)	
5. A living-donor kidney transplant may strengthen the relationship between the donor and recipient.	DDKT	8 (2)	55 (10)	254 (46)	77 (14)	158 (29)	<0.001
	LDKT	13 (2)	65 (10)	314 (48)	198 (30)	69 (11)	
6. Approaching a potential donor who then says no will change the relationship between the two people.	DDKT	47 (9)	185 (34)	85 (16)	33 (6)	200 (36)	0.001
	LDKT	91 (14)	235 (36)	96 (15)	14 (2)	222 (34)	
7. Asking someone to donate makes the recipient seem selfish.	DDKT	45 (8)	204 (37)	120 (22)	41 (8)	139 (25)	0.45
	LDKT	68 (10)	256 (39)	145 (22)	38 (6)	151 (23)	
8. It is acceptable for a parent to receive a kidney from his/her child (over 18 years old).	DDKT	23 (4)	45 (8)	292 (53)	106 (19)	86 (16)	0.002
	LDKT	17 (3)	40 (6)	365 (56)	169 (26)	68 (10)	
9. Decisions about donation should be made by the donor alone. The recipient should not ask for a kidney.	DDKT	19 (4)	112 (20)	203 (37)	127 (23)	90 (16)	<0.001
	LDKT	42 (6)	121 (18)	213 (32)	220 (33)	62 (9)	
10. Since the donor operation is not risk free, someone who needs a kidney transplant should wait for a kidney from someone who has died.	DDKT	87 (16)	311 (56)	52 (9)	10 (2)	92 (17)	<0.001
	LDKT	265 (40)	336 (51)	5 (0.8)	8 (1)	44 (7)	

[a] DDKT = deceased-donor kidney transplant; LDKT = living-donor kidney transplant.

Table 3. Strength of agreement and likelihood of being an LDKT recipient over a DDKT recipient.

Belief Statement	Association between Agreement with Statement and Likelihood of Being an LDKT Recipient over a DDKT Recipient		Interpretation
	Unadjusted OR (95% CI)	Adjusted OR [a] (95% CI)	
1. It is morally acceptable to take a kidney from a healthy person.	1.47 (1.26–1.71)	1.47 (1.29–1.68)	Agreement with statement predicts being an LDKT recipient
2. Donors often agree to donate due to feelings of guilt or family pressure.	0.56 (0.45–0.70)	0.57 (0.45–0.73)	Disagreement with statement predicts being an LDKT recipient
3. Donating a kidney is a rewarding experience for the live donors.	1.56 (1.24–1.94)	1.42 (1.13–1.78)	Agreement with statement predicts being an LDKT recipient
4. Donating a kidney to someone requires an extremely close personal relationship.	0.97 (0.84–1.13)	0.94 (0.79–1.12)	
5. A living-donor kidney transplant may strengthen the relationship between the donor and recipient.	1.42 (1.20–1.68)	1.45 (1.21–1.74)	Agreement with statement predicts being an LDKT recipient
6. Approaching a potential donor who then says no will change the relationship between the two people.	0.69 (0.62–0.78)	0.62 (0.55–0.71)	Disagreement with statement predicts being an LDKT recipient
7. Asking someone to donate makes the recipient seem selfish.	0.88 (0.75–1.02)	0.86 (0.71–1.04)	
8. It is acceptable for a parent to receive a kidney from his/her child (over 18 years old).	1.31 (1.10–1.56)	1.29 (1.04–1.60)	Agreement with statement predicts being an LDKT recipient
9. Decisions about donation should be made by the donor alone. The recipient should not ask for a kidney.	1.09 (0.98–1.21)	1.05 (0.95–1.19)	
10. Since the donor operation is not risk free, someone who needs a kidney transplant should wait for a kidney from someone who has died.	0.36 (0.27–0.47)	0.38 (0.27–0.54)	Disagreement with statement predicts being an LDKT recipient

[a] Adjusted for sex, 10-year age-group, ethnicity (White and Black, Asian and Minority Ethnic (BAME) groups), religion (No religion, Christian, Other), university education (university education or no university education.

3.3.3. Education

For two of the ten statements, a greater proportion of those who did not go to university disagreed with the statement compared to those who did: statement (5)—'A living-donor kidney transplant may strengthen the relationship between the donor and recipient' (13% vs. 7%, chi^2 $p = 0.008$), and statement (6)—'Approaching a potential donor who then says no will change the relationship between the two people' (49% versus 42%, chi^2 p-value 0.03). For statement (9)—'Decisions about donation should be made by the donor alone. The recipient should not ask for a kidney'—individuals without a university degree were more likely to agree than those with (66% versus 58%, chi^2 p-value 0.04).

Individuals without a university degree indicated greater uncertainty with respect to statement (7)—'Asking someone to donate makes the recipient seem selfish'—with a higher proportion selecting 'Don't know' compared to those with a university degree (26% versus 18%, chi^2 p-value 0.01).

3.3.4. Ethnicity

The majority of both white and non-white individuals agreed with statement (1) regarding the moral acceptability of taking a living-donor transplant (89% and 81%), but of the remainder, non-white individuals were more likely to select 'Don't know' than white individuals (13% versus 6%, chi^2 p value = 0.002). Statement (10)—'Since the donor operation is not risk free, someone who needs a kidney transplant should wait for a kidney from someone who has died'—generated the greatest ethnic difference in opinion: non-white individuals were less likely to say they disagreed with this statement (69% versus 85%) and more likely to indicate that they did not know (21% versus 9%, chi^2 $p < 0.001$).

3.3.5. Religion

For statement (1)—'It is morally acceptable to take a kidney from a healthy person'—a greater proportion of people from the 'Other religions' group selected 'Don't know' (13%) compared to those of no religion (5%) and Christians (7%) (Chi^2 $p = 0.01$). Similarly, for statement (3)—'Donating a kidney is a rewarding experience for the live donors'—individuals from the group comprising religions other than Christianity were less likely to agree, and more likely to select 'Don't know' (24%) compared to those of no religion (19%) and Christians (11%) (Chi^2 $p < 0.001$). For statement (10)—'Since the donor operation is not risk free, someone who needs a kidney transplant should wait for a kidney from someone who has died'—a smaller proportion of people in the 'Other religions' group said that they disagreed with this statement (65%) compared to people of no religion (89%) or Christians (89%), and a greater proportion selected 'Don't know' (24%) compared to Christians (10%) and people with no religion (8%) (chi^2 $p < 0.001$).

For statement (6)—'Approaching a potential donor who then says no will change the relationship between the two people'—a slightly greater proportion of Christians (49%) disagreed with the statement compared those of 'Other religions' (43%) or none (42%) (chi^2 $p = 0.008$).

4. Discussion

In this questionnaire-based case–control study, we compared the beliefs of LDKT and DDKT recipients about the acceptability of living kidney donation and transplantation. We found no evidence that DDKT recipients hold strong beliefs against living-donor kidney transplantation. Rather, DDKT recipients hold similar beliefs to LDKT recipients, but report less conviction and greater uncertainty. We did not investigate the source of beliefs in this questionnaire, but it would be interesting to investigate whether the greater uncertainty in the DDKT respondents influences or reflects the beliefs of family members and potential donors. Uncertainty may reflect differing or conflicting beliefs within a family regarding the acceptability of living-donor kidney transplantation.

We aimed to identify groups with beliefs against living-donor kidney transplantation that may explain observed sex, age, ethnic and socioeconomic disparities in the uptake of LDKTs. Overall, we did not find any evidence of significant difference in the direction of belief with sex, age, ethnicity, religion or education. This suggests that inequality in LDKT uptake associated with sex, age, ethnic, or socioeconomic position is not explained by disproportionately high numbers of individuals in these groups holding beliefs that are incompatible with living-donor kidney transplantation.

BAME group ethnicity and having a religious affiliation other than Christianity were both associated with greater uncertainty regarding a number of belief statements. BAME individuals were particularly uncertain as to whether one should wait for a DDKT, given that living kidney donation is not risk free. Uncertainty regarding organ donation and transplantation has previously been reported in qualitative research amongst certain ethnic and religious groups, attributed specifically to uncertainty regarding religious edicts [31,32]. One qualitative study from the Netherlands identified a lack of awareness about the 'official' position of an individual's religion regarding living organ donation within communities, and confusion due to differing interpretations of religious texts [32]. Research from the USA has shown that, amongst church-attending African-American individuals without kidney disease, 37% disagreed with living donation [33], and members of the clergy were more likely to express reservations about living donation than deceased donation (33.3% versus 16.7%) [33]. These studies suggest that faith leaders might play an important educational role, that their opinion might be influential, and that clarity over the position of the religion on living-donation needs to be made explicit [32–34]. To this end, during the preparation of this manuscript, a new fatwa clarifying Islamic approval of living and deceased organ donation and transplantation was published in the UK [35].

Older people reported greater uncertainty in their beliefs about the impact of donation on the family, and whether asking is selfish on the recipient's part. Older people have been reported as being unhappy to accept an organ from a younger living donor [36,37], in part due to parents believing they should protect their children from harm [36,37]. This belief regarding the acceptability of living-donor kidney transplantation might be influenced by clinicians: research from the USA has suggested that eligible older people with kidney disease are less likely to be encouraged to seek a transplant by their nephrologists [38].

Our findings suggest that the majority of DDKT recipients believe living kidney donation and living-donor kidney transplantation are acceptable, appropriate and justifiable. The majority of demographic groups believe that there are benefits from LDKTs to both the donor and the recipient. Given these beliefs, it suggests that there is capacity to increase LDKT activity in the UK. There should be no assumption that people of certain groups (BAME or older people) have strong beliefs against an LDKT—but rather, any uncertainty should be taken as an opportunity to engage in discussion. Attitudes towards living kidney donation are often open to change and, accordingly, can be influenced [39]. Conversations with religious leaders may help to overcome specific uncertainties regarding a particular religion's position on living donation [34,35].

The belief statements in this study were first developed and used in a Canadian population [29]. LDKT recipients and wait-listed patients surveyed in Canada were found to have the same direction of response as LDKT recipients and DDKT recipients in the UK for all statements except for Statements (4) and (10). For Statement (4)—'Donating a kidney to someone requires an extremely close personal relationship'—69% Canadian LDKT recipients agreed or strongly agreed with this statement, compared to 26% of UK LDKT recipients. For statement (10)—'Since the donor operation is not risk free, someone who needs a kidney transplant should wait for a kidney from someone who has died'—a greater proportion of UK DDKT recipients disagreed with this statement when compared to Canadian wait-listed patients (72% versus 52%). These differences may reflect transplant practice and beliefs changing over time, since the Canadian study was undertaken over 15 years earlier. However, these differences may in part explain why the UK's LDKT activity is greater than Canada's [40], and this requires further investigation.

In our study, statement (10)—'Since the donor operation is not risk free, someone who needs a kidney transplant should wait for a kidney from someone who has died'—generated the most difference in opinion; therefore, how beliefs will change with the UK's move to an opt-out deceased-donation law in 2020 will need to be investigated.

This was a large, multicentre study. To our knowledge, this is the first quantitative study to investigate beliefs about living-donor kidney transplantation amongst transplant recipients. The questionnaire was evaluated in cognitive interviews prior to use, validated and then piloted [26]. The proportion of missing data was small. However, the study has limitations: (i) Although our response rate was reasonable for an unincentivized postal survey, and compares to the response rate of other postal surveys in the UK [41,42] and that of previous a previous European transplant survey [43], there is a risk of self-selection bias. We have reported in our results that our population appeared population representative (Table S2). In addition, we compared our findings to those from the Access to Transplantation and Transplant Outcome Measures (ATTOM) study (which had 72% participation), and found the same effect sizes between socioeconomic position and likelihood of an LDKT (see Table S4) providing further evidence our sample is fairly representative of the total population of such patients. (ii) A total of 14% of participants were from BAME groups—this is not a surprising finding as in the UK between 2013 and 2017 BAME individuals comprised 17% of LDKT recipients and 27% of LDKT kidney transplant recipients [44], but this did prevent the analysis of individual ethnic groups (e.g., Asian, Black, Chinese).

The questionnaire was administered to LDKT and DDKT transplant recipients, both of whom have experienced transplantation; thus in the analyses examining the relationship between beliefs and transplant type, one might expect responses to be subject to a range of cognitive biases, including justifying their decision, and endowment effects. However, evidence against a significant endowment effect on the direction of belief includes the finding that the majority of DDKT recipients expressed positive beliefs about living donation and transplantation. Were there significant endowment effects, we would not have expected the majority of DDKT recipients to express positive beliefs about LDKTs. Cognitive biases do not explain the differences in beliefs between different demographic groups.

5. Conclusions

The majority of both DDKT and LDKT recipients across all demographic groups reported holding positive beliefs about living donation and transplantation. This encouraging finding suggests that, at least on the part of the transplant candidate, beliefs that are incompatible with LDKT are not a major barrier to living-donor transplantation in the UK, and that there is capacity to increase LDKT activity.

Author Contributions: Conceptualization, P.K.B., Y.B.-S., C.T.; Methodology, P.K.B., Y.B.-S., S.M.; Software, P.K.B.; Formal analysis, P.K.B., S.M.; Investigation, P.K.B.; Data curation, P.K.B.; Writing—original draft preparation, P.K.B.; Writing—review and editing, P.K.B., S.M., F.J.M.F.D., Y.B.-S., C.T., F.J.C.; Supervision, Y.B.-S., C.T., F.J.C.; Project administration, P.K.B.; Funding acquisition, P.K.B. All authors have read and agreed to the published version of the manuscript.

Acknowledgments: The authors would like to thank all the study participants, the participating centre research nurses and coordinators (Hugh Murtagh, Nina Bleakley, Mary Dutton, Kulli Kuningas, Cecilio Bing Andujar, Ann-Marie O'Sullivan, Nicola Johnson, Kieron Clark, Thomas Walters, Mary Quashie-Akponeware, Jane Turner, Gillian Curry, Hannah Beer, Lynn.D Langhorne, Sarah Brand, Maria Weetman, Molly Campbell, Megan Bennett, Sharirose Abat, and Agyapong Kwame Ansu) and the local collaborators who facilitated the study (Sarah Heap, Mysore Phanish, Shafi Malik, Aisling Courtney, Adnan Sharif, Nicholas Torpey, Refik Gökmen, Michael Picton, Linda Bisset, Edward Sharples, and Simon Curran).

References

1. Cecka, J. Living donor transplants. *Clin. Transplant.* **1995**, *10*, 363–377.
2. Terasaki, P.; Cecka, J.; Gjertson, D.; Takemoto, S. High survival rates of kidney transplants from spousal and living unrelated donors. *N. Engl. J. Med.* **1995**, *333*, 333–336. [CrossRef] [PubMed]
3. Laupacis, A.; Keown, P.; Pus, N.; Krueger, H.; Ferguson, B.; Wong, C.; Muirhead, N. A study of the quality of life and cost-utility of renal transplantation. *Kidney Int.* **1996**, *50*, 235–242. [CrossRef] [PubMed]
4. Cecka, J. The OPTN/UNOS Renal Transplant Registry. *Clin. Transpl.* **2005**, 1–16.
5. Roodnat, J.I.; van Riemsdijk, I.C.; Mulder, P.G.H.; Doxiadis, I.; Claas, F.H.J.; Ijzermans, J.N.M.; van Gelder, T.; Weimar, W. The superior results of living-donor renal transplantation are not completely caused by selection or short cold ischemia time: A single-center, multivariate analysis. *Transplantation* **2003**, *75*, 2014–2018. [CrossRef]
6. Statistics and Clinical Audit: NHS Blood and Transplant Organ Donation and Transplantation Activity Report 2013/14. Available online: https://nhsbtdbe.blob.core.windows.net/umbraco-assets-corp/1286/activity_report_2013_14.pdf (accessed on 20 December 2019).
7. Barnieh, L.; Manns, B.; Klarenbach, S.; McLaughlin, K.; Yilmaz, S.; Hemmelgarn, B. A description of the costs of living and standard criteria deceased donor kidney transplantation. *Am. J. Transplant.* **2011**, *11*, 478–488. [CrossRef]
8. Smith, C.; Woodward, R.; Cohen, D.; Singer, G.; Brennan, D.; Lowell, J.; Howard, T.; Schnitzler, M. Cadaveric versus living donor kidney transplantation: A Medicare payment analysis. *Transplantation* **2000**, *69*, 311–314. [CrossRef]
9. Maggiore, U.; Budde, K.; Heemann, U.; Hilbrands, L.; Oberbauer, R.; Oniscu, G.; Pascual, J.; Schwartz Sorensen, S.; Viklicky, O.; Abramowicz, D. Long-term risks of kidney living donation: Review and position paper by the ERA-EDTA DESCARTES working group. *Nephrol. Dial. Transplant.* **2017**, *32*, 216–223. [CrossRef]
10. Muzaale, A.D.; Massie, A.B.; Wang, M.; Montgomery, R.; McBride, M.; Wainright, J.; Segev, D. Risk of end-stage renal disease following live kidney donation. *JAMA* **2014**, *311*, 579–586. [CrossRef]
11. Massie, A.; Muzaale, A.; Luo, X.; Chow, E.; Locke, J.; Nguyen, A.; Henderson, M.; Snyder, J.; Segev, D. Quantifying Postdonation Risk of ESRD in Living Kidney Donors. *J. Am. Soc. Nephrol.* **2017**, *28*, 2749–2755. [CrossRef]
12. Segev, D.L.; Muzaale, A.D.; Caffo, B.S.; Mehta, S.; Singer, A.; Taranto, S.; McBride, M.; Montgomery, R. Perioperative mortality and long-term survival following live kidney donation. *JAMA* **2010**, *303*, 959–966. [CrossRef] [PubMed]
13. Lumsdaine, J.A.; Wray, A.; Power, M.J.; Jamieson, N.V.; Akyol, M.; Andrew Bradley, J.; Forsythe, J.L.R.; Wigmore, S.J. Higher quality of life in living donor kidney transplantation: Prospective cohort study. *Transpl. Int.* **2005**, *18*, 975–980. [CrossRef] [PubMed]
14. Johnson, E.; Anderson, J.; Jacobs, C.; Suh, G.; Humar, A.; Suhr, B.; Kerr, S.; AJ, M. Long-term follow-up of living kidney donors: Quality of life after donation. *Transplantation* **1999**, *67*, 717–721. [CrossRef] [PubMed]
15. Statistics and Clinical Audit: NHS Blood and Transplant Organ Donation and Transplantation Activity Report 2017/18. Available online: https://nhsbtdbe.blob.core.windows.net/umbraco-assets-corp/12300/transplant-activity-report-2017-2018.pdf (accessed on 20 December 2019).
16. Udayaraj, U.; Ben-Shlomo, Y.; Roderick, P.; Casula, A.; Dudley, C.; Collett, D.; Ansell, D.; Tomson, C.; Caskey, F. Social Deprivation, Ethnicity, and Uptake of Living Kidney Donor Transplantation in the United Kingdom. *Transplantation* **2012**, *93*, 610–616. [CrossRef] [PubMed]
17. Wu, D.; Robb, M.; Watson, C.; Forsythe, J.; Tomson, C.; Cairns, J.; Roderick, P.; Johnson, R.; Ravanan, R.; Fogarty, D.; et al. Barriers to living donor kidney transplantation in the United Kingdom: A national observational study. *Nephrol. Dial. Transplant.* **2017**, *32*, 890–900. [CrossRef] [PubMed]
18. Kayler, L.; Rasmussen, C.; Dykstra, D.; Ojo, A.; Port, F.; Wolfe, R.; Merion, R. Gender imbalance and outcomes in living donor renal transplantation in the United States. *Am. J. Transplant.* **2003**, *3*, 452–458. [CrossRef] [PubMed]
19. Ojo, A.; Port, F. Influence of race and gender on related donor renal transplantation rates. *Am. J. Kidney Dis.* **1993**, *22*, 835–841. [CrossRef]
20. Lentine, K.; Kasiske, B.; Levey, A.; Adams, P.; Alberú, J.; Bakr, M.; Gallon, L.; Garvey, C.; Guleria, S.; Li, P.; et al. KDIGO Clinical Practice Guideline on the Evaluation and Care of Living Kidney Donors. *Transplantation* **2017**, *101*, S1–S109. [CrossRef]

21. Karet Frankl, F.; Coward, R.; Gallagher, H.; Hilton, R.; Loud, F.; Modi, K.; Ormandy, P.; Woolf, A. *UK Renal Research Strategy*; UK Kidney Research Consortium: Cambridgeshire, UK, 2016; Available online: https://kidneyresearchuk.org/wp-content/uploads/2019/02/KR9501-UKRRS-Booklet-V8-WEB.pdf (accessed on 20 December 2019).
22. Rodrigue, J.; Kazley, A.; Mandelbrot, D.; Hays, R.; LaPointe Rudow, D.; Baliga, P. Living Donor Kidney Transplantation: Overcoming Disparities in Live Kidney Donation in the US-Recommendations from a Consensus Conference. *Clin. J. Am. Soc. Nephrol.* **2015**, *10*, 1687–1695. [CrossRef]
23. Martínez-Alarcón, L.; Ríos, A.; Conesa, C.; Alcaraz, J.; González, M.J.; Ramírez, P.; Parrilla, P. Attitude of kidney patients on the transplant waiting list toward related-living donation. A reason for the scarce development of living donation in Spain. *Clin. Transplant.* **2006**, *20*, 719–724. [CrossRef]
24. Zimmerman, D. The influence of socio-demographic factors, treatment perceptions and attitudes to living donation on willingness to consider living kidney donor among kidney transplant candidates. *Nephrol. Dial. Transplant.* **2006**, *21*, 2569–2576. [CrossRef] [PubMed]
25. *StataCorp 2017*; Release 15; Stata Statistical Software; StataCorp LLC: College Station, TX, USA, 2017.
26. Bailey, P.; Tomson, C.; Ben-Shlomo, Y. What factors explain the association between socioeconomic deprivation and reduced likelihood of live-donor kidney transplantation? A questionnaire based pilot case-control study. *BMJ Open* **2016**, *6*. [CrossRef]
27. Harris, P.; Taylor, R.; Thielke, R.; Payne, J.; Gonzalez, N.; Conde, J. Research electronic data capture (REDCap)–a metadata-driven methodology and workflow process for providing translational research informatics support. *J. Biomed. Inform.* **2009**, *42*, 377–381. [CrossRef] [PubMed]
28. Stothers, L.; Gourlay, W.; Liu, L. Attitudes and predictive factors for live kidney donation: A comparison of live kidney donors versus nondonors. *Kidney Int.* **2005**, *67*, 1105–1111. [CrossRef] [PubMed]
29. Gourlay, W.; Stothers, L.; Liu, L. Attitudes and predictive factors for live kidney donation in British Columbia. A comparison of recipients and wait-list patients. *Can. J. Urol.* **2005**, *12*, 2511–2520. [PubMed]
30. O'Brien, R.; Potter-Collins, A. *2011 Census Analysis: Ethnicity and Religion of the non-UK Born Population in England and Wales: 2011*; Office for National Statistics: South Wales, UK, 2015. Available online: https://www.ons.gov.uk/peoplepopulationandcommunity/culturalidentity/ethnicity/articles/2011censusanalysisethnicityandreligionofthenonukbornpopulationinenglandandwales/2015-06-18 (accessed on 20 December 2019).
31. Irving, M.; Tong, A.; Jan, S.; Cass, A.; Rose, J.; Chadban, S.; Allen, R.; Craig, J.; Wong, G.; Howard, K. Factors that influence the decision to be an organ donor: A systematic review of the qualitative literature. *Nephrol. Dial. Transplant.* **2012**, *27*, 2526–2533. [CrossRef] [PubMed]
32. Ismail, S.; Massey, E.; Luchtenburg, A.; Claassens, L.; Zuidema, W.; Busschbach, J.; Weimar, W. Religious attitudes towards living kidney donation among Dutch renal patients. *Med. Health Care Philos.* **2012**, *15*, 221–227. [CrossRef]
33. Locke, J.; Qu, H.; Shewchuk, R.; Mannon, R.; Gaston, R.; Segev, D.; Mannon, E.; Martin, M. Identification of strategies to facilitate organ donation among African Americans using the nominal group technique. *Clin. J. Am. Soc. Nephrol.* **2015**, *10*, 286–293. [CrossRef]
34. Afzal Aghaee, M.; Dehghani, M.; Sadeghi, M.; Khaleghi, E. Awareness of Religious Leaders' Fatwa and Willingness to Donate Organ. *Int. J. Organ Transplant. Med.* **2015**, *6*, 158–164.
35. *New Fatwa to Clarify Lslamic Position on Organ Donation*; NHS Blood and Transplant: Filton, UK, 19 June 2019; Available online: https://www.organdonation.nhs.uk/get-involved/news/new-fatwa-published-to-clarify-islamic-position-on-organ-donation/ (accessed on 20 December 2019).
36. Hanson, C.; Chadban, S.; Chapman, J.; Craig, J.; Wong, G.; Ralph, A.; Tong, A. The Expectations and Attitudes of Patients with Chronic Kidney Disease Toward Living Kidney Donor Transplantation: A Thematic Synthesis of Qualitative Studies. *Transplantation* **2015**, *99*, 540–554. [CrossRef]
37. Gordon, E. "They don't have to suffer for me": Why dialysis patients refuse offers of living donor kidneys. *Med. Anthropol. Q.* **2001**, *15*, 245–267. [CrossRef] [PubMed]
38. Gordon, E.; Sehgal, A. Patient-nephrologist discussions about kidney transplantation as a treatment option. *Adv. Ren. Replace. Ther.* **2000**, *7*, 177–183. [CrossRef] [PubMed]
39. Hilhorst, M.; Kranenburg, L.; Busschbach, J. Should health care professionals encourage living kidney donation? *Med. Health Care Philos.* **2007**, *10*, 81–90. [CrossRef] [PubMed]
40. International Registry in Organ Donation and Transplantation (IRODaT) Database. Available online: http://www.irodat.org/?p=database (accessed on 20 December 2019).

41. Robb, K.; Gatting, L.; Wardle, J. What impact do questionnaire length and monetary incentives have on mailed health psychology survey response? *Br. J. Health Psychol.* **2017**, *22*, 671–685. [CrossRef] [PubMed]
42. Harrison, S.; Henderson, J.; Alderdice, F.; Quigley, M. Methods to increase response rates to a population-based maternity survey: A comparison of two pilot studies. *BMC Med. Res. Methodol.* **2019**, *19*, 65. [CrossRef] [PubMed]
43. Slaats, D.; Lennerling, A.; Pronk, M.; van der Pant, K.; Dooper, I.; Wierdsma, J.; Schrauwers, C.; Maple, H.; van de Wetering, J.; Weimar, W.; et al. Donor and Recipient Perspectives on Anonymity in Kidney Donation From Live Donors: A Multicenter Survey Study. *Am. J. Kidney Dis.* **2018**, *71*, 52–64. [CrossRef] [PubMed]
44. Organ Donation and Transplantation Data for Black, Asian and Minority Ethnic (BAME) Communities. NHS Blood and Transplant. Report for 2017/2018 (1 April 2013–31 March 2018). Available online: https://nhsbtdbe.blob.core.windows.net/umbraco-assets-corp/12048/bame-organ-donation-and-transplantation-data-2017-18.pdf (accessed on 20 December 2019).

10

Targeted Urine Metabolomics for Monitoring Renal Allograft Injury and Immunosuppression in Pediatric Patients

Tara K. Sigdel, Andrew W. Schroeder †, Joshua Y. C. Yang †, Reuben D. Sarwal, Juliane M. Liberto and Minnie M. Sarwal *

Division of Transplant Surgery, Department of Surgery, University of California San Francisco, San Francisco, CA 94143, USA; tara.sigdel@ucsf.edu (T.K.S.); andrew.schroeder@ucsf.edu (A.W.S.); joshua.yang@alumni.ucsf.edu (J.Y.C.Y.); reuben.sarwal@ucsf.edu (R.D.S.); jlibert7@jhmi.edu (J.M.L.)

* Correspondence: minnie.sarwal@ucsf.edu

† Authors contributed equally.

Abstract: Despite new advancements in surgical tools and therapies, exposure to immunosuppressive drugs related to non-immune and immune injuries can cause slow deterioration and premature failure of organ transplants. Diagnosis of these injuries by non-invasive urine monitoring would be a significant clinical advancement for patient management, especially in pediatric cohorts. We investigated the metabolomic profiles of biopsy matched urine samples from 310 unique kidney transplant recipients using gas chromatography–mass spectrometry (GC-MS). Focused metabolite panels were identified that could detect biopsy confirmed acute rejection with 92.9% sensitivity and 96.3% specificity (11 metabolites) and could differentiate BK viral nephritis (BKVN) from acute rejection with 88.9% sensitivity and 94.8% specificity (4 metabolites). Overall, targeted metabolomic analyses of biopsy-matched urine samples enabled the generation of refined metabolite panels that non-invasively detect graft injury phenotypes with high confidence. These urine biomarkers can be rapidly assessed for non-invasive diagnosis of specific transplant injuries, opening the window for precision transplant medicine.

Keywords: kidney transplantation; metabolomics; immunosuppression; urine; acute rejection; immunosuppression; allograft

---

1. Introduction

Kidney transplantation (KTx) is the preferred method of treatment for end-stage kidney failure [1]. Increasing the longevity of transplanted kidneys is critical because of the shortage of available kidneys and kidney donors [2]. While improved short-term survival of the transplanted kidney has been attributed to better immunosuppressive drugs and sophistication in organ procurement and surgical methods [3], long-term survival outcomes have largely remained limited and unchanged [4]. Currently used methods of KTx monitoring, such as patient serum creatinine and proteinuria, are neither sufficiently sensitive nor specific to detect early-stage injury and only detect advanced and often irreversible tissue injury [5]. Additionally, kidney biopsies cannot easily be used to predict injury [6,7]. Over recent years, the application of high throughput technologies towards a more discovery-based approach for correlative biomarkers of graft injury have utilized sequencing [8] gene expression, proteomic [9–14], and metabolomic methods [15,16]. Many of these approaches show background signals of other clinical confounders, such as immunosuppression exposure [17], and thus require the application of more customized and robust analytical techniques for improving the diagnostic accuracy of biomarkers in blood and urine to reflect different transplant (Tx) injury phenotypes [18–20].

In this study, we hypothesized that the recipient's immune response towards the graft induces immunological and downstream metabolic changes at the time of specific injuries, such as acute rejection (AR), which result in perturbations in specific urine metabolite concentrations. We also hypothesized that specific metabolic pathways are injury-specific such that a panel of metabolites can be used as a surrogate biomarker to monitor KTx injuries. In this report, we present our findings from a comprehensive targeted metabolomics analysis of urine collected from pediatric KTx patients. These samples have been biopsy matched, providing an accurate phenotype characterization, and enabling exploration of metabolic pathways associated with KTx dysfunction.

2. Experimental Section

2.1. Patients and Samples

Biobanked urine samples available in the Sarwal lab from previously funded studies were screened for matching biopsy data on the day of urine collection. Out of a total of 2016 biobanked urine samples collected between 2006 and 2009, 770 were biopsy-matched, of which 326 unique and clinically annotated urine samples were included in the first part of this study. These patients were on calcineurin inhibitor (CNI) based immunosuppression (IS). All urine samples were stored at −80 °C with urine processing techniques, procedures, and conditions in which we have previously shown negligible degradation of urine components [11].

All samples from our biobank were matched with transplant biopsies; all biopsies were read by a central pathologist and scored by the Banff and Chronic Allograft Damage Index (CADI) [21–23] as acute cellular or humoral rejection with clinical graft dysfunction, and tubulitis and/or vasculitis on histology (AR; $n = 106$) [24], stable with no histological or clinical graft injury (stable graft function (STA); $n = 111$), interstitial fibrosis and tubular atrophy (IFTA; $n = 71$) [25], and BK viral nephritis with SV40 staining on histology, with/without clinical graft dysfunction (BK viral nephritis (BKVN); $n = 22$). Intragraft C4d stains were performed to assess for antibody-mediated rejection (ABMR). AR was defined, at minimum, by the following criteria: (i) TCMR consisting of either a tubulitis (t) score > 2 accompanied by an interstitial inflammation score > 2 or vascular changes (v) score > 0; (ii) C4d-positive ABMR consisting of positive donor-specific antibodies (DSAs) with a glomerulitis (g) score > 0 or peritubular capillaritis score (ptc) > 0 or v > 0 with unexplained acute tubular necrosis/thrombotic microangiopathy (ATN/TMA) with C4d = 2; or (iii) C4d-negative ABMR consisting of positive DSA with unexplained ATN/TMA with g + ptc ≥ 2 and C4d = 0 or 1. Stable allografts were defined by an absence of substantial injury on the matched biopsy pathology and definitions of the inflammation or i score and the tubulitis or t score. IFTA used standard pathology definitions as described by the Banff schema on the paired biopsies from each individual urine sample.

This study was conducted in accordance with the relevant guidelines and regulations as approved by the University of California San Francisco (UCSF) Human Research Protection Program Institutional Review Board (IRB) under IRB #14-13573. All patients provided written informed consent. In cases of pediatric and young adult patients, written informed consent was obtained from a parent and/or legal guardian to participate in the research, in full adherence to the Declaration of Helsinki. The clinical and research activities being reported are consistent with the Principles of the Declaration of Istanbul as outlined in the 'Declaration of Istanbul on Organ Trafficking and Transplantation Tourism'. As such, no organs or tissues were procured from prisoners. All organs or tissues were procured from the Departments of Surgery at either UCSF or Stanford University.

2.2. Urine Collection, Initial Processing, Storage, and GC/MS-TOF Analysis

Second morning void mid-stream urine (50–100 mL) was collected in sterile containers and was centrifuged at 2000× *g* for 20 min at room temperature within 1 h of collection. Specifically, the urine specimens were collected in sterile polypropylene collection tubes that are leak-resistant with a sterility seal. Processing of the urine was done all in one bath with sterile polypropylene plastic tubes. The supernatant was separated from the pellet containing any particulate matter including cells and cell debris. The pH of the supernatant was adjusted to 7.0 with Tris-HCL and stored at −80 °C in polypropylene plastic tubes until further analysis. The identification of metabolites followed the well-established FiehnLib protocol [26]. In brief, all metabolite reference standards underwent a two-step derivatization procedure following the previously published protocol [27]. The derivatization of urine metabolites procedure has been described previously [27]. Briefly, neat urine samples were lyophilized without further pretreatment after our initial finding of severe alterations using urease treatments. To the dried samples, 20 µL of 40 mg/mL methoxylamine hydrochloride in pyridine was added, and samples were agitated at 30 °C for 30 min. Subsequently, 180 µL of trimethylsilylating agent *N*-methyl-*N*-trimethylsilyltrifluoroacetamide (MSTFA) was added, and samples were agitated at 37 °C for 30 min. GC–MS analysis was performed using an Agilent 6890 N gas chromatograph (Atlanta, GA, USA) interfaced to a time-of-flight (TOF) Pegasus III mass spectrometer (Leco, St. Joseph, MI, USA) [27]. Automated injections were performed with a programmable robotic Gerstel MPS2 multipurpose sampler (Mülheim an der Ruhr, Germany). The GC was fitted with both an Agilent injector and a Gerstel temperature-programmed injector, cooled injection system (model CIS 4), with a Peltier cooling source. An automated liner exchange (ALEX) designed by Gerstel was used to eliminate cross-contamination from sample matrix occurring between sample runs. Multiple baffled liners for the GC inlet were deactivated with 1 µL injections of MSTFA. The Agilent injector temperature was held constant at 250 °C while the Gerstel injector was programmed (initial temperature 50 °C, hold 0.1 min, and increased at a rate of 10 °C/s to a final temperature of 330 °C, hold time 10 min). Injections of 1 µL were made in split (1:5) mode (purge time 120 s, purge flow 40 mL/min). Chromatography was performed on a Rtx-5Sil MS column (30 m × 0.25 mm inner diameter (i.d.), 0.25 µm film thickness) with an Integra-Guard column (Restek, Bellefonte, PA, USA). Helium carrier gas was used at a constant flow of 1 mL/min. The GC oven temperature program was initially 50 °C with a 1-min hold time and ramping at 20 °C/min to a final temperature of 330 °C with a 5-min hold time before cool-down for a 20 min run time. MS parameters were based on Autotune using FC43 (Perfluorotributylamine) with manufacturer-specific tune settings. Transfer line temperature was 250 °C and electron impact ionization was set at 70 eV. Filament source temperature was at 250 °C and TOF at room temperature. After a solvent delay of 350 s, mass spectra were acquired at 20 scans/s with a mass range of 50 to 500 *m/z*. Initial peak detection and mass spectrum deconvolution were performed with Leco Chroma-TOF software (version 2.25, Leco) and samples were exported to the netCDF format for further data evaluation with MZmine [28] and XCMS [29].

2.3. *Raw Data Processing and Statistics*

All chromatograms were assessed in the same manner by software packages MZmine [28] and XCMS [29]. These packages performed peak finding in an automated and unbiased way using the common MS netCDF file format that enables a unique way of data export irrespective of different instrument platforms. For the raw GC–MS data, the netCDF export function from the Leco ChromaTOF software was used. For MZmine, the *m/z* bin size was set to 0.01, the chromatographic threshold level was set to 0.5, the absolute intensity threshold was set to 2500, the tolerance in *m/z* values was set to 0.5, the tolerance in intensity was set to 1.0, and the minimum peak length was set to 2 s.

The raw data was normalized using urine creatinine, as an internal control, measured as a part of urine metabolome assessment and quantile normalization for batch correction. Moreover, 310 biopsy-matched urine samples, with resulting panels of 266 metabolites, were used for the analyses of both post-transplant injury classification and significant metabolite selection. Non-parametric imputation was applied to these samples via the missForest algorithm [30]. If more there was missing data on more than one-third of the metabolites, these samples were excluded. Sixteen samples met this criterion.

Clustering was performed and visualized with Morpheus (Broad Institute) using average linkage hierarchical clustering. The log-transformed data was median centered, per metabolite, prior to clustering for better visualization. One minus Pearson's correlation was used for the similarity metric. A fire color scheme was used in heat maps of the metabolites. Z-score analysis scaled each metabolite according to a reference distribution.

To evaluate the performance of the classification models, these 310 samples were randomly assigned to training (75%) and test (25%) sets. To avoid overfitting, 10-fold cross-validation was performed for models on the training set. The primary statistical learning method used for allograft outcome classification was Random Forests [31] via the randomForest package in R. Significant metabolites were selected from the Random Forests model using the VSURF package in R [32]. Additionally, for visualization of significant metabolites, volcano plots were produced using variable importance values derived from Random Forests models as a significance measure. Metabolite selection was done by Bonferroni-corrected *p*-value in addition to VSURF to display a traditional volcano plot and directly compare VSURF to traditional t-testing methods and their resulting metabolite lists. These variable importance scores are defined as the mean percentage decrease in classification accuracy of the model if the metabolite data were to be randomly permuted rather than taken as quantified (a higher score denotes a higher variable importance). Comparison of classification models was done by computing and plotting area under the curve (AUC) from the receiver operating characteristic (ROC) using the pROC package in R. Statistical comparison between full and abbreviated metabolite models to assess diagnostic accuracy similarity was carried out using the DeLong's test [33]. Given that certain clinical data variables were significantly different between groups, these variables were reviewed for any association with particular variable differences within or between groups and their impact on metabolite signatures of different transplant phenotypes. Analysis was performed using the R statistical software version 3.4.3. MetaboAnalyst (www.metaboanalyst.ca) was used to perform targeted pathway and enrichment analysis [34].

2.4. Data Availability

The datasets generated during and analyzed during the current study are not publicly available due to legacy IRB consent restrictions on public sharing of data from these patient populations but are available from the corresponding author on reasonable request.

3. Results

3.1. Metabolites in Urine Are Perturbed in Different Transplant Injuries in Kidney Transplantation

We processed 326 urine samples for a targeted metabolomics assay that identified 266 metabolites. Figure 1 summarizes the study. Sixteen samples had missing data on more than one third of total metabolites identified following a tool called MissForest on non-parametric missing value imputation for mixed-type data [30]. Metabolomics data on the remaining 310 biopsy-matched urine samples was used for the analyses of both post-Tx injury detection and associated metabolic pathways and their enrichment. Baseline characteristics of the study subjects is provided in Table 1.

The data was used for supervised clustering to generate a heat map (Figure 2A) and z-score plot (Figure 2B). The heatmap shows heterogeneity in overall metabolome data across urine samples from different phenotypes. In the z-score plot, stable-based z-scores were plotted for each of the 266 metabolites. The plots revealed robust metabolic alterations in AR (z-score range: −4.2 to 800.5) and IFTA (z-score range: −3.8 to 265.4) compared to fewer changes in BKVN samples (z-score range: −3.4 to 116.9).

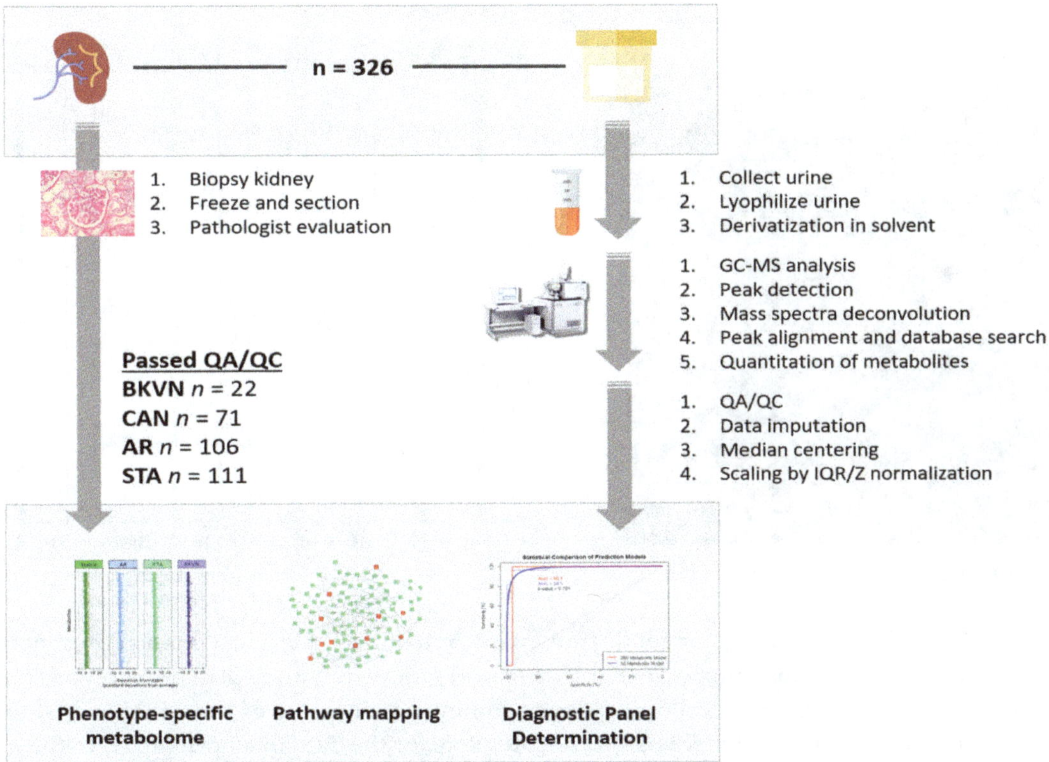

Figure 1. Sample selection and study schematic of the study. Summary outlining study samples, assay platform, study phenotypes, analysis, and results.

Table 1. Patient demographic data for the discovery cohort.

Phenotype	AR	STA	IFTA	BKVN	*p*-Value
Number of Patients	106	111	71	22	
Maintenance (% Steroid-free)	63.2%	50.5%	56.3%	36.4%	0.078
Recipient Gender (% M)	64.2%	58.6%	67.6%	59.1%	0.002
Recipient Age * (years)	13 ± 5 (14; 2–21)	14 ± 5 (15; 1–21)	10 ± 6 (10; 1–20)	14 ± 5 (17; 1–18)	0.003
Donor Gender (% M)	46.2%	52.3%	52.1%	72.7%	0.123
Donor Age * (years)	29 ± 11 (29; 4–50)	30 ± 10 (28; 14–51)	30 ± 10 (32; 12–50)	28 ± 10 (29; 16–49)	0.353
Month post-Tx (mean ± SD)	71 ± 32	15 ± 24	23 ± 32	8 ± 7	0.311
Donor Source (%): 1 = Living Related 2 = Living Unrelated 3 = Deceased	 1 = 24.5% 2 = 40.6% 3 = 34.0%	 1 = 37.8% 2 = 8.1% 3 = 44.1%	 1 = 43.7% 2 = 8.5% 3 = 47.9%	 1 = 9.1% 2 = 31.8% 3 = 54.5%	
Recipient Race (%): 1 = Caucasian 2 = Asian 3 = African American 4 = Hispanic 5 = Mixed and Others	 1 = 42.5% 2 = 5.7% 3 = 16.0% 4 = 7.5% 5 = 12.3%	 1 = 43.2% 2 = 4.5% 3 = 18.0% 4 = 2.7% 5 = 16.2%	 1 = 50.7% 2 = 7.0% 3 = 18.3% 4 = 5.6% 5 = 9.9%	 1 = 27.3% 2 = 0.0% 3 = 13.6% 4 = 18.2% 5 = 0.0%	
HLA Mismatch	4.64 ± 1.41	4.15 ± 1.35	3.62 ± 1.67	4.80 ± 1.15	0.245
eGFR	75.3 ± 42.3	95.4 ± 28.5	104.1 ± 36.7	N/A #	0.171

* Age in years: mean ± SD (median; range). AR, acute rejection; STA, stable graft function; IFTA, interstitial fibrosis and tubular atrophy; BKVN, BK virus nephropathy. # Estimated glomerular filtration rate (eGFR) data were unavailable for BKVN samples. Immunosuppression consisted of Tacrolimus and Mycophenolate Mofetil for all patients, with maintenance steroids for those on steroid-based immunosuppression. All patients received IL2R monoclonal antibody (Daclizumab) induction; steroid-based patients received this for 2 months and steroid-free patients received this for 6 months. Most patients were unsensitized and recipients for first allografts, with 4 repeat transplants. Of the 106 AR, 29 were ABMR. The clinical data variables that were significantly different between groups were assessed for any statistical association with their impact on metabolite signatures of different transplant phenotypes and were not found to be significant.

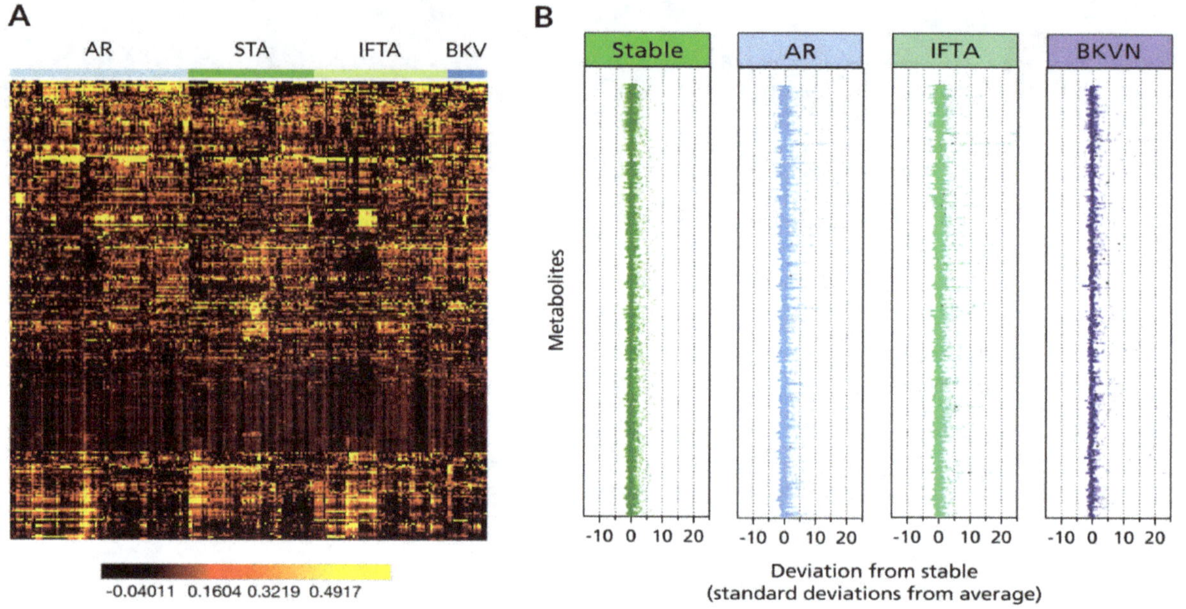

Figure 2. Metabolomic profiling of renal transplant outcomes. (**A**) Heat map representation of unsupervised hierarchical clustering by metabolite (rows) grouped by transplant phenotype (columns). Shades of black to red to orange to yellow represent continuous increases of a metabolite relative to the median metabolite levels (see color scale). (**B**) z-score plots for the data in a normalized to the mean of the stable phenotype urine samples (truncated at 25 s.d. for clarity).

3.2. Metabolite Marker Panel for Alloimmune Injury

Applying the VSURF method, a panel of 9 metabolites (Table 2) were selected out of 266 to accurately classify post-Tx alloimmune injury, combining the output from samples with either acute or chronic alloimmune injury (AR/IFTA) versus stable (STA) samples. The resulting model had a 95% accuracy of correctly discriminating between the two outcome groups (AUC = 0.950, sensitivity = 95.3%, specificity = 75.9%). This lower specificity is likely due to within group heterogeneity between AR and IFTA phenotypes. The 9 metabolite VSURF model was nearly identical in accuracy to the full 266-metabolite model, which had an AUC of 0.954. This difference in AUC values was not significant using DeLong's test ($p = 0.731$), meaning there is no significant change in classification accuracy between the full and abbreviated metabolite models (Figure 3A). This suggests that no diagnostic accuracy is lost in using the abbreviated metabolite model.

Table 2. Transplant phenotype-specific metabolite markers.

Injury-Specific ($n = 9$)	AR ($n = 11$)	BKVN ($n = 5$)
Glycine	Glycine	Arabinose
N-methylalanine	Glutaric acid	2-hydroxy-2-methylbutanoic acid
Adipic acid	Adipic acid	Hypoxanthine
Glutaric acid	Inulobiose	Benzyl alcohol
Inulobiose	Threose	*N*-acetyl-D-mannosamine
Threitol	Sulfuric acid	
Isothreitol	Taurine	
Sorbitol	*N*-methylalanine	
Isothreonic acid	Asparagine	
	5-aminovaleric acid lactam	
	Myo-inositol	

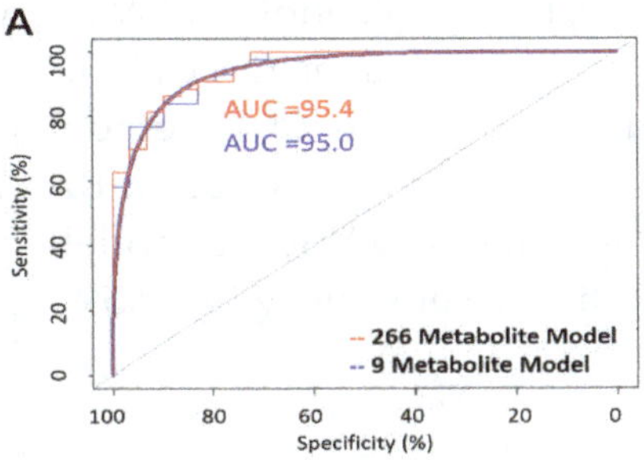

Injury Markers	*p*-value
glycine	6.54×10^{-10}
N-methylalanine	1.39×10^{-06}
adipic acid	4.60×10^{-03}
glutaric acid	1.32×10^{-06}
inulobiose	2.80×10^{-12}
threitol	4.33×10^{-08}
isothreitol	4.18×10^{-01}
sorbitol	1.32×10^{-02}
isothreonic acid	6.43×10^{-04}

Comparison of renal injury-specific metabolite models			
	AUC	Se/Sp	PPV/NPV
266 met. model	95.4	97.7/72.4	84.0/95.5
9 met. model	95.0	95.3/75.9	85.4/91.7

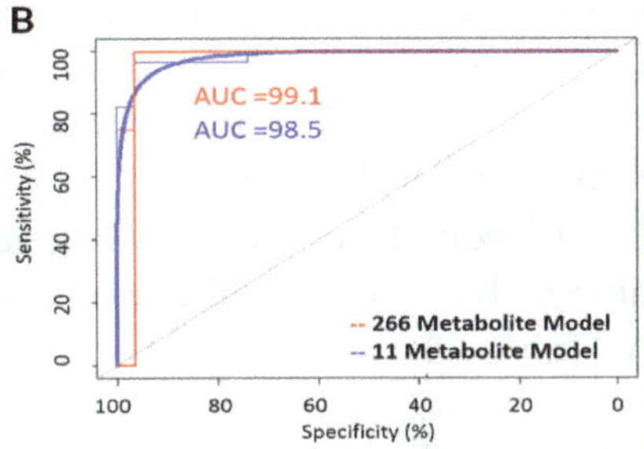

AR Markers	*p*-value
glycine	6.54×10^{-10}
glutaric acid	1.32×10^{-06}
adipic acid	4.60×10^{-03}
inulobiose	2.80×10^{-12}
threose	2.90×10^{-02}
sulfuric acid	5.23×10^{-06}
taurine	2.22×10^{-10}
N-methylalanine	1.39×10^{-06}
asparagine	1.21×10^{-02}
5-aminovaleric acid lactame	2.98×10^{-05}
myo-inositol	7.76×10^{-07}

Comparison AR-specific metabolite models			
	AUC	Se/Sp (%)	PPV/NPV (%)
266 met. model	99.1	85.7/96.3	96.0/86.7
11 met. model	98.5	92.9/96.3	96.3/92.9

Figure 3. Identification of potential biomarker panel of metabolites for KTx alloimmune injury and acute rejection using VSURF method. (**A**) Two receiver operating characteristic (ROC) curves representing classification accuracies and a statistical comparison of the full and sparse RF models for alloimmune injury and the table displaying classification accuracy on the test set. The metabolites in the panel are listed on the right-hand side (**B**) Two ROC curves representing classification accuracies and a statistical comparison of the full and sparse Random Forests (RF) models for acute rejection (AR) injury and the bottom table displaying classification accuracy on the test set. The metabolites in the panel are listed on the right-hand side.

3.3. Metabolite Marker Panel for Acute Rejection

In order to identify a metabolite marker panel specific to acute rejection of KTx, we applied VSURF exclusively to the AR and STA urine metabolome datasets (n = 217). The resulting model contained 11 metabolites (Table 2) for AR detection. The ROC analysis resulted with an AUC of 0.985 with 92.9% sensitivity and 96.3% specificity (Figure 3B). Individual distributions for the three most significant metabolites, glycine, *N*-methylalanine, and inulobiose, are presented in the form of bean plots (Figure 4).

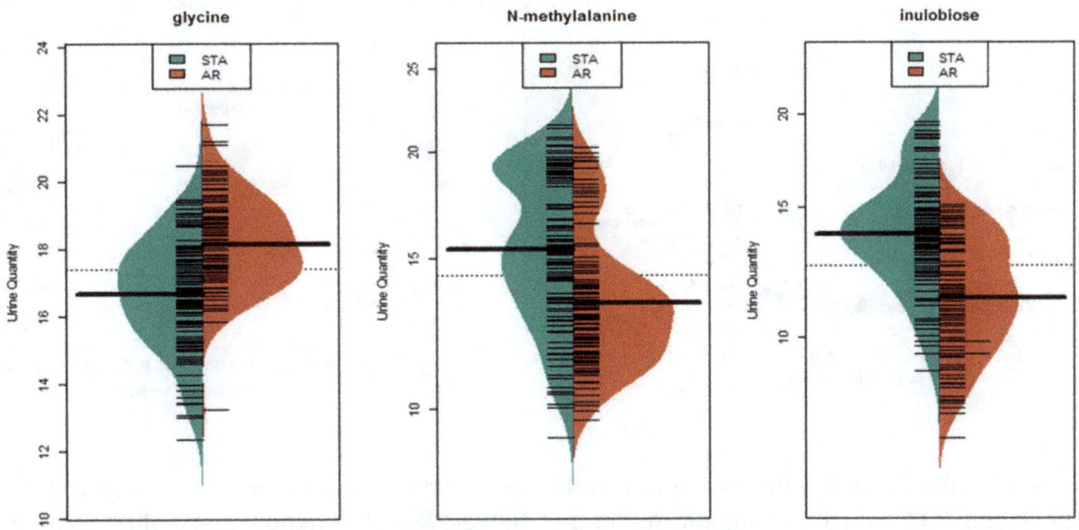

Figure 4. Significantly altered metabolites in AR versus STA. Bean plots demonstrating distribution of the 3 most significant metabolites in AR comparing to STA. The bold horizontal line represents mean value for each group.

3.4. Metabolite Marker Panel for BK Virus Nephritis

In order to identify BKVN-specific metabolites, we used VSURF on 22 BKVN urine and 288 non-BKVN urine that included AR, IFTA, and STA urine. The resulting VSURF panel contained 5 metabolites, Arabinose, 2-hydroxy-2-methylbutanoic acid, hypoxanthine, benzyl alcohol, and *N*-acetyl-D-mannosamine (Table 2) for BKVN classification with 72.7% sensitivity and 96.2% specificity (Table S1). When we confined our analysis to only BKVN vs. STA, VSURF resulted in a panel of 4 metabolites, arabinose, 2-hydroxy-2-methylbutanoic acid, octadecanol, and phosphate. For this panel, BKVN classification was 88.9% sensitive and 94.8% specific (Table S2). The 4-metabolite VSURF model had accuracy comparable to that of the full 266-metabolite model, which had a sensitivity of 87.5% and specificity of 93.2% (Table S3).

3.5. Metabolic Pathways Associated with Graft Injury

To explore metabolite significance by both statistical significance and magnitude of fold change in the injury group, a volcano plot with Random Forests (RF) importance score was generated (Figure 5A) that shows the relative importance of the metabolite in terms of RF score for AR-specific panel. Additionally, a volcano plot with fold changes (increased or decreased) and corresponding *p*-values displayed the significance of the various metabolites in AR (Figure S1). The plot reveals metabolites of increasing significance relative to the Random Forests classification model. Some metabolites from the 9-metabolite marker panel for alloimmune injury and the 11-metabolite marker panel for AR are among the very highly perturbed metabolites. The metabolites significantly perturbed in KTx injury with *p*-value < 0.001 ($n = 42$) were analyzed for metabolic pathway enrichment with MetaboAnalyst. Pathway analysis for enrichment identified nitrogen metabolism, ascorbate, and aldarate metabolism, and amino sugar and nucleotide sugar metabolism as the three most significantly enriched pathways (Figure 5B).

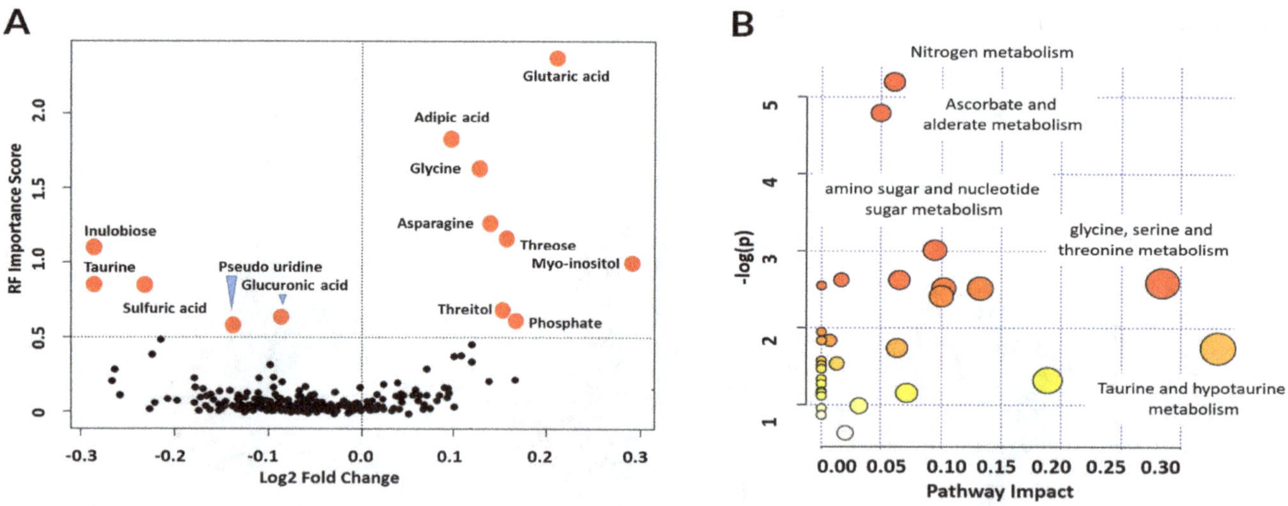

Figure 5. Metabolites and pathways significantly perturbed in KTx alloimmune injury. (**A**) Volcano plot displaying fold change and significance of metabolites. Red dots denote metabolites significant at a Random Forests importance score greater than 0.5. The right half displays metabolites in the injury group with a higher signature relative to the stable group. Some metabolites from the 9-metabolite marker panel for alloimmune injury and the 11-metabolite marker panel for AR are among the very highly perturbed metabolites labeled in red dots. (**B**) Enrichment analysis of metabolic pathways using significantly altered metabolites showed enrichment in nitrogen metabolism ($p = 0.0055$), ascorbate and aldarate metabolism ($p = 0.0083$), and amino sugar and nucleotide sugar metabolism ($p = 0.05$) as significantly enriched pathways. The y-axis represents the *p*-values as the negative of their natural logarithm.

4. Discussion

Sophisticated interrogation of urine through advanced technologies for kidney diseases is important as urine provides an attractive alternative biospecimen [35] and unlike invasive biopsies, urine metabolite changes can be diagnostic of advanced tissue injury. Additionally, our data suggest that these urine panels can have much greater sensitivity and specificity over measured serum creatinine [35–39]. Molecular perturbations in the kidney have been previously shown to occur much earlier than both histological changes and clinical alterations in kidney function, and previously published studies confirm that urine is an excellent mirror of these intra-graft molecular changes [11,35,40–49]. In this comprehensive study, we had access to a unique resource of over 300 biopsy matched urine samples archived from kidney transplant patients transplanted at multiple transplant centers, mapped with detailed clinical demographics, which enhanced the results obtained from the urine metabolomic studies conducted in this study.

Prior studies, using different assay platforms, have evaluated the urine metabolome for assessing kidney transplant injury [43,50–52]. Wang et al. [50] applied matrix-assisted laser desorption/ionization Fourier transform mass spectrometry (MALDI-FTMS) for studying acute tubular injury, Blydt-Hanson et al. [51] used liquid chromatography tandem mass spectrometry for studying transplant rejection, Dieme et al. [52] used GC-MS to study the metabolic effects of calcineurin inhibitor drugs in kidney transplant patients, Ho et al. [53] used LC-MS for analysis of alloimmune injury, and Suhre et al. [43] applied LC-MS and GC-MS. Most of these studies have larger metabolite diagnostic panels and only few studies have urine samples that are all biopsy-matched, resulting in little overlap across the identified panels to date. Using all biopsy-matched urine samples matched with pathologist blinded biopsy evaluations, GC-MS, and custom informatics analyses using nonlinear, nonparametric machine learning model development, we were able to greatly refine, as well as cross-validate the performance of small panels of urine metabolites for AR and BKVN. These clinical phenotypes are often difficult to distinguish even by biopsy, and pose a clinical challenge for patient management, specifically concerning the decision between immunosuppression augmentation (in AR) or minimization (in BKVN). In addition to selecting the most informative metabolites to provide discriminant diagnostic models for biopsy matched transplant injury categories, we have also tried to better understand the biological mechanisms that some of the metabolites suggest are dysregulated in transplant injury, using panels in this study and other published studies on the urine metabolome.

Many of the metabolites that we identified as correlated with transplant injury have previously been associated with changes in renal physiology. Taurine is a key metabolite that was included in our AR specific panel and was found to have significantly reduced levels in urine during rejection. Taurine plays a role in different physiologic and biologic processes in the kidney as reflected in urinary excretion patterns. Taurine participates in several physiological functions in the kidney [54–56], such as its role in the renal cell cycle and apoptosis. It also functions as an osmolyte during the stress response. Therefore, the changes in urinary taurine levels seen in this study may relate to the higher burden of tissue injury in AR, and its lower levels in the kidney may reflect a failure in protecting the kidney during immune-mediated damage [57]. The low level of taurine in urine during rejection may reflect a combination of decreased production in the kidney and perturbed osmolar reabsorption of taurine in the medulla [58].

Myo-inositol was found to be a significant biomarker in our model and had been previously shown by Dieme et al. [52] and Suhre et al. [43] to be relevant to and increased in transplant rejection. Urinary myo-inositol was the most important metabolite for discriminating between AR, STA, and IFTA phenotypes in our models. Myo-inositol is an osmolyte of the renal medulla that plays an important role in protecting renal cells from hyperosmotic stress [59]. It is enriched under hyperosmotic conditions via the sodium/myo-inositol cotransporter in the thick ascending limb of the loop of Henle [60]. The kidney is the most important organ for myo-inositol metabolism given that there is high expression of its associated enzymes, L-myo-inositol-1-phosphate synthetase, and myo-inositol oxygenase, in the renal parenchyma [61]. Inhibition of myo-inositol transport has been shown to cause acute renal failure in rats [62]. Furthermore, it has recently been shown through urine metabolomics profiling of humans that increased levels of myo-inositol are significantly associated with kidney disease and inversely proportional to eGFR [63]. It has also been shown to be elevated in the plasma metabolomic profiles of patients with end-stage renal disease [50,61]. These studies suggest an essential role of myo-inositol in renal physiology. Thus, its higher levels in AR may relate to the severity or progression of rejection. In looking at known perturbations in gene expression levels in AR [14] we observed that the sodium-myo-inositol transporter (SMIT), encoded by *SLC5A3*, is located in the thick ascending limb and functions to reabsorb myo-inositol into the renal medullary cells under conditions of hypertonicity [64]. Thus, perturbations of this transporter may be a key mechanism for acute rejection related tissue injury, mediated by hyperosmolar stress [63]. Given that patients with AR may have preserved kidney graft function and stable serum creatinine levels, the utility of this biomarker may be confounded given its correlation with eGFR. Further studies are needed to further validate role of myo-inositol in the progression of rejection.

These are first observations, should be consolidated with more integrative analysis of multi-omic datasets, and could be further aided by spatial metabolomics. Use of metabolomics for kidney disease outcomes generally could complement diagnostics made using other modalities, including gene expression, cell-free DNA, and proteomics [65–69].

This study benefits from the evaluation of the human urine metabolome in different geographic and demographic cohorts, as the samples came from enrolled patients at Stanford and UCSF. The diversity of patient samples supports the robustness and clinical utility of the described metabolite panels. Translation of these biomarker panels to clinical practice can be done by GC-MS/TOF based assays that are readily available in most commercial labs. Despite the fact that we have analyzed urine from a diverse population and using two different immunosuppressive drugs, additional independent validation studies that allow for prospective clinical testing and application of these metabolite panels will be required to validate the performance of these biomarker panels for diagnostic transplant monitoring. This is important because the diversity of the cohort also introduces many factors that are known to affect the metabolic profiles of patients, such as age, gender, BMI, diet, exercise, comorbidities, and even the time of day as a function of the circadian rhythm [70]. In our cohorts, age and gender were significantly different and as would be expected from a pediatric population, they had few comorbidities. A future study consisting of a larger cohort size that collected these additional details would help to delineate the effects of these parameters on the metabolic profiles. Furthermore, we note that storage length is known to affect the metabolites present and detected in urine studies. While our urine samples were stored at −80 °C, this may have influenced the distribution of the metabolites in the samples. Future work should be done to compare biobanked samples versus freshly collected samples to delineate any potential differences in the metabolomic profile.

There are a number of additional limitations to this study. We note that certain patient subsets, such as the BKVN arm had a relatively smaller number of patients (n = 22), and this warrants further investigation with a larger number of samples to validate the results. We also note that all samples AR samples used were collected at the time of the rejection, rather than before, and thus we could not assess the predictive value of metabolite alterations in transplant rejection. We believe this would be a useful area of future study, as predictive signatures of rejection prior to clinical AR (e.g., picking up subclinical AR) would be valuable to prevent further decline of kidney function [71].

Nevertheless, urinary metabolite profiles provide an exciting opportunity for rapid bedside–to-bench screening for risk assessment, improved immunosuppression titration, and rejection prevention to ultimately improve transplant and patient outcomes. With the increasing number of studies in this space [43,72], a comprehensive metabolomics picture of allograft outcomes can be created and further contribute to the care management of transplant patients.

Author Contributions: Conceptualization, project administration, funding acquisition, supervision, and resources, T.K.S. and M.M.S.; visualization, T.K.S., A.W.S., and J.Y.C.Y.; methodology, software, validation, formal analysis, investigation, data curation, writing—original draft preparation, and writing—review and editing by all authors. All authors have read and agreed to the published version of the manuscript.

Acknowledgments: We are grateful for the help from physicians, clinical coordinators, research personnel, patients, and patient families. We are grateful to Maggie Kerwin for proofreading while revising the manuscript.

References

1. Abecassis, M.; Bartlett, S.T.; Collins, A.J.; Davis, C.L.; Delmonico, F.L.; Friedewald, J.J.; Hays, R.; Howard, A.; Jones, E.; Leichtam, A.B.; et al. Kidney transplantation as primary therapy for end-stage renal disease: A National Kidney Foundation/Kidney Disease Outcomes Quality Initiative (NKF/KDOQITM) conference. *Clin. J. Am. Soc. Nephrol. CJASN* **2008**, *3*, 471–480. [CrossRef] [PubMed]
2. Pomfret, E.A.; Sung, R.S.; Allan, J.; Kinkhabwala, M.; Melancon, J.K.; Roberts, J.P. Solving the organ shortage crisis: The 7th annual American Society of Transplant Surgeons' State-of-the-Art Winter Symposium. *Am. J. Transplant.* **2008**, *8*, 745–752. [CrossRef] [PubMed]
3. Meier-Kriesche, H.U.; Schold, J.D.; Srinivas, T.R.; Kaplan, B. Lack of improvement in renal allograft survival despite a marked decrease in acute rejection rates over the most recent era. *Am. J. Transplant.* **2004**, *4*, 378–383. [CrossRef] [PubMed]
4. Gaston, R.S. Improving Long-Term Outcomes in Kidney Transplantation: Towards a New Paradigm of Post-Transplant Care in the United States. *Trans. Am. Clin. Climatol. Assoc.* **2016**, *127*, 350–361. [PubMed]
5. Nasr, M.; Sigdel, T.; Sarwal, M. Advances in diagnostics for transplant rejection. *Expert Rev. Mol. Diagn.* **2016**, *16*, 1121–1132. [CrossRef]
6. Loupy, A.; Haas, M.; Solez, K.; Racusen, L.; Glotz, D.; Seron, D.; Nankivell, B.J.; Colvin, R.B.; Afrouzian, M.; Akalin, E.; et al. The Banff 2015 Kidney Meeting Report: Current Challenges in Rejection Classification and Prospects for Adopting Molecular Pathology. *Am. J. Transplant.* **2017**, *17*, 28–41. [CrossRef]
7. Filler, G.; Bendrick-Peart, J.; Christians, U. Pharmacokinetics of mycophenolate mofetil and sirolimus in children. *Ther. Drug Monit.* **2008**, *30*, 138–142. [CrossRef]
8. Yang, J.Y.; Sarwal, M.M. Transplant genetics and genomics. *Nat. Rev. Genet.* **2017**, *18*, 309–326. [CrossRef]
9. Reeve, J.; Bohmig, G.A.; Eskandary, F.; Einecke, G.; Lefaucheur, C.; Loupy, A.; Halloran, P.F. The MMDx-Kidney Study Group. Assessing rejection-related disease in kidney transplant biopsies based on archetypal analysis of molecular phenotypes. *JCI Insight* **2017**, *2*, 1–14. [CrossRef]
10. Roedder, S.; Sigdel, T.; Salomonis, N.; Hsieh, S.; Dai, H.; Bestard, O.; Metes, D.; Zeevi, A.; Gritsh, A.; Cheeseman, J.; et al. The kSORT assay to detect renal transplant patients at high risk for acute rejection: Results of the multicenter AART study. *PLoS Med.* **2014**, *11*, e1001759. [CrossRef]
11. Sigdel, T.K.; Salomonis, N.; Nicora, C.D.; Ryu, S.; He, J.; Dinh, V.; Orton, D.J.; Moore, R.J.; Hsieh, S.C.; Dai, H.; et al. The identification of novel potential injury mechanisms and candidate biomarkers in renal allograft rejection by quantitative proteomics. *Mol. Cell. Proteom. MCP* **2014**, *13*, 621–631. [CrossRef] [PubMed]
12. Khatri, P.; Roedder, S.; Kimura, N.; De Vusser, K.; Morgan, A.A.; Gong, Y.; Fischbein, M.P.; Robbins, R.C.; Naesens, M.; Bute, A.J.; et al. A common rejection module (CRM) for acute rejection across multiple organs identifies novel therapeutics for organ transplantation. *J. Exp. Med.* **2013**, *210*, 2205–2221. [CrossRef] [PubMed]
13. Yang, J.Y.; Sigdel, T.K.; Sarwal, M.M. Self-antigens and rejection: A proteomic analysis. *Curr. Opin. Organ Transplant.* **2016**, *21*, 362–367. [CrossRef] [PubMed]
14. Sarwal, M.; Chua, M.S.; Kambham, N.; Hsieh, S.C.; Satterwhite, T.; Masek, M.; Salvatierra, O., Jr. Molecular heterogeneity in acute renal allograft rejection identified by DNA microarray profiling. *N. Engl. J. Med.* **2003**, *349*, 125–138. [CrossRef] [PubMed]
15. Erpicum, P.; Hanssen, O.; Weekers, L.; Lovinfosse, P.; Meunier, P.; Tshibanda, L.; Ktzesinski, J.M.; Hustinx, R.; Jouret, F. Non-invasive approaches in the diagnosis of acute rejection in kidney transplant recipients, part II: Omics analyses of urine and blood samples. *Clin. Kidney J.* **2017**, *10*, 106–115. [CrossRef]
16. Wishart, D.S. Metabolomics: A complementary tool in renal transplantation. *Contrib. Nephrol.* **2008**, *160*, 76–87.

17. Klawitter, J.; Klawitter, J.; Kushner, E.; Jonscher, K.; Bendrick-Peart, J.; Leibfritz, D.; Christians, U.; Schmitz, V. Association of immunosuppressant-induced protein changes in the rat kidney with changes in urine metabolite patterns: A proteo-metabonomic study. *J. Proteome Res.* **2010**, *9*, 865–875. [CrossRef]
18. Bouatra, S.; Aziat, F.; Mandal, R.; Guo, A.C.; Wilson, M.R.; Knox, C.; Bjorndahl, T.C.; Krishamurthy, R.; Saleem, F.; Liu, P.; et al. The human urine metabolome. *PLoS ONE* **2013**, *8*, e73076. [CrossRef]
19. Bohra, R.; Klepacki, J.; Klawitter, J.; Klawitter, J.; Thurman, J.; Christians, U. Proteomics and metabolomics in renal transplantation-quo vadis? *Transpl. Int.* **2013**, *26*, 225–241. [CrossRef]
20. Gromski, P.S.; Muhamadali, H.; Ellis, D.I.; Xu, Y.; Correa, E.; Turner, M.L.; Goodacre, R. A tutorial review: Metabolomics and partial least squares-discriminant analysis-a marriage of convenience or a shotgun wedding. *Anal. Chim. Acta* **2015**, *879*, 10–23. [CrossRef]
21. Racusen, L.C.; Halloran, P.F.; Solez, K. Banff 2003 meeting report: New diagnostic insights and standards. *Am. J. Transplant.* **2004**, *4*, 1562–1566. [CrossRef] [PubMed]
22. Racusen, L.C.; Solez, K.; Colvin, R.B.; Bonsib, S.M.; Castro, M.C.; Cavallo, T.; Croker, B.P.; Demetris, A.J.; Drachenberg, C.B.; Fogo, A.B.; et al. The Banff 97 working classification of renal allograft pathology. *Kidney Int.* **1999**, *55*, 713–723. [CrossRef] [PubMed]
23. Solez, K.; Colvin, R.B.; Racusen, L.C.; Haas, M.; Sis, B.; Mengel, M.; Halloran, P.F.; Baldwin, W.; Banfi, G.; Collins, A.B.; et al. Banff 07 classification of renal allograft pathology: Updates and future directions. *Am. J. Transplant.* **2008**, *8*, 753–760. [CrossRef] [PubMed]
24. Nankivell, B.J.; Alexander, S.I. Rejection of the kidney allograft. *N. Engl. J. Med.* **2010**, *363*, 1451–1462. [CrossRef]
25. Fletcher, J.T.; Nankivell, B.J.; Alexander, S.I. Chronic allograft nephropathy. *Pediatric Nephrol.* **2009**, *24*, 1465–1471. [CrossRef]
26. Kind, T.; Wohlgemuth, G.; Lee, D.Y.; Lu, Y.; Palazoglu, M.; Shahbaz, S.; Fiehn, O. FiehnLib: Mass spectral and retention index libraries for metabolomics based on quadrupole and time-of-flight gas chromatography/mass spectrometry. *Anal. Chem.* **2009**, *81*, 10038–10048. [CrossRef] [PubMed]
27. Kind, T.; Tolstikov, V.; Fiehn, O.; Weiss, R.H. A comprehensive urinary metabolomic approach for identifying kidney cancerr. *Anal. Biochem.* **2007**, *363*, 185–195. [CrossRef] [PubMed]
28. Katajamaa, M.; Miettinen, J.; Oresic, M. MZmine: Toolbox for processing and visualization of mass spectrometry based molecular profile data. *Bioinformatics* **2006**, *22*, 634–636. [CrossRef]
29. Smith, C.A.; Want, E.J.; O'Maille, G.; Abagyan, R.; Siuzdak, G. XCMS: Processing mass spectrometry data for metabolite profiling using nonlinear peak alignment, matching, and identification. *Anal. Chem.* **2006**, *78*, 779–787. [CrossRef]
30. Stekhoven, D.J.; Buhlmann, P. MissForest-non-parametric missing value imputation for mixed-type data. *Bioinformatics* **2012**, *28*, 112–118. [CrossRef]
31. Breiman, L. Random forests. *Mach. Learn.* **2001**, *45*, 5–32. [CrossRef]
32. Genuer, R.; Poggi, J.M.; Tuleau-Malot, C. VSURF: An R Package for Variable Selection Using Random Forests. *R. J.* **2015**, *7*, 19–33. [CrossRef]
33. Delong, E.R.; Delong, D.M.; Clarkepearson, D.I. Comparing the Areas under 2 or More Correlated Receiver Operating Characteristic Curves-a Nonparametric Approach. *Biometrics* **1988**, *44*, 837–845. [CrossRef] [PubMed]
34. Chong, J.; Soufan, O.; Li, C.; Caraus, I.; Li, S.; Bourque, G.; Wishart, D.S.; Xia, J. MetaboAnalyst 4.0: Towards more transparent and integrative metabolomics analysis. *Nucleic Acids Res.* **2018**, *46*, W486–W494. [CrossRef]
35. Nissaisorakarn, V.; Lee, J.R.; Lubetzky, M.; Suthanthiran, M. Urine biomarkers informative of human kidney allograft rejection and tolerance. *Hum. Immunol.* **2018**, *79*, 343–355. [CrossRef] [PubMed]
36. Sigdel, T.K.; Kaushal, A.; Gritsenko, M.; Norbeck, A.D.; Qian, W.J.; Xiao, W.; Camp, D.G.; Smith, R.D.; Sarwal, M.M. Shotgun proteomics identifies proteins specific for acute renal transplant rejection. *Proteom. Clin. Appl.* **2010**, *4*, 32–47. [CrossRef]
37. Sigdel, T.K.; Lee, S.; Sarwal, M.M. Profiling the proteome in renal transplantation. *Proteom. Clin. Appl.* **2011**, *5*, 269–280. [CrossRef]
38. Sigdel, T.K.; Sarwal, M.M. The proteogenomic path towards biomarker discovery. *Pediatric Transplant.* **2008**, *12*, 737–747. [CrossRef]
39. Sigdel, T.K.; Sarwal, M.M. Recent advances in biomarker discovery in solid organ transplant by proteomics. *Expert Rev. Proteom.* **2011**, *8*, 705–715. [CrossRef]

40. Sigdel, T.K.; Gao, Y.; He, J.; Wang, A.; Nicora, C.D.; Fillmore, T.L.; Shi, T.; Webb-Robertson, B.J.; Smith, R.D.; Qian, W.J.; et al. Mining the human urine proteome for monitoring renal transplant injury. *Kidney Int.* **2016**, *89*, 1244–1252. [CrossRef] [PubMed]
41. Sigdel, T.K.; Ng, Y.W.; Lee, S.; Nicora, C.D.; Qian, W.J.; Smith, R.D.; Qian, W.J.; Salvatierra, O.; Camp, D.G.; Sarwal, M.M. Perturbations in the urinary exosome in transplant rejection. *Front. Med.* **2014**, *1*, 57. [CrossRef] [PubMed]
42. Sigdel, T.K.; Vitalone, M.J.; Tran, T.Q.; Dai, H.; Hsieh, S.C.; Salvatierra, O.; Sarwal, M.M. A rapid noninvasive assay for the detection of renal transplant injury. *Transplantation* **2013**, *96*, 97–101. [CrossRef] [PubMed]
43. Suhre, K.; Schwartz, J.E.; Sharma, V.K.; Chen, Q.; Lee, J.R.; Muthukumar, T.; Dadhania, D.M.; Ding, R.; Ikle, D.H.; Bridges, N.D.; et al. Urine Metabolite Profiles Predictive of Human Kidney Allograft Status. *J. Am. Soc. Nephrol. JASN* **2016**, *27*, 626–636. [CrossRef]
44. Fairchild, R.L.; Suthanthiran, M. Urine CXCL10/IP-10 Fingers Ongoing Antibody-Mediated Kidney Graft Rejection. *J. Am. Soc. Nephrol. JASN* **2015**, *26*, 2607–2609. [CrossRef]
45. Li, B.; Hartono, C.; Ding, R.; Sharma, V.K.; Ramaswamy, R.; Qian, B.; Serur, D.; Mouradian, J.; Schwartz, J.E.; Suthanthiran, M. Noninvasive diagnosis of renal-allograft rejection by measurement of messenger RNA for perforin and granzyme B in urine. *N. Engl. J. Med.* **2001**, *344*, 947–954. [CrossRef] [PubMed]
46. Li, R.; Guo, L.X.; Li, Y.; Chang, W.Q.; Liu, J.Q.; Liu, L.F.; Xin, G.Z. Dose-response characteristics of Clematis triterpenoid saponins and clematichinenoside AR in rheumatoid arthritis rats by liquid chromatography/mass spectrometry-based serum and urine metabolomics. *J. Pharm. Biomed. Anal.* **2017**, *136*, 81–91. [CrossRef] [PubMed]
47. Schaub, S.; Mayr, M.; Honger, G.; Bestland, J.; Steiger, J.; Regeniter, A.; Mihatsch, M.J.; Wilkins, J.A.; Rush, D.; Nickerson, P. Detection of subclinical tubular injury after renal transplantation: Comparison of urine protein analysis with allograft histopathology. *Transplantation* **2007**, *84*, 104–112. [CrossRef]
48. Schaub, S.; Rush, D.; Wilkins, J.; Gibson, I.W.; Weiler, T.; Sangster, K.; Nicolle, L.; Karpinski, M.; Jeffery, J.; Nickerson, P. Proteomic-based detection of urine proteins associated with acute renal allograft rejection. *J. Am. Soc. Nephrol. JASN* **2004**, *15*, 219–227. [CrossRef]
49. Torng, S.; Rigatto, C.; Rush, D.N.; Nickerson, P.; Jeffery, J.R. The urine protein to creatinine ratio (P/C) as a predictor of 24-hour urine protein excretion in renal transplant patients. *Transplantation* **2001**, *72*, 1453–1456. [CrossRef]
50. Choi, J.Y.; Yoon, Y.J.; Choi, H.J.; Park, S.H.; Kim, C.D.; Kim, I.S.; Kwon, T.H.; Do, J.Y.; Kim, S.H.; Ryu, D.H.; et al. Dialysis modality-dependent changes in serum metabolites: Accumulation of inosine and hypoxanthine in patients on haemodialysis. *Nephrol. Dial. Transpl.* **2011**, *26*, 1304–1313. [CrossRef]
51. Blydt-Hansen, T.D.; Sharma, A.; Gibson, I.W.; Mandal, R.; Wishart, D.S. Urinary metabolomics for noninvasive detection of borderline and acute T cell-mediated rejection in children after kidney transplantation. *Am. J. Transplant.* **2014**, *14*, 2339–2349. [CrossRef]
52. Dieme, B.; Halimi, J.M.; Emond, P.; Buchler, M.; Nadal-Desbarat, L.; Blasco, H.; Guellec, C.L. Assessing the metabolic effects of calcineurin inhibitors in renal transplant recipients by urine metabolic profiling. *Transplantation* **2014**, *98*, 195–201. [CrossRef] [PubMed]
53. Ho, J.; Sharma, A.; Mandal, R.; Wishart, D.S.; Wiebe, C.; Storsley, L.; Karpinski, M.; Gibson, I.M.; Nickerson, P.W.; Rush, D.N. Detecting Renal Allograft Inflammation Using Quantitative Urine Metabolomics and CXCL10. *Transplant. Direct* **2016**, *2*, e78. [CrossRef] [PubMed]
54. Hoffman, N.E.; Iser, J.H.; Smallwood, R.A. Hepatic bile acid transport: Effect of conjugation and position of hydroxyl groups. *Am. J. Physiol* **1975**, *229*, 298–302. [CrossRef]
55. Chesney, R.W.; Han, X.; Patters, A.B. Taurine and the renal system. *J. Biomed. Sci.* **2010**, *17* (Suppl. 1):S4, 1–10. [CrossRef] [PubMed]
56. Trachtman, H.; Sturman, J.A. Taurine: A therapeutic agent in experimental kidney disease. *Amino Acids* **1996**, *11*, 1–13. [CrossRef] [PubMed]
57. Trachtman, H.; Futterweit, S.; Prenner, J.; Hanon, S. Antioxidants reverse the antiproliferative effect of high glucose and advanced glycosylation end products in cultured rat mesangial cells. *Biochem. Biophys. Res. Commun.* **1994**, *199*, 346–352. [CrossRef]
58. Dantzler, W.H.; Silbernagl, S. Renal tubular reabsorption of taurine, gamma-aminobutyric acid (GABA) and beta-alanine studied by continuous microperfusion. *Pflug. Arch.* **1976**, *367*, 123–128. [CrossRef]

59. Brocker, C.; Thompson, D.C.; Vasiliou, V. The role of hyperosmotic stress in inflammation and disease. *Biomol. Concepts* **2012**, *3*, 345–364. [CrossRef]
60. Yorek, M.A.; Dunlap, J.A.; Lowe, W.L., Jr. Osmotic regulation of the Na+/myo-inositol cotransporter and postinduction normalization. *Kidney Int.* **1999**, *55*, 215–224. [CrossRef]
61. Niewczas, M.A.; Sirich, T.L.; Mathew, A.V.; Skupien, J.; Mohney, R.P.; Warram, J.H.; Smiles, A.; Huang, X.; Walker, W.; Byun, J.; et al. Uremic solutes and risk of end-stage renal disease in type 2 diabetes: Metabolomic study. *Kidney Int.* **2014**, *85*, 1214–1224. [CrossRef] [PubMed]
62. Kitamura, H.; Yamauchi, A.; Sugiura, T.; Matsuoka, Y.; Horio, M.; Tohyama, M.; Shimada, S.; Imai, E.; Hori, M. Inhibition of myo-inositol transport causes acute renal failure with selective medullary injury in the rat. *Kidney Int.* **1998**, *53*, 146–153. [CrossRef] [PubMed]
63. Gil, R.B.; Ortiz, A.; Sanchez-Nino, M.D.; Markoska, K.; Schepers, E.; Vanholder, R.; Glorieux, G.; Schmitt-Kopplin, P.; Heinzmann, S.S. Increased urinary osmolyte excretion indicates chronic kidney disease severity and progression rate. *Nephrol. Dial. Transplant.* **2018**, *33*, 2156–2164. [CrossRef] [PubMed]
64. Burg, M.B.; Ferraris, J.D. Intracellular organic osmolytes: Function and regulation. *J. Biol. Chem.* **2008**, *283*, 7309–7313. [CrossRef] [PubMed]
65. Yang, J.Y.C.; Sarwal, R.; Ky, K.; Dong, V.; Stoller, M.; Sarwal, M.; Chi, T. Non-Radiologic Assessment of Kidney Stones by KIT, a Spot Urine Assay. *Br. J. Urol. Int.* **2020**, *125*, 732–738. [CrossRef]
66. Yang, J.Y.C.; Sarwal, R.D.; Fervenza, F.C.; Sarwal, M.M.; Lafayette, R.A. Noninvasive Urinary Monitoring of Progression in IgA Nephropathy. *Int. J. Mol. Sci.* **2019**, *20*, 4463. [CrossRef]
67. Sigdel, T.K.; Yang, J.Y.C.; Bestard, O.; Schroeder, A.; Hsieh, S.-C.; Liberto, J.M.; Qamm, I.; Geraedts, A.C.M.; Sarwal, M.M. A urinary Common Rejection Module (uCRM) score for non-invasive kidney transplant monitoring. *PLoS ONE* **2019**, *7*, 1–15. [CrossRef]
68. Sigdel, T.; Yang, J.; Bestard, O.; Hsieh, S.; Roedder, S.; Damm, I.; Liberto, J.; Nandoe, S.; Sarwal, M. A Non-Invasive Urinary Common Rejection Module (uCRM) Gene Expression Score Quantifies and Differentiates Kidney Transplant Injury. *Am. J. Transplant.* **2017**. [CrossRef]
69. Yang, J.Y.C.; Sarwal, R.D.; Sigdel, T.K.; Damm, I.; Rosenbaum, B.; Liberto, J.M.; Chan-on, C.; Arreola-Guerra, J.M.; Alberu, J.M.; Vincenti, F.; et al. A urine score for noninvasive accurate diagnosis and prediction of kidney transplant rejection. *Sci. Transl. Med.* **2020**, *12*, 1–11. [CrossRef]
70. Bi, H.; Guo, Z.; Jia, X.; Liu, H.; Ma, L.; Xue, L. The key points in the pre-analytical procedures of blood and urine samples in metabolomics studies. *Metabolomics* **2020**, *16*, 1–15. [CrossRef]
71. Moreso, F.; Carrera, M.; Goma, M.; Hueso, M.; Sellares, J.; Martorell, J.; Grinyó, J.M.; Serón, D. Early subclinical rejection as a risk factor for late chronic humoral rejection. *Transplantation* **2012**, *93*, 41–46. [CrossRef] [PubMed]
72. Bassi, R.; Niewczas, M.A.; Biancone, L.; Bussolino, S.; Merugumala, S.; Tezza, S.; D'Addio, F.; Nasr, M.B.; Valderrama-Vasquez, A.; Usuelli, V. Metabolomic profiling in individuals with a failing kidney allograft. *PLoS ONE* **2017**, *12*, 1–14. [CrossRef] [PubMed]

11

Degree of Glomerulosclerosis in Procurement Kidney Biopsies from Marginal Donor Kidneys and their Implications in Predicting Graft Outcomes

Wisit Cheungpasitporn [1,*], Charat Thongprayoon [2,*], Pradeep K Vaitla [1], Api Chewcharat [2], Panupong Hansrivijit [3], Felicitas L. Koller [4], Michael A Mao [5], Tarun Bathini [6], Sohail Abdul Salim [1], Sreelatha Katari [7], Lee S Cummings [7], Eddie Island [7], Jameson Forster [7] and Napat Leeaphorn [7,*]

1 Division of Nephrology, Department of Medicine, University of Mississippi Medical Center, Jackson, MS 39216, USA; pvaitla@umc.edu (P.K.V.); sohail3553@gmail.com (S.A.S.)
2 Division of Nephrology and Hypertension, Mayo Clinic, Rochester, MN 55905, USA; chewcharat.api@mayo.edu
3 Department of Internal Medicine, University of Pittsburgh Medical Center Pinnacle, Harrisburg, PA 17105, USA; hansrivijitp@upmc.edu
4 Department of Transplant and Hepatobiliary Surgery, University of Mississippi Medical Center, Jackson, MS 39216, USA; fkoller@umc.edu
5 Division of Nephrology, Division of Nephrology and Hypertension, Mayo Clinic, Jacksonville, FL 32224, USA; mao.michael@mayo.edu
6 Department of Internal Medicine, University of Arizona, Tucson, AZ 85721, USA; tarunjacobb@gmail.com
7 Renal Transplant Program, School of Medicine/Saint Luke's Health System, University of Missouri-Kansas City, Kansas City, MO 64110, USA; skatari@saint-lukes.org (S.K.); lscummings@saint-lukes.org (L.S.C.); eisland@saint-lukes.org (E.I.); jforster@saint-lukes.org (J.F.)
* Correspondence: wcheungpasitporn@gmail.com (W.C.); charat.thongprayoon@gmail.com (C.T.); napat.leeaphorn@gmail.com (N.L.)

Abstract: Background: This study aimed to assess the association between the percentage of glomerulosclerosis (GS) in procurement allograft biopsies from high-risk deceased donor and graft outcomes in kidney transplant recipients. **Methods:** The UNOS database was used to identify deceased-donor kidneys with a kidney donor profile index (KDPI) score > 85% from 2005 to 2014. Deceased donor kidneys were categorized based on the percentage of GS: 0–10%, 11–20%, >20% and no biopsy performed. The outcome included death-censored graft survival, patient survival, rate of delayed graft function, and 1-year acute rejection. **Results:** Of 22,006 kidneys, 91.2% were biopsied showing 0–10% GS (58.0%), 11–20% GS (13.5%), >20% GS (19.7%); 8.8% were not biopsied. The rate of kidney discard was 48.5%; 33.6% in 0–10% GS, 68.9% in 11–20% GS, and 77.4% in >20% GS. 49.8% of kidneys were discarded in those that were not biopsied. Death-censored graft survival at 5 years was 75.8% for 0–10% GS, 70.9% for >10% GS, and 74.8% for the no biopsy group. Among kidneys with >10% GS, there was no significant difference in death-censored graft survival between 11–20% GS and >20% GS. Recipients with >10% GS had an increased risk of graft failure (HR = 1.27, $p < 0.001$), compared with 0–10% GS. There was no significant difference in patient survival, acute rejection at 1-year, and delayed graft function between 0% and 10% GS and >10% GS. **Conclusion:** In >85% KDPI kidneys, our study suggested that discard rates increased with higher percentages of GS, and GS >10% is an independent prognostic factor for graft failure. Due to organ shortage, future studies are needed to identify strategies to use these marginal kidneys safely and improve outcomes.

Keywords: procurement kidney biopsy; glomerulosclerosis; kidney transplantation; transplantation; outcomes

1. Introduction

In the United States, more than 90,000 patients with end-stage kidney disease (ESKD) are currently waiting for a kidney transplant [1,2]. A significant gap between the number of kidney transplant candidates and donors remains an ongoing problem, resulting in a median wait time exceeding four years [3–6]. This delay has a dramatic impact on ESKD patients on the transplant waiting list, as their survival is, on average, below 40% after 5 years on dialysis [7]. Despite the severe organ shortage, a significant number of procured organs are discarded every year [8,9].

The shortage of deceased donor organs continues to be a problem in kidney transplantation despite the implementation of expanded criteria donor (ECD) programs in 2002 to increase the use of organs from donors with ≥60 years or comorbidities [10]. In 2013, the United Network of Organ Sharing (UNOS) Kidney Transplantation Committee approved a new allocation policy based on the kidney donor profile index (KDPI), a percentile score that compares an organ to previously recovered kidneys and signifies donor factors affecting transplant function [11]. KDPI >85% kidneys, previously designated as expanded criteria donor (ECD) kidneys, are offered to patients who have consented to accept a non-ideal renal allograft, thereby increasing access to earlier kidney transplantation [11]. Unfortunately, the discard rate for KDPI >85% kidneys continues to be high, close to 50% under the new kidney allocation system (KAS). The major determinants of discarded kidneys are donor comorbidities and procurement wedge biopsy findings, especially the percentage of glomerulosclerosis (GS) [8,12–16].

Despite conflicting evidence regarding the prognostic capability of histologic findings for differentiating donor kidneys at greater risk of inferior outcomes [17–19], the use of procurement biopsies has become an increasingly common practice, particularly in KDPI >85% kidneys in which 95% of recovered kidneys were biopsied [9,18,20]. The percentage of GS is commonly the primary biopsy information reviewed because it provides a convenient cutoff for offer turndowns [8,21,22]. This is in spite of studies noting that the percentage of GS has failed to consistently predict graft outcomes [18,21,23–29].

The aim of this study is to explore the association between the percentage of GS and graft outcomes in kidney transplant recipients who received KDPI >85% kidneys between 1 January 2005 to 2 December 2014 using the Organ Procurement and Transplantation Network (OPTN)/UNOS database.

2. Methods

2.1. Data Source and Study Population

We used the OPTN/UNOS database to identify deceased-donor kidneys recovered from January 1, 2005 to December 2, 2014 (before implementation of the kidney allocation system). The study was exempt from the institutional review board due to the publicly available nature of the de-identified database of the OPTN/UNOS database. All data used in the analysis were provided by UNOS through the Standard Transplant Analysis and Research (STAR) database. The database is a de-identified, patient-level data source that contains donor, waitlist, and transplant recipient variables derived from UNet forms for any transplant in the United States after October 1, 1987. KDPI (reference year of 2017) was calculated based on donor factors to summarize the likelihood of graft failure after deceased donor kidney transplant. Higher KDPI scores are associated with shorter estimated graft function. Although the KDPI was not formally introduced into allocation policy until implementation of the new kidney allocation system (KAS) on December 2014, the OPTN/UNOS database has KDPI values for 99% of all deceased donor recipients who underwent kidney transplantation during the study period. To assess the predictive value of procurement biopsy GS percentage in high-risk deceased donors, we only included deceased-donor kidneys with a KDPI score > 85%. We excluded recovered kidneys for dual-kidney transplant and kidneys from donors with body weight < 20 kg. Subsequently, we assess the post-transplant outcomes based on GS percentage in deceased-donor kidney transplant recipients who received kidney with KDPI > 85%. We excluded patients undergoing kidney re-transplants or multi-organ transplant from the analysis.

2.2. Outcomes

We categorized deceased donor kidneys into four groups based on the percentage of GS: 0–10%, 11–20%, >20% and no biopsy performed. We investigated the kidney discard rates and post-transplant deceased donor allograft outcomes based on GS groups. The primary outcome was death-censored graft survival. Death-censored graft survival began at kidney transplant, was followed until graft failure, defined as the requirement of renal replacement therapy and/or kidney re-transplant, and was censored at death or the end of study (6 September 2018), whichever was earlier. The secondary outcomes were patient survival, rate of delayed graft function, and 1-year acute rejection. Delayed graft function was defined as a requirement of dialysis within the first week of transplantation. As there was no statistical difference in any post-transplant outcomes between 11–20% and >20% GS (Table S1), we combined these two groups together (>10% GS) when assessing post-transplant outcomes.

2.3. Covariates

Donor-related factors included donor age, sex, race, diabetes mellitus, hypertension, body mass index, the last serum creatinine before kidney procurement, donation after cardiac death, hepatitis C virus (HCV) antibody status, cause of death, and machine perfusion. Recipient-related factors included recipient age, sex, race, body mass index, diabetes mellitus, preemptive transplant, dialysis duration, and panel reactive antibody. Transplant-related factors included HLA-DR mismatch, cold ischemic time, transplant period, and induction therapy.

2.4. Statistical Analysis

Baseline characteristics were described using mean ± standard deviation (SD) for continuous variables or frequencies with percentage for categorical variables. Continuous variables were compared between GS groups using the student's *t*-test or ANOVA, as appropriate. Categorical variables were compared between GS groups using the Chi-squared test. Patient survival and death-censored graft survival outcomes were estimated using the Kaplan–Meier method with significance tested using the log-rank test. The associations of the GS percentage group with death-censored graft failure and patient mortality was assessed using Cox proportional hazards analysis. The proportional hazards assumption was tested using Schoenfeld residuals ($p = 0.29$). Because the OPTN/UNOS database did not specify the date of occurrence, the associations of the GS percentage group with delayed graft function and 1-year acute rejection were assessed using logistic regression analysis. Multivariable analysis was performed to adjust for covariates associated with outcomes of interest with $p < 0.05$ in univariate analysis. All *p*-values were two-tailed, and *p*-values of <0.05 were considered significant. Stata version 13 (StataCorp, College Station, TX, USA) was used for all statistical analyses.

3. Results

3.1. Kidney Procurement Cohort and Rate of Kidney Discard

During the study period, 25,154 kidneys were recovered from deceased donors with KDPI > 85%. A total of 3014 kidneys recovered for dual-kidney transplant and 134 kidneys from donors with a body weight < 20 kg were excluded. A total of 22,006 kidneys with KDPI > 85% were included in the kidney procurement cohort. Of these kidneys, 58.0% had 0–10% GS, 13.5% had 11–20% GS, 19.7% had >20% GS, and 8.8% had no kidney biopsy performed (Figure S1). Overall, the rate of kidney discard was 48.5%; 33.6% in 0–10% GS, 68.9% in 11–20% GS, and 77.4% in >20% GS. 49.8% kidneys were discarded in the no kidney biopsy group.

3.2. Kidney Transplant Recipient Cohort

In this cohort of 22,006 deceased donor kidneys with KDPI > 85%, 10,662 kidneys were discarded. After excluding 1032 recipients with prior kidney transplants or undergoing multi-organ transplant, a total of 10,312 recipients with donor KDPI > 85% were included in the post-transplant outcome analysis. Of these patients, 75.6% had 0–10% GS, 11.9% had 11–20% GS, 4.9% had >20% GS, and 7.6% had no kidney biopsy performed (Figure S2). The median (IQR) number of glomeruli in each kidney biopsy was 47 (IQR: 28, 69). There was no association between KDPI and percent of GS ($p = 0.70$). The donor, recipient, and transplant-related characteristics stratified by percent of GS are shown in Table 1.

Table 1. Characteristics of donors, recipients, and transplant according to percent GS in transplanted allograft.

	Glomerulosclerosis				
	0–10%	**11–20%**	**>20%**	**No-Biopsy**	***p*-Value**
N	7796	1230	500	786	
Donor					
Age (years)	60.7 ± 7.1	60.5 ± 6.9	60.6 ± 6.7	58.5 ± 7.4	<0.001
Male (%)	46.7	41.1	46.4	36.6	<0.001
Black (%)	28.8	29.5	25.2	30.0	0.26
Diabetes (%)	26.5	34.2	30.6	20.2	<0.001
Hypertension (%)	79.0	81.8	80.8	73.8	<0.001
BMI (kg/m^2)	28.8 ± 6.9	29.2 ± 7.5	29.2 ± 7.5	27.3 ± 6.5	<0.001
Creatinine (mg/dL) before kidney procurement	1.2 ± 1.0	1.2 ± 0.6	1.2 ± 0.5	1.2 ± 1.0	0.04
Donor after cardiac death (%)	10.0	7.1	6.8	4.6	<0.001
HCV antibody positive (%)	5.8	2.4	2.8	12.9	<0.001
Cause of death (%)					
Cerebrovascular accident	78.1	79.4	83.0	82.8	0.002
Machine perfusion (%)	49.9	51.2	47.8	19.5	<0.001
Expanded criteria donor (%)	85.4	87.7	86.4	75.5	<0.001
Recipient					
Age (years)	61.5 ± 9.8	62.4 ± 9.6	61.6 ± 9.8	59.9 ± 10.6	0.001
Male (%)	64.0	63.1	63.2	63.9	0.92
Black (%)	36.4	36.8	40.6	33.3	0.07
BMI	27.9 ± 5.3	28.4 ± 5.5	27.5 ± 5.0	27.6 ± 5.4	0.001
Diabetes (%)	47.2	46.8	48.8	47.1	0.90
Dialysis duration (%)					
Preemptive	9.8	8.9	9.8	9.0	0.70
<1 years	8.7	8.1	7.0	9.5	0.41
1–3 years	29.6	26.7	30.8	30.7	0.13
>3 years	49.4	54.0	48.4	46.8	0.006
PRA (%)					
<10	81.7	84.7	81.8	78.1	0.003
10–60	12.0	9.8	12.6	15.0	0.005
>60	5.9	4.6	4.4	5.7	0.21
Missing	0.5	0.9	1.2	1.2	0.01
Transplant					
HLA DR mismatch (%)					
0	8.2	7.2	7.8	8.9	0.42
1	39.0	36.3	38.4	36.9	0.27
2	52.8	56.5	53.8	54.2	0.12
Cold ischemic time (hours)	19.5 ± 9.4	20.5 ± 9.5	19.8 ± 9.1	15.7 ± 9.2	<0.001
Transplant period					
2005–2007	28.6	22.7	35.0	45.2	<0.001
2008–2010	33.8	31.6	35.6	27.4	0.001
2011–2014	37.6	45.7	29.4	27.5	<0.001
Induction therapy (%)					
Thymoglobulin	46.1	52.3	51.4	47.3	<0.001
Alemtuzumab	14.7	13.5	16.0	9.5	0.001
Basiliximab	18.9	19.2	17.2	24.7	0.001
Other induction	7.6	8.1	5.2	7.1	0.19
No induction	16.3	11.0	13.4	15.0	<0.001

GS, glomerulosclerosis; HCV, hepatitis C virus; BMI, body mass index; PRA, panel reactive antibody; HLA, human leukocyte antigen.

3.3. Baseline Characteristics Based on Percentages of Glomerulosclerosis

Table 2 summarizes and compares donor, recipient, and transplant-related characteristics between 0–10% and >10% GS allograft groups. Kidneys donors with >10% GS had a higher prevalence of female sex, diabetes and hypertension. Kidney donors with 0–10% GS had a higher prevalence of donation after cardiac death and positive hepatitis C antibody. Recipients of kidneys with GS > 10% were older and had longer dialysis vintage, whereas recipients of kidneys with 0–10% GS had higher panel reactive antibodies. Kidney transplants with >10% GS had more HLA DR mismatch, cold ischemic time, and thymoglobulin induction. Kidney transplants with 0–10% GS had more transplants without induction therapy.

Table 2. Comparison of donors, recipients, and transplant characteristics between GS 0–10% and GS > 10% transplanted allografts.

	Glomerulosclerosis		
	0–10%	**>10%**	***p*-Value**
N	7796	1730	
Donor			
Age (years)	60.7 ± 7.1	60.5 ± 6.8	0.18
Male (%)	46.7	42.7	0.002
Black (%)	28.8	28.3	0.66
Diabetes (%)	26.5	33.1	<0.001
Hypertension (%)	79.0	81.5	0.02
BMI (kg/m^2)	28.8 ± 6.9	29.2 ± 7.5	0.04
Creatinine (mg/dL) before kidney procurement	1.2 ± 1.0	1.2 ± 0.6	0.85
Donor after cardiac death (%)	10.0	7.0	<0.001
HCV antibody positive (%)	5.8	2.5	<0.001
Cause of death (%)			
Cerebrovascular accident	78.1	80.4	0.04
Machine perfusion (%)	49.9	50.2	0.82
Expanded criteria donor (%)	85.4	87.3	0.04
Recipient			
Age (years)	61.5 ± 9.8	62.2 ± 9.6	0.003
Male (%)	64.0	63.1	0.48
Black (%)	36.4	37.9	0.26
BMI	27.9 ± 5.3	28.1 ± 5.4	0.35
Diabetes (%)	47.2	47.4	0.86
Dialysis duration (%)			
Preemptive	9.8	9.1	0.40
<1 years	8.7	7.8	0.25
1–3 years	29.6	27.9	0.16
>3 years	49.4	52.4	0.02
PRA (%)			
<10	81.7	83.9	0.03
10–60	12.0	10.6	0.10
>60	5.9	4.6	0.03
Missing	0.5	1.0	0.01
Transplant			
HLA DR mismatch (%)			
0	8.2	7.4	0.30
1	39.0	36.9	0.10
2	52.8	55.7	0.03
Cold ischemic time (hours)	19.5 ± 9.4	20.3 ± 9.4	<0.001
Transplant period			
2005–2007	28.6	26.2	0.05
2008–2010	33.8	32.8	0.40
2011–2014	37.6	41.0	0.008
Induction therapy (%)			
Thymoglobulin	46.1	52.0	<0.001
Alemtuzumab	14.7	14.2	0.59
Basiliximab	18.9	18.6	0.79
Other induction	7.6	7.3	0.67
No induction	16.3	11.7	<0.001

GS, glomerulosclerosis; HCV, hepatitis C virus; BMI, body mass index; PRA, panel reactive antibody; HLA, human leukocyte antigen.

3.4. *Post-Transplant Outcomes Based on Percentages of Glomerulosclerosis*

The median (IQR) follow-up was 4.87 (2.90, 7.02) years after kidney transplant. During follow-up, 3015 (29.2%) patients had allograft failure, and 4433 (43.0%) patients died. A total of 1443 (14.0%) patients had acute rejection within one year, and 3436 (33.3%) patients had delayed graft function. Figure 1 compares death-censored graft survival between 0–10% and >10% GS. Graft survival rate at 5 years was 75.8% for 0–10% GS and 70.9% for >10% GS ($p < 0.001$).

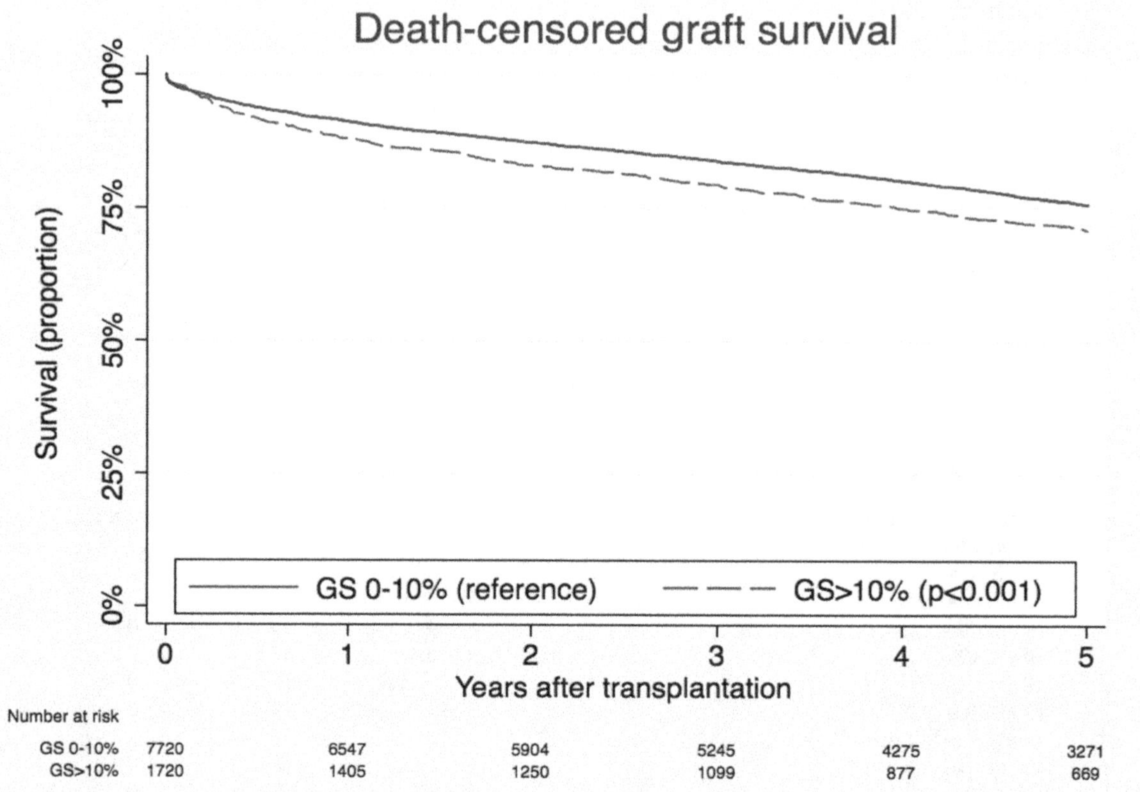

Figure 1. Kaplan–Meier death-censored graft survival curves between 0–10% and >10% allograft glomerulosclerosis (GS) groups.

In unadjusted analysis, kidneys with >10% GS were associated with a 24% higher risk of graft failure compared to kidneys with 0–10% GS (HR 1.24; 95% CI 1.13–1.36, $p < 0.001$). After adjusting for baseline donor, recipient, and transplant-related factors, kidneys with >10% GS remained significantly associated with a 27% higher risk of graft failure compared to kidneys with 0–10% GS (HR 1.27; 95% CI 1.15–1.40, $p < 0.001$) (Table S2). Of note, there was no difference in death-censored graft survival between 11–20% GS and >20% GS (Figure 2 and Table S1). There was no significant difference in patient survival (HR 1.03; 95% CI 0.96–1.12, $p = 0.40$), rate of acute rejection at 1-year (HR 1.13; 95% CI 0.97–1.31, $p = 0.11$), and rate of delayed graft function (HR 1.10; 95% CI 0.98–1.23, $p = 0.11$) between 0–10% GS and >10% GS (Table S2).

We examined the graft outcomes of >85% KDPI kidney with a low degree of GS, compared with 71–85% KDPI kidneys. The death-censored graft survival at 5 years in >85% KDPI kidneys with 0–10% GS was inferior to in 71–85% KPDI kidneys (75.8% vs. 81.2%; $p < 0.001$), as shown in Figure 3.

3.5. *Characteristics and Outcomes of Kidneys with No Biopsy Performed*

Kidneys donors with no biopsy performed were younger, more were female, and had a greater prevalence of positive hepatitis C antibody, but had a lower prevalence of diabetes, hypertension, body weight, donation after cardiac death, use of machine perfusion, and expanded criteria donation when compared with kidneys with 0–10% GS (Table 1). Graft survival rate at 5 years was comparable between 0% and 10% GS and the no biopsy group (75.8% vs. 74.8%; $p = 0.62$), as shown in Figure 2.

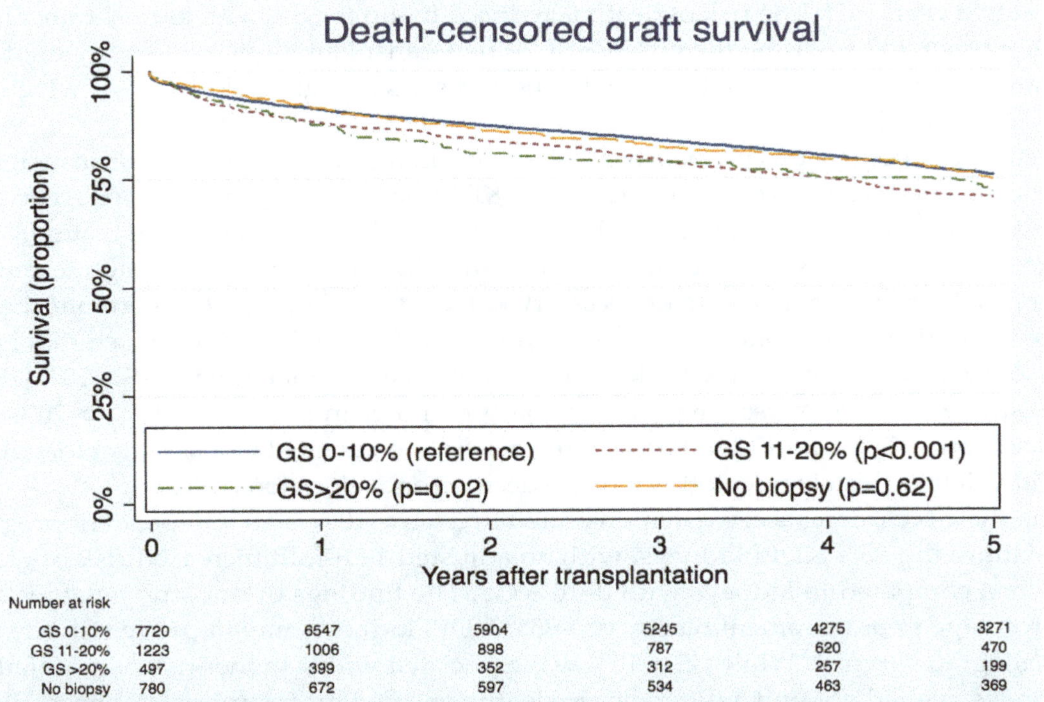

Figure 2. Kaplan–Meier death-censored graft survival curves according to percent glomerulosclerosis (GS) in allografts.

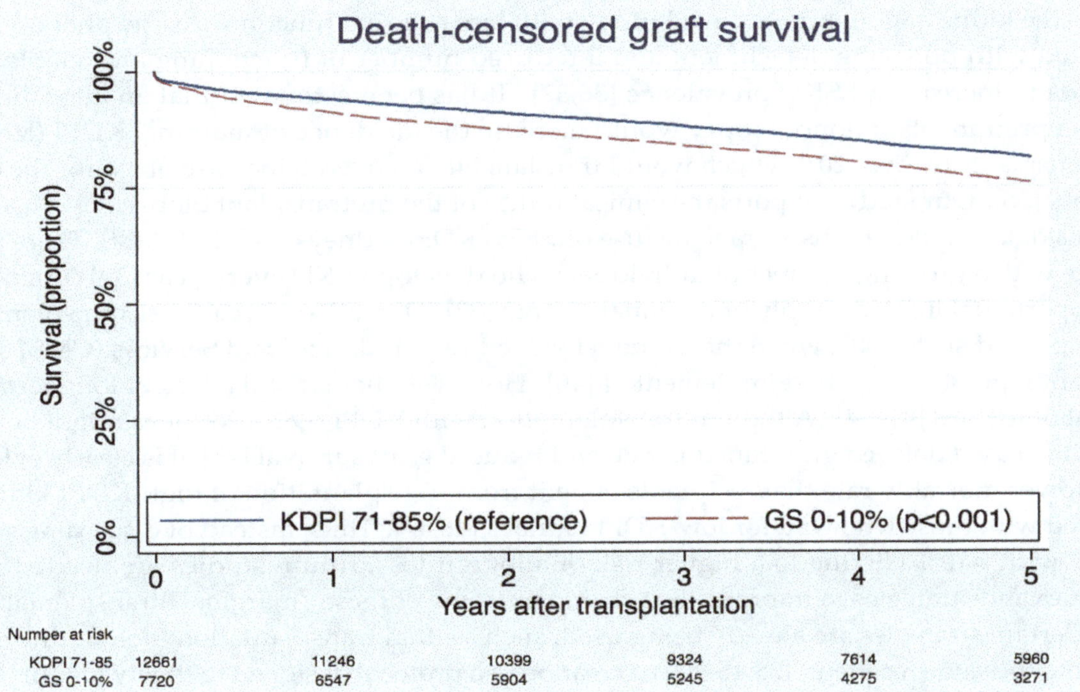

Figure 3. Kaplan–Meier death-censored graft survival curves between the kidney donor profile index (KDPI) 71–85% group and the KDPI >85% with 0–10% percent glomerulosclerosis (GS) group.

4. Discussion

Over 700,000 patients in the United States have ESKD, with the United States having the second-highest incidence rate of treated ESKD in the world [30]. Despite an improvement in dialysis care over the last 15 years, the overall survival on dialysis remains dismal with 22% at one year, 43% at three years and 58% at five years [31]. The risk of death is reduced by up to 66% with kidney transplantation [31]. A major limitation to increasing the number of kidney transplantations is the number of donors. It is thus of paramount importance to decrease the discard rates of high KDPI kidneys, which is estimated to be as high as 50% [8,32].

Our study showed that procurement biopsies are becoming increasingly common in marginal deceased donors in the United States. Ninety-one percent of KDPI >85% kidneys were biopsied on procurement during this study period compared to 85% between 2000 and 2003 in the United States [33]. The utility of procurement biopsies has been debated as they can delay decisions, require high resources, prolong duration of cold ischemia, and lead to unnecessary kidney discard [21,22]. Furthermore, the reliability of GS degree in predicting graft outcomes has been questioned [8,32]. While several studies have reported increased delayed graft function risk, leading to poor outcomes in kidneys with GS > 20% [19,25,28,34,35], and other studies have conversely reported similar prognoses in kidneys with GS > 20% compared to kidneys with lower GS [24,26,27,29]. Banff guidelines for procurement biopsies therefore discourage the use of rigidly defined histologic cutoffs for organ decision and allocation [19].

Using the UNOS database, we demonstrated that GS > 10% is an independent prognostic factor for graft failure in >85% KDPI kidneys, with an adjusted 1.28-fold increased risk of graft failure at 5 years when compared to kidneys with 0–10% GS. The findings of our study suggest that the use of GS percentage in procurement biopsy of >85% KDPI kidneys may improve risk stratification for recipient allograft survival. While GS > 10% was associated with a higher risk of graft failure in >85% KDPI kidneys, we did not find a difference in death-censored graft survival between allografts with 11–20% GS and >20% GS. This may suggest that >10% GS in procurement biopsies can potentially be utilized as a cutoff for risk prediction in clinical practice. Given that the presence of GS > 10% in >85% KDPI kidneys had no significant impact on delayed graft function rate, acute rejection, or patient survival, the underlying explanation for higher graft failure in GS > 10% kidneys is likely due to the progressive kidney aging process in a kidney with less residual function. As the phenotype of GS is associated with podocyte detachment and a reduced number of functioning and viable glomeruli, this leads to increasing ESKD prevalence [36,37]. It has been estimated that an allocation strategy based on pretransplant donor biopsy would increase the incidence of marginal KDPI (80% to 100%) renal transplants by over 20%, which would translate into an overall increase of 4% for the entire pool of donors [38]. Our study supports the clinical utility of the pretransplant biopsy.

This data should not discourage the use of >85% KDPI kidneys with >10% GS. There is an organ shortage with a growing number of individuals who develop ESKD every year [39] combined with a non-proportional limited supply of potential donors [32]. Overall, one-year post-transplant outcomes have improved since 2007, when the Centers for Medicare and Medicaid Services (CMS) solid organ transplant regulation was first implemented [40]. However, there is still a lack of long term graft and survival outcomes [41–44]. Although transplantation with KDPI > 85% kidneys might be associated with an increased delayed graft function rate and reduced graft survival [45], it is clearly evident based on the lower mortality rate that recipients benefit from transplantation of high-KDPI kidneys when compared with those who wait for low-KDPI kidneys [46,47]. Thus, instead of discarding >85% KDPI kidneys with >10% GS due to a higher risk of allograft loss, future studies are needed to identify techniques and strategies to improve the use and outcome of these "marginal" transplantable kidneys safely. Certain strategies are already being used, such as dual transplantation (both kidneys from one donor into the same recipient) [38,48–52] or creation of a protocol designed to timely identify and match suitable patient characteristics with these "marginal" kidneys (e.g., balancing the number of viable nephrons supplied within the graft versus the metabolic demand of the recipient [32]). For example, a >85% KDPI kidney with >10% GS recovered from a female donor with a low BMI may not be the best option for a male candidate with a BMI>35 kg/m^2 [53]; further studies are needed to identify other patient and donor characteristics that would yield optimal outcomes.

Although our study aimed to assess the impact of GS degree on >85% KDPI graft outcomes, the findings of our study cannot be generalized to lower KDPI kidneys. We did compare graft outcomes between KDPI >85% kidneys with 0–10% GS to the overall KDPI 71–85% kidneys. This demonstrated that graft outcomes of KDPI >85% kidneys with 0–10% GS were inferior to KDPI 71–85% kidneys, suggesting a stronger impact of KDPI-related factors on graft outcomes over the percentage of GS on procurement biopsies. As KDPI is comprised of several clinically important donor characteristics that impact outcomes [11], it is hypothesized that these characteristics would similarly have an impact on biopsy pathology that is not limited to GS. Thus, GS percentage should not be used in isolation from other biopsy findings for individualized organ acceptance decisions. In addition, the impact GS on graft outcomes of lower KDPI scores remains unclear, since many lower KDPI kidneys are not biopsied [17–19].

Although our study using the UNOS database is among the largest cohorts investigating procurement biopsies with KDPI > 85%, there are some major limitations. First, there is a lack of uniform criteria for procuring, processing and interpreting procurement graft biopsies [19,54]. Core needle biopsies (during reperfusion) are usually superior to wedge biopsies (during procurement), as wedge biopsies primarily obtain sub capsular tissue, which can overestimate the amount of GS [24,26,32]. Specimens are frozen sections as opposed to paraffin-embedded tissue obtained for regular kidney biopsies or biopsies at reperfusion [21,32]. Procurement biopsies are also often interpreted by on-call general pathologists rather than nephro-pathologists. Unfortunately, the numbers of glomeruli in samples or type of pathologist were not reported in the registry. Thus, more studies aimed at optimizing assessment of procurement biopsy samples to optimally allocate organs are needed. Second, data on other important biopsy parameters in the UNOS database, such as interstitial fibrosis, tubular atrophy, and arteriosclerosis, were limited. Only 30 patients in our cohort had available reports on the degree of interstitial fibrosis, tubular atrophy, or arteriosclerosis. Therefore, future studies evaluating the predictive role of a complete histological evaluation [55], including glomerular, tubular, interstitial, and vascular compartments of >85% KDPI kidneys, are required. Furthermore, GS percentage was reported in the database as 0–10%, 11–20%, and >20%. Thus, kidney transplant outcomes using a higher cut-off of GS percentage could not be evaluated and required future studies. Furthermore, given the differences between procurement biopsies and reperfusion biopsies [18], the findings of our study cannot be generalized to reperfusion biopsies for >85% KDPI kidneys. Finally, the registry may be subjected to selection bias. Kidneys from donors that did not undergo biopsy tended to have less unfavorable clinical characteristics, than those with biopsy as demonstrated in our study (kidney donors in the no biopsy group were younger and had a lower prevalence of diabetes and hypertension), and thus had comparable graft survival rate when compared to the 0–10% GS group, but superior to the >10% GS group. Kidneys with a higher degree of GS were likely to be more carefully selected for unreported factors, including other biopsy characteristics. Alternatively, the kidney discards in each GS percentage cohort may have been impacted by other non-reported factors that influenced study outcomes.

In conclusion, we demonstrated that procurement biopsies for >85% KDPI kidneys are very commonly obtained in the United States, at a rate of 91.2%. A higher percentage of GS in >85% KDPI kidney biopsies are associated with an increased discard rate. Among KDPI >85% kidneys, GS >10% is an independent risk factor for allograft failure. However, graft survival from 0–10% GS kidneys is still inferior to kidneys with KDPI 71–85%, suggesting a stronger impact of KDPI on graft outcomes. Instead of discarding kidneys, future studies are needed to identify strategies to optimally utilize these "marginal" kidneys safely.

Author Contributions: Conceptualization, W.C., C.T., P.K.V., S.K., L.S.C., E.I., J.F. and N.L.; Data curation, W.C. and N.L.; Formal analysis, W.C., A.C. and N.L.; Investigation, W.C., C.T. and N.L.; Methodology, W.C., C.T. and N.L.; Project administration, T.B.; Resources, T.B. and N.L.; Software, N.L.; Supervision, C.T., F.L.K., M.A.M., T.B., S.A.S., S.K., L.S.C., E.I., J.F. and N.L.; Validation, W.C., C.T., A.C., P.H., F.L.K., M.A.M., S.A.S. and N.L.; Visualization, W.C. and C.T.; Writing—original draft, W.C.; Writing—review & editing, W.C., C.T., P.K.V., A.C., P.H., F.L.K., M.A.M., T.B., S.A.S., S.K., L.S.C., E.I., J.F. and N.L. W.C., C.T., P.K.V., A.C., P.H., F.L.K., M.A.M., T.B., S.A.S., S.K., L.S.C., E.I., J.F. and N.L. All authors have read and agreed to the published version of the manuscript.

Acknowledgments: None. All authors had access to the data and played essential roles in writing of the manuscript.

References

1. Hart, A.; Smith, J.M.; Skeans, M.A.; Gustafson, S.K.; Wilk, A.R.; Robinson, A.; Wainright, J.L.; Haynes, C.R.; Snyder, J.J.; Kasiske, B.L. OPTN/SRTR 2016 annual data report: Kidney. *Am. J. Transp.* **2018**, *18*, 18–113. [CrossRef] [PubMed]
2. Papadopoulos, E.B.; Ladanyi, M.; Emanuel, D.; Mackinnon, S.; Boulad, F.; Carabasi, M.H.; Castro-Malaspina, H.; Childs, B.H.; Gillio, A.P.; Small, T.N.; et al. Infusions of donor leukocytes to treat Epstein-Barr virus-associated lymphoproliferative disorders after allogeneic bone marrow transplantation. *N. Engl. J. Med.* **1994**, *330*, 1185–1191. [CrossRef]
3. Gupta, M.; Abt, P.L. Trends among kidney transplant candidates in the United States: Sifting through the tea leaves. *Am. J. Transp.* **2019**, *19*, 313–314. [CrossRef] [PubMed]
4. Cecka, J.M. Kidney transplantation in the United States. *Clin. Transp.* **2008**, 1–18.
5. Andre, M.; Huang, E.; Everly, M.; Bunnapradist, S. The UNOS renal transplant registry: Review of the last decade. *Clin Transp.* **2014**, 1–12.
6. Hart, A.; Smith, J.M.; Skeans, M.A.; Gustafson, S.K.; Stewart, D.E.; Cherikh, W.S.; Wainright, J.L.; Kucheryavaya, A.; Woodbury, M.; Snyder, J.J.; et al. OPTN/SRTR 2015 annual data report: Kidney. *Am. J. Transp.* **2017**, *17*, 21–116. [CrossRef]
7. United States Renal Data System. *2015 USRDS Annual Data Report: Epidemiology of Kidney Disease in the United States*; National Institutes of Health, National Institute of Diabetes and Digestive: Bethesda, MD, USA, 2015.
8. Mohan, S.; Chiles, M.C.; Patzer, R.E.; Pastan, S.O.; Husain, S.A.; Carpenter, D.J.; Dube, G.K.; Crew, R.J.; Ratner, L.E.; Cohen, D.J. Factors leading to the discard of deceased donor kidneys in the United States. *Kidney Int.* **2018**, *94*, 187–198. [CrossRef]
9. Lentine, K.L.; Naik, A.S.; Schnitzler, M.A.; Randall, H.; Wellen, J.R.; Kasiske, B.L.; Marklin, G.; Brockmeier, D.; Cooper, M.; Xiao, H.; et al. Variation in use of procurement biopsies and its implications for discard of deceased donor kidneys recovered for transplantation. *Am. J. Transp.* **2019**, *19*, 2241–2251. [CrossRef]
10. Metzger, R.A.; Delmonico, F.L.; Feng, S.; Port, F.K.; Wynn, J.J.; Merion, R.M. Expanded criteria donors for kidney transplantation. *Am. J. Transp.* **2003**, *4*, 114–125. [CrossRef]
11. Israni, A.K.; Salkowski, N.; Gustafson, S.; Snyder, J.J.; Friedewald, J.J.; Formica, R.N.; Wang, X.; Shteyn, E.; Cherikh, W.; Stewart, D.; et al. New national allocation policy for deceased donor kidneys in the United States and possible effect on patient outcomes. *J. Am. Soc. Nephrol.* **2014**, *25*, 1842–1848. [CrossRef]
12. Hart, A.; Smith, J.M.; Skeans, M.A.; Gustafson, S.K.; Wilk, A.R.; Castro, S.; Robinson, A.; Wainright, J.L.; Snyder, J.J.; Kasiske, B.L.; et al. OPTN/SRTR 2017 annual data report: Kidney. *Am. J. Transp.* **2019**, *19*, 19–123. [CrossRef] [PubMed]
13. Reese, P.P.; Harhay, M.N.; Abt, P.L.; Levine, M.H.; Halpern, S.D. New solutions to reduce discard of kidneys donated for transplantation. *J. Am. Soc. Nephrol.* **2016**, *27*, 973–980. [CrossRef] [PubMed]
14. Bae, S.; Massie, A.B.; Luo, X.; Anjum, S.; Desai, N.M.; Segev, D.L. Changes in discard rate after the introduction of the kidney donor profile index (KDPI). *Am. J. Transp.* **2016**, *16*, 2202–2207. [CrossRef] [PubMed]
15. Narvaez, J.R.F.; Nie, J.; Noyes, K.; Leeman, M.; Kayler, L.K. Hard-to-place kidney offers: Donor- and system-level predictors of discard. *Am. J. Transp.* **2018**, *18*, 2708–2718. [CrossRef]
16. Cohen, J.B.; Shults, J.; Goldberg, D.S.; Abt, P.L.; Sawinski, D.L.; Reese, P.P. Kidney allograft offers: Predictors of turndown and the impact of late organ acceptance on allograft survival. *Am. J. Transp.* **2018**, *18*, 391–401. [CrossRef] [PubMed]

17. Mohan, S.; Campenot, E.; Chiles, M.C.; Santoriello, D.; Bland, E.; Crew, R.J.; Rosenstiel, P.; Dube, G.; Batal, I.; Radhakrishnan, J.; et al. Association between reperfusion renal allograft biopsy findings and transplant outcomes. *J. Am. Soc. Nephrol.* **2017**, *28*, 3109–3117. [CrossRef]
18. Carpenter, D.; Husain, S.A.; Brennan, C.; Batal, I.; Hall, I.E.; Santoriello, D.; Rosen, R.; Crew, R.J.; Campenot, E.; Dube, G.K.; et al. Procurement biopsies in the evaluation of deceased donor kidneys. *Clin. J. Am. Soc. Nephrol.* **2018**, *13*, 1876–1885. [CrossRef]
19. Liapis, H.; Gaut, J.P.; Klein, C.; Bagnasco, S.; Kraus, E.; Farris, A.B., 3rd; Honsova, E.; Perkowska-Ptasinska, A.; David, D.; Goldberg, J.; et al. Banff histopathological consensus criteria for preimplantation kidney biopsies. *Am. J. Transp.* **2017**, *17*, 140–150. [CrossRef]
20. Hall, I.E.; Parikh, C.R.; Schroppel, B.; Weng, F.L.; Jia, Y.; Thiessen-Philbrook, H.; Reese, P.P.; Doshi, M.D. Procurement biopsy findings versus kidney donor risk index for predicting renal allograft survival. *Transp. Direct* **2018**, *4*, e373. [CrossRef]
21. Kasiske, B.L.; Stewart, D.E.; Bista, B.R.; Salkowski, N.; Snyder, J.J.; Israni, A.K.; Crary, G.S.; Rosendale, J.D.; Matas, A.J.; Delmonico, F.L. The role of procurement biopsies in acceptance decisions for kidneys retrieved for transplant. *Clin. J. Am. Soc. Nephrol.* **2014**, *9*, 562–571. [CrossRef]
22. Stewart, D.E.; Garcia, V.C.; Rosendale, J.D.; Klassen, D.K.; Carrico, B.J. Diagnosing the decades-long rise in the deceased donor kidney discard rate in the United States. *Transplantation* **2017**, *101*, 575–587. [CrossRef] [PubMed]
23. Wang, C.J.; Wetmore, J.B.; Crary, G.S.; Kasiske, B.L. The donor kidney biopsy and its implications in predicting graft outcomes: A systematic review. *Am. J. Transp.* **2015**, *15*, 1903–1914. [CrossRef]
24. Sung, R.S.; Christensen, L.L.; Leichtman, A.B.; Greenstein, S.M.; Distant, D.A.; Wynn, J.J.; Stegall, M.D.; Delmonico, F.L.; Port, F.K. Determinants of discard of expanded criteria donor kidneys: Impact of biopsy and machine perfusion. *Am. J. Transp.* **2008**, *8*, 783–792. [CrossRef] [PubMed]
25. Escofet, X.; Osman, H.; Griffiths, D.F.; Woydag, S.; Adam Jurewicz, W. The presence of glomerular sclerosis at time zero has a significant impact on function after cadaveric renal transplantation. *Transplantation* **2003**, *75*, 344–346. [CrossRef] [PubMed]
26. Malek, S.K. Procurement biopsies in kidneys retrieved for transplantation. *Clin. J. Am. Soc. Nephrol.* **2014**, *9*, 443–444. [CrossRef]
27. Bajwa, M.; Cho, Y.W.; Pham, P.T.; Shah, T.; Danovitch, G.; Wilkinson, A.; Bunnapradist, S. Donor biopsy and kidney transplant outcomes: An analysis using the organ procurement and transplantation network/united network for organ sharing (OPTN/UNOS) database. *Transplantation* **2007**, *84*, 1399–1405. [CrossRef]
28. Edwards, E.B.; Posner, M.P.; Maluf, D.G.; Kauffman, H.M. Reasons for non-use of recovered kidneys: The effect of donor glomerulosclerosis and creatinine clearance on graft survival. *Transplantation* **2004**, *77*, 1411–1415. [CrossRef]
29. Cicciarelli, J.; Cho, Y.; Mateo, R.; El-Shahawy, M.; Iwaki, Y.; Selby, R. Renal biopsy donor group: The influence of glomerulosclerosis on transplant outcomes. *Transplant. Proc.* **2005**, *37*, 712–713. [CrossRef]
30. Barlesi, F.; Vansteenkiste, J.; Spigel, D.; Ishii, H.; Garassino, M.; de Marinis, F.; Özgüroğlu, M.; Szczesna, A.; Polychronis, A.; Uslu, R.; et al. Avelumab versus docetaxel in patients with platinum-treated advanced non-small-cell lung cancer (JAVELIN Lung 200): An open-label, randomised, phase 3 study. *Lancet Oncol.* **2018**, *19*, 1468–1479. [CrossRef]
31. Hanna, R. Acute kidney injury after pembrolizumab-induced adrenalitis and adrenal insufficiency. *Case Rep. Nephrol. Dial.* **2018**, *8*, 238. [CrossRef]
32. Angeletti, A.; Cravedi, P. Making procurement biopsies important again for kidney transplant allocation. *Nephron* **2019**, *142*, 34–39. [CrossRef] [PubMed]
33. Cecka, J.M.; Cohen, B.; Rosendale, J.; Smith, M. Could more effective use of kidneys recovered from older deceased donors result in more kidney transplants for older patients? *Transplantation* **2006**, *81*, 966–970. [CrossRef] [PubMed]
34. Gaber, L.W.; Moore, L.W.; Alloway, R.R.; Amiri, M.H.; Vera, S.R.; Gaber, A.O. Glomerulosclerosis as a determinant of posttransplant function of older donor renal allografts. *Transplantation* **1995**, *60*, 334–339. [CrossRef] [PubMed]
35. Randhawa, P.S.; Minervini, M.I.; Lombardero, M.; Duquesnoy, R.; Fung, J.; Shapiro, R.; Jordan, M.; Vivas, C.; Scantlebury, V.; Demetris, A. Biopsy of marginal donor kidneys: Correlation of histologic findings with graft dysfunction. *Transplantation* **2000**, *69*, 1352–1357. [CrossRef]

36. Hodgin, J.B.; Bitzer, M.; Wickman, L.; Afshinnia, F.; Wang, S.Q.; O'Connor, C.; Yang, Y.; Meadowbrooke, C.; Chowdhury, M.; Kikuchi, M.; et al. Glomerular aging and focal global glomerulosclerosis: A podometric perspective. *J. Am. Soc. Nephrol.* **2015**, *26*, 3162–3178. [CrossRef]
37. Rowland, J.; Akbarov, A.; Maan, A.; Eales, J.; Dormer, J.; Tomaszewski, M. Tick-tock chimes the kidney clock—From biology of renal ageing to clinical applications. *Kidney Blood Press. Res.* **2018**, *43*, 55–67. [CrossRef]
38. Gandolfini, I.; Buzio, C.; Zanelli, P.; Palmisano, A.; Cremaschi, E.; Vaglio, A.; Piotti, G.; Melfa, L.; La Manna, G.; Feliciangeli, G.; et al. The Kidney Donor Profile Index (KDPI) of marginal donors allocated by standardized pretransplant donor biopsy assessment: Distribution and association with graft outcomes. *Am. J. Transp.* **2014**, *14*, 2515–2525. [CrossRef]
39. McCullough, K.P.; Morgenstern, H.; Saran, R.; Herman, W.H.; Robinson, B.M. Projecting ESRD incidence and prevalence in the United States through 2030. *J. Am. Soc. Nephrol.* **2019**, *30*, 127–135. [CrossRef]
40. Jay, C.; Schold, J.D. Measuring transplant center performance: The goals are not controversial but the methods and consequences can be. *Curr. Transp.* **2017**, *4*, 52–58. [CrossRef]
41. Thongprayoon, C.; Hansrivijit, P.; Leeaphorn, N.; Acharya, P.; Torres-Ortiz, A.; Kaewput, W.; Kovvuru, K.; Kanduri, S.R.; Bathini, T.; Cheungpasitporn, W. Recent advances and clinical outcomes of kidney transplantation. *J. Clin. Med.* **2020**, *9*, 1193. [CrossRef]
42. Thongprayoon, C.; Kaewput, W.; Kovvuru, K.; Hansrivijit, P.; Kanduri, S.R.; Bathini, T.; Chewcharat, A.; Leeaphorn, N.; Gonzalez-Suarez, M.L.; Cheungpasitporn, W. Promises of big data and artificial intelligence in nephrology and transplantation. *J. Clin. Med.* **2020**, *9*, 1107. [CrossRef] [PubMed]
43. Leeaphorn, N.; Thongprayoon, C.; Chon, W.J.; Cummings, L.S.; Mao, M.A.; Cheungpasitporn, W. Outcomes of kidney retransplantation after graft loss as a result of BK virus nephropathy in the era of newer immunosuppressant agents. *Am. J. Transp.* **2020**, *20*, 1334–1340. [CrossRef] [PubMed]
44. Cheungpasitporn, W.; Kremers, W.K.; Lorenz, E.; Amer, H.; Cosio, F.G.; Stegall, M.D.; Gandhi, M.J.; Schinstock, C.A. De novo donor-specific antibody following BK nephropathy: The incidence and association with antibody-mediated rejection. *Clin. Transp.* **2018**, *32*, e13194. [CrossRef] [PubMed]
45. Zens, T.J.; Danobeitia, J.S.; Leverson, G.; Chlebeck, P.J.; Zitur, L.J.; Redfield, R.R.; D'Alessandro, A.M.; Odorico, S.; Kaufman, D.B.; Fernandez, L.A. The impact of kidney donor profile index on delayed graft function and transplant outcomes: A single-center analysis. *Clin. Transp.* **2018**, *32*, e13190. [CrossRef] [PubMed]
46. Jay, C.L.; Washburn, K.; Dean, P.G.; Helmick, R.A.; Pugh, J.A.; Stegall, M.D. Survival benefit in older patients associated with earlier transplant with high KDPI kidneys. *Transplantation* **2017**, *101*, 867–872. [CrossRef]
47. Massie, A.B.; Luo, X.; Chow, E.K.; Alejo, J.L.; Desai, N.M.; Segev, D.L. Survival benefit of primary deceased donor transplantation with high-KDPI kidneys. *Am. J. Transp.* **2014**, *14*, 2310–2316. [CrossRef]
48. Ruggenenti, P.; Silvestre, C.; Boschiero, L.; Rota, G.; Furian, L.; Perna, A.; Rossini, G.; Remuzzi, G.; Rigotti, P. Long-term outcome of renal transplantation from octogenarian donors: A multicenter controlled study. *Am. J. Transp.* **2017**, *17*, 3159–3171. [CrossRef]
49. Moore, P.S.; Farney, A.C.; Sundberg, A.K.; Rohr, M.S.; Hartmann, E.L.; Iskandar, S.S.; Gautreaux, M.D.; Rogers, J.; Doares, W.; Anderson, T.K.; et al. Dual kidney transplantation: A case-control comparison with single kidney transplantation from standard and expanded criteria donors. *Transplantation* **2007**, *83*, 1551–1556. [CrossRef]
50. Gill, J.; Cho, Y.W.; Danovitch, G.M.; Wilkinson, A.; Lipshutz, G.; Pham, P.T.; Gill, J.S.; Shah, T.; Bunnapradist, S. Outcomes of dual adult kidney transplants in the United States: An analysis of the OPTN/UNOS database. *Transplantation* **2008**, *85*, 62–68. [CrossRef]
51. Remuzzi, G.; Cravedi, P.; Perna, A.; Dimitrov, B.D.; Turturro, M.; Locatelli, G.; Rigotti, P.; Baldan, N.; Beatini, M.; Valente, U.; et al. Long-term outcome of renal transplantation from older donors. *N. Engl. J. Med.* **2006**, *354*, 343–352. [CrossRef]
52. Lee, K.W.; Park, J.B.; Cha, S.R.; Lee, S.H.; Chung, Y.J.; Yoo, H.; Kim, K.; Kim, S.J. Dual kidney transplantation offers a safe and effective way to use kidneys from deceased donors older than 70 years. *BMC Nephrol.* **2020**, *21*, 3. [CrossRef] [PubMed]
53. Foley, D.P.; Sawinski, D. Personalizing donor kidney selection: Choosing the right donor for the right recipient. *Clin. J. Am. Soc. Nephrol.* **2019**, *15*, 418–420. [CrossRef] [PubMed]
54. Naesens, M. Zero-time renal transplant biopsies: A comprehensive review. *Transplantation* **2016**, *100*, 1425–1439. [CrossRef] [PubMed]

12

Altered Gut Microbial Fermentation and Colonization with *Methanobrevibacter smithii* in Renal Transplant Recipients

Tim J. Knobbe [1,*], Rianne M. Douwes [1], Daan Kremer [1], J. Casper Swarte [1,2], Michele F. Eisenga [1], António W. Gomes-Neto [1], Marco van Londen [1], Frans T. M. Peters [2], Hans Blokzijl [2], Ilja M. Nolte [3], Wouter H. Hendriks [4], Hermie J. M. Harmsen [5] and Stephan J. L. Bakker [1]

1 Department of Internal Medicine, Division of Nephrology, University Medical Center Groningen, University of Groningen, 9700 RB Groningen, The Netherlands; r.m.douwes@umcg.nl (R.M.D.); d.kremer@umcg.nl (D.K.); j.c.swarte@umcg.nl (J.C.S.); m.f.eisenga@umcg.nl (M.F.E.); a.w.gomes.neto@umcg.nl (A.W.G.-N.); m.van.londen@umcg.nl (M.v.L.); s.j.l.bakker@umcg.nl (S.J.L.B.)

2 Department of Gastroenterology and Hepatology, University Medical Center Groningen, University of Groningen, 9700 RB Groningen, The Netherlands; f.t.m.peters@umcg.nl (F.T.M.P.); h.blokzijl@umcg.nl (H.B.)

3 Department of Epidemiology, University Medical Center Groningen, University of Groningen, 9700 RB Groningen, The Netherlands; i.m.nolte@umcg.nl

4 Department of Animal Sciences, Wageningen University & Research centre, 6708 PB Wageningen, The Netherlands; wouter.hendriks@wur.nl

5 Department of Medical Microbiology, University Medical Center Groningen, University of Groningen, 9700RB Groningen, The Netherlands; h.j.m.harmsen@umcg.nl

* Correspondence: t.j.knobbe@umcg.nl

Abstract: Renal transplant recipients (RTRs) often suffer from posttransplant diarrhea. The observed dysbiosis in RTR may influence the fermentation processes in the gut. In this study, we aimed to investigate whether fermentation differs between RTRs and healthy controls (HCs), by measuring breath H_2 and CH_4 concentrations. Additionally, we determined the fecal presence of the methanogen *Methanobrevibacter smithii* (*M. smithii*), which plays a main role in the process of methanogenesis. Data from the TransplantLines Biobank and Cohort Study (NCT03272841) was used. A total of 142 RTRs and 77 HCs were included. Breath H_2 concentrations in RTRs were not significantly different from HCs. Breath CH_4 concentrations in RTRs were significantly lower compared with HCs (median [interquartile range (IQR)] 7.5 [3.9–10.6] ppm vs. 16.0 [8.0–45.5] ppm, $p < 0.001$). *M. smithii* was less frequently present in the feces of RTRs compared to HCs (28.6% vs. 86.4% resp., $p < 0.001$). Our findings regarding the altered methanogenesis in the gut of RTRs show similarities with previous results in inflammatory bowel disease patients. These findings provide novel insight into the alterations of fermentation after renal transplantation, which may contribute to understanding the occurrence of posttransplant diarrhea.

Keywords: posttransplant diarrhea; methanogenesis; *Methanosphaera stadtmanae*; mucins; sulfate-reducing bacteria

---

1. Introduction

Renal transplantation is the preferred treatment for patients with end-stage renal disease [1–3]. Part of its success has been made possible by improved therapeutic options, such as ameliorations in surgical techniques and perioperative care [4]. Despite the success of transplantation, the burden of morbidity in renal transplant recipients (RTRs) remains high [5].

Patients often experience gastrointestinal complaints such as diarrhea, which is associated with premature kidney allograft failure and mortality, and which affects quality of life [5,6]. This posttransplant diarrhea is believed to be non-infectious and induced by the use of medication [5,7]. Recently, a study in RTRs showed that dysbiosis in the gut might cause or contribute to this posttransplant diarrhea [7]. Lee et al. demonstrated in this study that the gut microbiota diversity of RTRs with diarrhea was significantly lower than in RTRs without diarrhea. In addition, RTRs with diarrhea had a lower diversity of commensal bacterial taxa in the gut, creating a dysfunctional metabolic state. These commensal bacterial taxa are important for the degradation of complex molecules such as complex carbohydrates. During this degradation, among many other molecules, short-chain fatty acids are produced, which contributes to overall gut health [8,9]. It has been proposed that posttransplant diarrhea might be the consequence of a diminished ability to digest complex sugars [7]. A proportion of complex polymers such as fibers escape digestion and absorption in the small bowel. These complex polymers are then fermented to short-chain fatty acids (acetate, butyrate and propionate) and gases (hydrogen (H_2) and carbon dioxide (CO_2)) [10].

In order to maintain fermentation, it is essential that H_2 concentration is reduced by H_2-consuming microorganisms [11]. H_2 can be used as an electron donor in sulfate respiration, methanogenesis or acetogenesis to produce hydrogen sulfide (H_2S), methane (CH_4) and acetate, respectively [12]. Production of H_2S is most favorable, followed by the production of CH_4 and acetate, respectively. However, for the production of H_2S, the presence of sulfate is necessary [13]. The production of CH_4 is performed by archaea. *Methanobrevibacter smithii* (*M. smithii*) and *Methanosphaera stadtmanae (M. stadtmanae)* are the two methanogens usually detected in the human gut. *M. smithii* is the predominant methanogen in the human colon [14]. Next to $H_{2,}$, formate can be used for the methanogenesis as well [15]. The produced CH_4 and the remaining H_2 are excreted in breath and flatus. Therefore, both gases can be measured in exhaled breath [13]. Measuring breath CH_4 concentrations is a simple way to investigate the metabolism of intestinal methanogens, since no significant catabolism elsewhere in the human body has been observed [12]. The presence of *M. smithii* can be measured in the feces, as has previously been performed in studies investigating patients suffering from inflammatory bowel disease (IBD) [12,16].

The dysbiosis in RTRs may influence the fermentation in the gut and the processes following fermentation, possibly leading to or contributing to posttransplant diarrhea. To gain more insight into pathogenesis of this diarrhea, we aimed to investigate the fermentation and methanogenesis in the gut in RTRs. Firstly, we aimed to investigate whether breath H_2 and CH_4 concentrations differ between RTRs and HCs. Secondly, we aimed to investigate whether the presence of *M. smithii* in feces differs between RTRs and HCs, and finally we aimed to identify the determinants of CH_4 production.

2. Methods

2.1. Study Population

For this study we used data from the TransplantLines Biobank and Cohort Study (ClinicalTrials.gov identifier: NCT03272841). A detailed description of the study design, inclusion and exclusion criteria has been described previously [17]. In addition to the standard protocol, we measured breath H_2 and CH_4 concentrations and analyzed the presence of *M. smithii* in feces for the current study. (Potential) living organ donors were used as a healthy control group for comparison. Our inclusion period was between February and December 2017. The study protocol has been approved by the Institutional Review Board (METc 2014/077) (METc UMCG), adheres to the UMCG Biobank Regulation, and is in accordance with the WMA Declaration of Helsinki and the Declaration of Istanbul [17].

2.2. Patient Comorbidities

Diabetes mellitus was defined according to the guidelines of the American Diabetes Association [18]. The estimated glomerular filtration rate (eGFR) was calculated using the serum creatinine-based chronic kidney disease epidemiology collaboration (CKD-EPI) formula. Data regarding the history of allograft rejection and primary renal disease before transplantation were retrieved from patients' medical files.

2.3. Breath H_2 and CH_4 Concentration Measurement

For H_2 and CH_4 measurements, breath samples were collected using a 50 cc syringe with an opening of 6 mm in diameter at approximately 40 cc with a 3-way-stopcock. Subjects were instructed to inhale normally and exhale fully in the syringe, with the plunger set at 50 cc and the 3-way stopcock open. After full expiration, the opening was immediately closed by the subject's finger, the plunger was set to 30 cc and the 3-way stopcock was closed. This resulted in breath samples that were not diluted by environmental air. Two breath samples were taken subsequently per study subject. Breath samples were analyzed within 12 h after sample collection. H_2, CH_4 and CO_2 measurements were performed using a solid-state gas-chromatography device (Breathtracker SC, QuinTron Instrument Company, Inc., Milwaukee, WI, USA). The device separates the components by the basic principle of gas chromatography, using room air as the carrier gas, which is pumped through the system by an internal circulating pump. H_2 and CH_4 are separated from all other reducing gases and from each other, and are carried past a solid-state sensor [19]. The sensors are reported to be affected only by reducing gases, so it is unaffected by other gases in the sample; it can also employ a CO_2 correction factor [19]. The analytical sensitivity is 1 ppm for H_2 and CH_4 and 0.1% for CO_2. The Breathtracker has a linear analytical range of 2–150 ppm for H_2, 2–75 ppm for CH_4 and 1000–70,000 ppm for CO_2. To ensure reliable breath measurements, study subjects were not allowed to smoke for at least one hour before the sample collection [20].

2.4. M. Smithii Measurement in Feces

Fecal samples were collected the day prior to the TransplantLines visit, using a FecesCatcher (TAG Hemi VOF, Zeijen, The Netherlands) and were immediately frozen after collection. The feces samples were transported in cold storage to the TransplantLines visit, and immediately stored at −80 °C (−112 °F) [17]. After thawing, DNA was extracted with the RBB and Qiagen method, as performed by Yu et al. with modifications described by de Goffau et al. [21,22]. To measure the quantity of *M. smithii*, real-time quantitative reverse transcription polymerase chain reaction (RT-PCR) (7500 real time PCR system, applied Biosystems, Thermo Fisher Scientific, Waltham, USA) was performed. Primers were taken as described by Johnston et al., and differentiation between *M. smithii* and other organisms in the sample was assessed using *nifH* genes [23]. The number of *nifH* genes are equal to the number of *M. smithii*, since only one gene of *nifH* is present in each *M. smithii* [24]. Analyses were performed using the Taqman machine and processed using SDSShell (Applied Biosystems, Thermo Fisher Scientific, Waltham, USA). The quantifiable presence of *M. smithii* was determined using a cycle threshold value. Values < 40 cycles were regarded as positive, and values ≥40 were regarded as negative. For analyses, CT-values ≥40 were regarded as negative and concentrations of *M. smithii* in these patients were regarded as 0 *M. smithii*/gram feces. A detailed method description is attached in Supplementary File 1.

2.5. Statistical Analyses

Statistical analyses were performed using the Statistical Package for the Social Sciences (SPSS) version 23.0 (IBM corp.; Armonk, NY, USA). In all analyses, $p < 0.05$ was regarded as statistically significant. Categorical variables are presented as n (%), normally distributed variables as mean ± standard deviation (SD) and non-normally distributed variables as median [interquartile range]. Normality was assessed using Q–Q plots. Differences between groups with normally distributed variables were assessed using independent T-tests. Non-normally distributed data were compared using the Mann–Whitney U test. Comparison of categorical variables was performed using a chi-square test for groups with $n \geq 5$ and a Fisher's exact test for groups with $n < 5$. For all other tests and visualizations, the mean of the duplicate measurements of the breath H_2 and CH_4 concentration in breath was used. To correct for environmental CH_4, 2 ppm was subtracted from each breath

CH_4-measurement [25,26]. Possible determinants of breath CH_4 were identified using univariable linear regression. All variables with a p-value <0.2 were included in a multivariable linear regression model run backward to identify the determinants of breath CH_4 production. Because H_2 is used by *M. smithii* for the conversion to CH_4, an interaction term of H_2 and *M. smithii* was added in the analysis. Log_{10} transformations were performed if necessary to reach conditions in all performed analyses.

3. Results

We included 219 study subjects, of whom 142 (64.8%) were RTRs and 77 (35.2%) were HCs. Among RTRs, 91 (64.1%) were male, and the mean age was 56.3 ± 13.7 years. Among HCs, 39 (50.6%) were male, and the mean age was 56.4 ± 10.6 years. Baseline characteristics are shown in Table 1. A Consort Flow diagram is presented to provide an overview of subgroups that were used in different analyses (Figure 1). Breath H_2 concentrations of the RTRs were not significantly different compared with HCs (Table 1). The RTRs had, however, lower breath CH_4 concentrations compared to the HCs (7.5 [3.9–10.6] ppm vs. 16.0 [8.0–45.5] ppm, $p < 0.001$). Data distributions of breath H_2 and CH_4 concentrations are shown in Supplementary File 2. Raw data are shown in the Supplementary data.

Table 1. Baseline characteristics.

Characteristics	Renal Transplant Recipients	Healthy Controls	p-Value
Number of subjects, *n* (%)	142 (64.8)	77 (35.2)	*n*/a
Fermentation parameters			
Breath H_2 concentration, ppm	11.3 [4.0–30.0]	10.5 [4.5–28.3]	0.9
Breath CH_4 concentration, ppm	7.5 [3.9–10.6]	16.0 [8.0–45.5]	<0.001
Quantifiable abundance of *M. smithii* in feces, *n* (valid %)	22 (28.6)	38 (86.4)	<0.001
Abundance of *M. smithii* in feces samples, *M. smithii*/gram	0.0 [0.0–4.0 × 10^5]	5.9 × 10^7 [1.2 × 10^6–8.9 × 10^8]	<0.001
Demographics			
Age, y	56.3 ± 13.7	56.4 ± 10.6	0.6
Number of males, *n* (%)	91 (64.1)	39 (50.6)	0.05
BMI, kg/m^2	28.0 ± 5.2	26.4 ± 3.8	0.01
Time since transplantation, y	1.0 [0.5–8.0]	-	n/a
Lifestyle parameters			
Current smokers, *n* (valid %)	23 (16.7)	14 (18.9)	0.4
Alcohol intake per day, units	0.0 [0.0–0.2]	0.25 [0.0-0.5]	0.003
Laboratory parameters			
Hemoglobin, g/dL	13.8 ± 1.9	14.4 ± 1.3	0.008
Hematocrit, L/L	0.42 ± 0.06	0.43 ± 0.04	0.2
Leukocytes, 10^9/L	7.4 ± 2.5	6.5 ± 1.9	<0.003
Platelets, 10^9/L	250.6 ± 78.4	261.2 ± 56.6	0.3
C-reactive protein, mg/L	2.3 [1.1–5.0]	1.2 [0.8–4.0]	0.035
Albumin, g/L	44.2 ± 3.1	45.4 ± 2.5	0.003
Glucose, mmol/L	6.0 ± 1.7	5.5 ± 0.7	0.005
HbA1c, mmol/mol	42.3 ± 7.8	36.9 ± 3.5	<0.001
eGFR, ml/min/1.73 m^2	49.8 ± 16.5	69.3 ± 18.7	<0.001
Creatinine, μmol/L	130 [103.0–156.8]	92.0 [81.0–106.0]	<0.001
Urea, mmol/L	9.4 ± 4.4	5.8 ± 1.6	<0.001
Medication use			
Antibiotics, *n* (%)	37 (16.9)	0 (0.0)	<0.001
Immunosuppressants, *n* (%)			
Prednisolone, *n* (%)	140 (98.6)	-	*n*/a
Mycophenolate mofetil, *n* (%)	112 (78.9)	-	*n*/a
Tacrolimus, *n* (%)	102 (71.8)	-	*n*/a

Table 1. *Cont.*

Characteristics	Renal Transplant Recipients	Healthy Controls	*p*-Value
Cyclosporine, *n* (%)	14 (9.9)	-	*n*/a
Everolimus, *n* (%)	7 (4.9)	-	*n*/a
Azathioprine, *n* (%)	10 (7.0)	-	*n*/a
Statins, *n* (%)	70 (49.3)	8 (10.4)	<0.001
Proton pump inhibitors, *n* (%)	108 (76.1)	0 (0.0)	<0.001
Insulin, *n* (%)	11 (7.8)	0 (0.0)	0.009
Biguanides, *n* (%)	7 (4.9)	0 (0.0)	0.09
Macrogol, *n* (%)	8 (5.6)	1 (1.3)	0.200
Lactulose, *n* (%)	2 (1.4)	0 (0.0)	0.500
Loperamide, *n* (%)	1 (0.7)	0 (0.0)	1.000
Antidepressants, *n* (%)	16 (7.3)	4 (5.2)	0.4
Primary renal disease before transplantation			
Unknown, *n* (%)	23 (16.2)	-	*n*/a
Inflammatory disease	55 (38.7)		
Congenital and hereditary kidney disease, *n* (%)	41 (28.9)	-	*n*/a
Renal vascular disease, excluding vasculitis, *n* (%)	13 (9.2)	-	*n*/a
Diabetic nephropathy, *n* (%)	10 (7.0)	-	*n*/a
Others			
Diabetes mellitus, *n* (%)	27 (19.0)	1 (1.3)	<0.001
History of allograft rejection, *n* (%)	14 (9.9)	-	*n*/a

Data are presented as mean ± standard deviation (SD), median with interquartile ranges (IQRs) or number with percentages (%). Abbreviations: BMI, body mass index; eGFR, estimated glomerular filtration rate; CH_4, methane; H_2, hydrogen; HbA1c, hemoglobin A1c; *M. smithii*, *Methanobrevibacter smithii*.

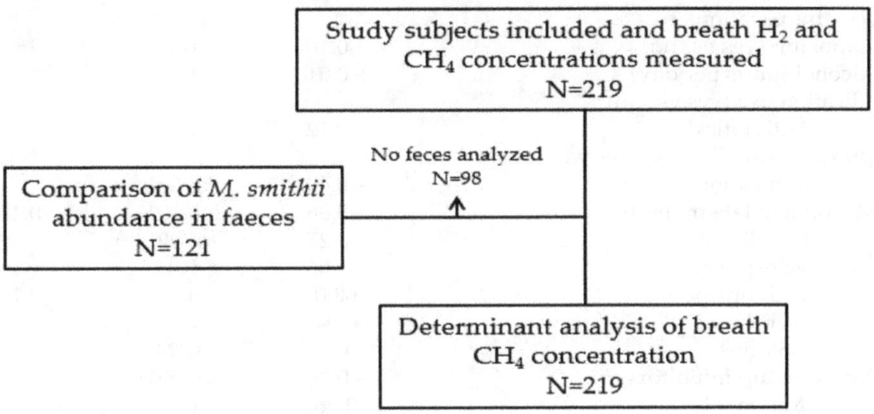

Figure 1. Consort flow diagram. Abbreviations: CH_4, methane; H_2, hydrogen; *M. smithii*, *Methanobrevibacter* smithii.

3.1. *M. Smithii in Feces*

The feces of 98 study subjects was not available for analysis. *M. smithii* abundance was analyzed in the feces samples of 77 RTRs and 44 HCs (i.e., 121 of 219 study subjects, see Figure 1). Among the RTRs, 22 (28.6%) had quantifiable concentrations of *M. smithii* in their stool samples. Among HCs, 38 (86.4%) had quantifiable concentrations of *M. smithii* in their feces samples. The median abundance of *M. smithii* in the feces of those study subjects was 5.9×10^7 [1.2×10^6–8.9×10^8] per gram feces. A quantifiable concentration of *M. smithii* was significantly less frequently observed in RTRs compared to HCs ((22 (28.6%) vs. 38 (86.4%) resp.; $p < 0.001$) (Table 1). In addition, the abundance of *M. smithii* was positively correlated with breath CH_4 concentrations ($r = 0.69$, $p < 0.001$).

3.2. Determinants of Breath CH_4

Determinants of breath CH_4 were analyzed using linear regression analysis in all 219 study subjects, and these results are presented in Table 2. Breath H_2 and the presence of a quantifiable abundance of *M. smithii* in feces were associated with higher breath CH_4 concentrations (standardized beta (st. β) 0.57, $p < 0.001$ and st. β 0.94, $p < 0.001$ resp.). A negative interaction was found between both determinants on breath CH_4 (st. β −0.51, $p = 0.001$), indicating that in the presence of *M. smithii* the magnitude of the correlation between H_2 and CH_4 in breath decreases from overt to virtually absent ($r = 0.88$, $p < 0.001$ vs. $r = 0.09$, $p = 0.5$ resp., Figure 2). In addition, the use of mycophenolate mofetil was associated with a lower breath CH_4 concentration (st. β −0.18, $p = 0.014$). The described determinants explained 55.0% of the total variation in breath CH_4 concentrations.

Table 2. Linear regression analysis of $\log_{10}$ breath CH_4 concentration.

	Univariable Linear Regression Analysis		Multivariable Linear Regression Analysis *	
	St. β	*p*-Value	St. β	*p*-Value
A medical history of renal transplantation (yes vs. no)	−0.42	<0.001		
Fermentation parameters				
$\log_{10}$ Breath H_2, ppm	0.32	<0.001	0.54	<0.001
Quantifiable abundance of *M. smithii* in feces (yes vs. no)	0.55	<0.001	0.95	<0.001
Interaction between $\log_{10}$ breath H_2 and *M. smithii* in feces	0.48	<0.001	−0.51	0.001
Demographics				
Age, y	0.07	0.3		
Gender (yes vs. no)	−0.02	0.7		
BMI, kg/m^2	−0.18	0.012		
eGFR, mL/min/1.73 m^2	0.25	<0.001		
Intoxications				
Smoking (yes vs. no)	−0.10	0.1		
Alcohol (units per day)	−0.01	0.9		
Medication use (yes vs. no)				
Antibiotics	−0.12	0.1		
Immunosuppressive medication (yes vs. no)				
Prednisolone	−0.40	<0.001		
Mycophenolate mofetil	−0.36	<0.001	−0.18	0.014
Tacrolimus	−0.27	<0.001		
Cyclosporine	−0.06	0.4		
Azathioprine	0.00	1.0	−0.10	0.1
Everolimus	0.04	0.5		
Statins	−0.15	0.024		
Proton pump inhibitors	−0.26	<0.001		
Macrogol	0.06	0.4		
Lactulose	0.10	0.1		
Loperamide	0.02	0.8		
Biguanide drugs	−0.04	0.6		
Insulin	−0.05	0.5		
Antidepressants	−0.14	0.044		
Primary renal disease of RTR (yes vs. no)				
Unknown	−0.04	0.6		
Inflammatory disease	0.02	0.8		
Congenital and hereditary kidney disease	0.00	1.0		
Renal vascular disease, excluding vasculitis	0.09	0.3		
Diabetes Mellitus	−0.08	0.3		
Others (yes vs. no)				
Suffering from Diabetes Mellitus	−0.06	0.4		
History of allograft rejection	−0.02	0.8		

Abbreviations: BMI, body mass index; eGFR, estimated glomerular filtration rate; CH_4, methane; H_2, hydrogen; *M. smithii*, *Methanobrevibacter smithii*; St. β, standardized beta. $R^2 = 0.550$. * Run backwards.

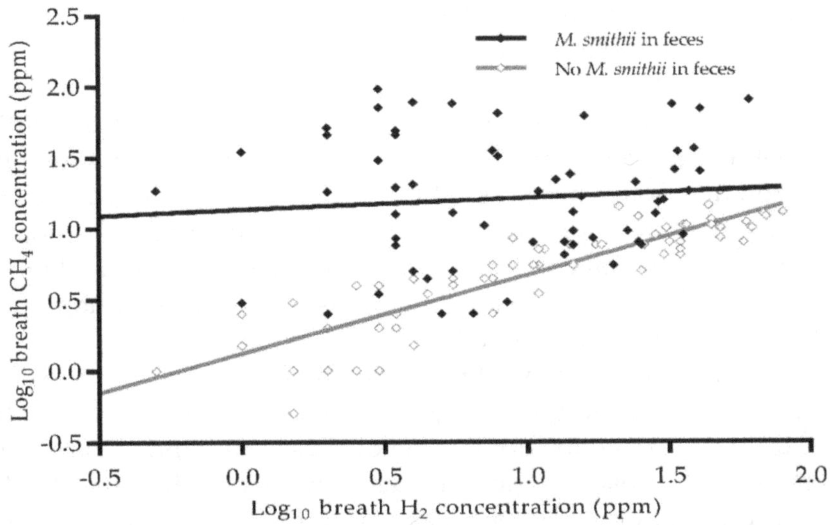

Figure 2. Scatterplot of $\log_{10}$ breath H_2 and CH_4 concentration by presence of *M. smithii* in feces. There is a difference between the relation between H_2 and CH_4 in subjects with and without *M. smithii*. Abbreviations: CH_4, methane; H_2, hydrogen; *M. smithii*, *Methanobrevibacter smithii*. $N = 121$. Pearson correlation in the absence of *M. smithii*, $r = 0.88$, $p < 0.001$. Pearson correlation in the presence of *M. smithii*, $r = 0.09$, $p = 0.5$.

4. Discussion

We have shown that although no significant difference in breath H_2 concentration was found between RTRs and HCs, breath CH_4 concentrations were significantly lower in the RTRs compared with the HCs. In addition, we found a significantly lower presence of *M. smithii* in the feces of RTRs compared with HCs. Breath H_2 and the presence of *M. smithii* in feces were associated with higher breath CH_4 concentrations. Moreover, the association between breath H_2 and CH_4 concentrations disappeared in presence of *M. smithii* in feces. Finally, mycophenolate mofetil was associated with a lower breath CH_4 concentration.

The reduced breath CH_4 concentration in RTRs compared to HCs which we observed might be explained by the reduced presence of *M. smithii* in the feces of RTRs, since *M. smithii* is the most abundant methanogen in the human gut [12]. One reason for the lower prevalence of *M. smithii* in the feces of RTRs may be the result of an increased presence or activity of sulfate-reducing bacteria (SRB). It has been described that a high concentration of either methanogens or sulfate-reducing bacteria is present in the feces of healthy individuals. These two groups of microorganisms appear to be competing for H_2, with the prevailing group becoming the predominant organism [27,28]. However, since no mechanism of direct competition between SRB, methanogens and acetogens has been observed, at this point it is impossible to predict any dominance of one of these hydrogenotrophs [29]. If the gut in RTRs is more colonized with SRB, or if these SRB are more active, more hydrogen sulfide (H_2S) is produced. H_2S is highly toxic to the colonocytes and impairs their metabolic function, especially the butyrate oxidation [30]. Butyrate has a known anti-inflammatory effect and several other health-promoting functions [31]. The presence of butyrate in the lumen and the oxidation by colonocytes are both involved in the regulation of water and sodium absorption from the colon [30]. SRB and the consequent disturbance of butyrate oxidation is believed to play a key role in the pathogenesis of IBD [12]. If SRB are indeed more present in RTRs, this might also be an explanatory factor for the occurrence of any of the gastrointestinal complaints of RTRs [16], especially since the butyrate concentration in RTRs seems to be lower due to the reduced prevalence of bacteria taxa that produce butyrate [7].

In addition, more colonization with SRB, and consequently more H_2S, may diminish the positive effects of the butyrate in the gut of RTRs. However, the presence of SRB was not measured in this study. Although our results regarding the decreased presence of *M. smithii* do support this hypothesis, future studies will have to further test this hypothesis.

Another reason for the lower prevalence of *M. smithii* in feces might be a lower presence of mucins in the gut of RTRs. We observed no significant correlation between breath H_2 and CH_4 concentrations in the presence of *M. smithii*. Therefore, the produced CH_4 by *M. smithii* may be derived from endogenous substrates such as mucins, formate or other unknown substrates [12,32]. Importantly, for mucins it has not yet been settled whether they contribute to methane production or rather inhibit it, or under which circumstances stimulation may shift towards inhibition [32,33]. Mucins cover the epithelium and form a protective layer in the gut, thereby providing a protective layer against pathogenic organisms [34]. Deficiencies of mucin in the intestinal barrier are associated with an abnormal mucosal inflammatory response, which is present in IBD [34]. The role of mucins in the fermentation processes in RTRs has, to our best knowledge, never been investigated.

We also observed a strong correlation between breath H_2 and CH_4 concentrations in the absence of *M. smithii* in feces (Figure 2). Possibly, other methanogens that flourish in the absence of *M. smithii* are more dependent upon H_2 concentrations. One of these methanogens might be *M. stadtmanae*, an archaeon that is the second most common archaeon in the healthy gut after *M. smithii* [35]. It is known that the CH_4 production by *M. stadtmanae* is highly dependent upon the presence of H_2 and methanol [36,37]. An increased prevalence of *M. stadtmanae* has been observed previously in IBD patients in a study by Lecours et al. [38]. Interestingly, it has been reported that *M. stadtmanae* can induce an inflammatory cytokine response from monocyte-derived dendritic cells, which may contribute to pathological conditions in the gut [39]. In order to gain more insight into gut health in RTRs, the prevalence of *M. stadtmanae* needs to be further investigated [12,39,40].

In addition, our study shows that patients using mycophenolate mofetil exhale lower concentrations of CH_4. Previous studies have shown that mycophenolate mofetil is associated with gastrointestinal injury and diarrhea, although any underlying mechanisms are incompletely understood [6]. Lower CH_4 levels are also associated with diarrhea [12]. Future studies may investigate whether methanogenesis plays a role in the association between mycophenolate mofetil and diarrhea.

Our observations are in line with previous studies in IBD patients [12,41]. This is interesting, since RTRs and IBD patients have similarities: both groups suffer from intestinal dysbiosis, often have diarrhea and often need to take immunosuppressive medication [38,42–44]. Scanlan et al. observed a significantly lower presence of methanogen-positive feces samples in patients suffering from ulcerative colitis compared to healthy controls (24% versus 48%). In addition, a lower presence of methanogens in patients suffering from Crohn's disease was observed (30% versus 48%), although this association was not statistically significant [41]. In another study by Ghavami et al., significantly higher amounts of *M. smithii* were found in the feces samples of HCs compared to IBD patients [16]. Our results suggest that the reduced colonization with *M. smithii*, and possibly the methanogenesis of IBD patients, might be comparable to RTRs.

It is known that CH_4 reduces inflammation, oxidative stress and apoptosis in the human body [45]. Our findings show significantly lower breath CH_4 concentrations in RTRs compared to HCs, while the protective properties of CH_4 appear especially important in RTRs in the context of (prevention of) renal rejection, inflammation and high levels of oxidative stress [46]. Future studies may further investigate the associations of (breath) CH_4 concentrations with patient outcomes, such as renal rejection. If the hypotheses regarding the protective properties of CH_4 are confirmed, the relatively low CH_4 levels in RTR may be a therapeutic target, since CH_4 concentrations in the body can be increased iatrogenically by inhalation or injection [47,48].

No difference in breath H_2 concentration was found in the current study. This is in line with other studies: the matter of hydrogenotrophics in the gut is highly complex, and is dependent upon many variables [49].

It is a limitation of our study that we did not measure mucin concentrations or potential colonization by SRB or *M. stadtmanae*. In addition, we did not measure H_2 and CH_4 concentrations in flatus, although it has been found that the concentration of both gases are higher in flatus than in breath when the concentrations are high [50]. No data regarding menopausal status was available in our study, although it is known that menopausal status does affect the gut microbiome [51]. Additionally, we did not measure breath H_2 and CH_4 concentrations and the abundance of *M. smithii* in the feces of RTRs before transplantation. Further limitations of our study are that it was performed in a single center, and that our RTRs were included at different time points after transplantation. Another limitation of this study is that for logistical reasons we were unable to analyze *M. smithii* in the feces of all our study subjects. In addition, although we measured the breath H_2 concentrations in the morning, shortly after breakfast, it was in a non-fasting state. Finally, the current study uses cross-sectional data, and therefore no conclusions regarding causal relationships can be drawn.

5. Conclusions

To the best of our knowledge, this is the first study to investigate both breath and feces samples in RTRs. The study shows that breath CH_4 concentration and the prevalence of *M. smithii* in feces are significantly lower in RTRs compared to HCs. Our findings regarding the altered methanogenesis in the gut of RTRs show significant similarities with previous results in IBD patients. We observed that in the absence of *M. smithii*, breath CH_4 production is highly dependent on H_2 concentration, while this is not the case in the presence of *M. smithii*. Apparently, methanogenesis differs significantly depending on presence of *M. smithii*. Finally, the use of mycophenolate mofetil was associated with methanogenesis. These findings provide novel insight into the alterations of fermentation after renal transplantation, which may contribute to the occurrence of posttransplant diarrhea. In addition, this study has raised important hypotheses regarding the potential role of SRB and *M. stadtmanae* in post-transplant diarrhea. Future studies are needed to investigate the role of SRB and *M. stadtmanae*. Additionally, future research may study whether altered methanogenesis is associated with clinical outcomes, such as posttransplant diarrhea.

Author Contributions: Data curation, T.J.K., R.M.D., M.F.E., A.W.G.-N., M.v.L., J.C.S. and S.J.L.B.; formal analysis T.J.K., R.M.D., D.K. and S.J.L.B.; methodology T.J.K., R.M.D., M.F.E., A.W.G.-N., M.v.L. and S.J.L.B.; writing—original draft preparation, T.J.K. and D.K.; writing—review and editing, T.J.K., R.M.D., D.K., J.C.S., M.F.E., A.W.G.-N., M.v.L., F.T.M.P., H.B., I.M.N., W.H.H., H.J.M.H. and S.J.L.B.; supervision, S.J.L.B. All authors have read and agreed to the published version of the manuscript.

References

1. Laupacis, A.; Keown, P.; Pus, N.; Krueger, H.; Ferguson, B.; Wong, C. MN A Study of Quality of Life and Cost Utility Analysis of Tx. *Kidney Int.* **1996**, *50*, 235–242. [CrossRef] [PubMed]
2. Jofré, R.; López-Gómez, J.M.; Moreno, F.; Sanz-Guajardo, D.; Valderrábano, F. Changes in quality of life after renal transplantation. *Am. J. Kidney Dis.* **1998**, *32*, 93–100. [CrossRef] [PubMed]
3. Wolfe, R.A.; Ashby, V.B.; Milford, E.L.; Ojo, A.O.; Ettenger, R.E.; Agodoa, L.Y.; Held, P.J.; Port, F. Comparison of mortality in all patients on dialysis, patients on dialysis awaiting transplantation, and recipients of a first cadaveric transplant. *N. Engl. J. Med.* **1999**, *341*, 1725–1730. [CrossRef]
4. Lamb, K.E.; Lodhi, S.; Meier-Kriesche, H.-U. Long-term renal allograft survival in the United States: A critical reappraisal. *Am. J. Transplant.* **2011**, *11*, 450–462. [CrossRef] [PubMed]
5. Bunnapradist, S.; Neri, L.; Wong, W.; Lentine, K.L.; Burroughs, T.E.; Pinsky, B.W.; Takemoto, S.K.; Schnitzler, M.A. Incidence and Risk Factors for Diarrhea Following Kidney Transplantation and Association With Graft Loss and Mortality. *Am. J. Kidney Dis.* **2008**, *51*, 478–486. [CrossRef]
6. Pant, C.; Deshpande, A.; Larson, A.; O'Connor, J.; Rolston, D.D.K.; Sferra, T.J. Diarrhea in solid-organ transplant recipients: A review of the evidence. *Curr. Med. Res. Opin.* **2013**, *29*, 1315–1328. [CrossRef]
7. Lee, J.R.; Magruder, M.; Zhang, L.; Westblade, L.F.; Satlin, M.J.; Robertson, A.; Edusei, E.; Crawford, C.; Ling, L.; Taur, Y.; et al. Gut microbiota dysbiosis and diarrhea in kidney transplant recipients. *Am. J. Transplant.* **2019**, *19*, 488–500. [CrossRef]
8. Ríos-Covián, D.; Ruas-Madiedo, P.; Margolles, A.; Gueimonde, M.; De los Reyes-Gavilán, C.G.; Salazar, N. Intestinal short chain fatty acids and their link with diet and human health. *Front. Microbiol.* **2016**, *7*, 185. [CrossRef]

9. Morrison, D.J.; Preston, T. Formation of short chain fatty acids by the gut microbiota and their impact on human metabolism. *Gut Microbes* **2016**, *7*, 189–200. [CrossRef]
10. Holscher, H.D. Dietary fiber and prebiotics and the gastrointestinal microbiota. *Gut Microbes* **2017**, *8*, 172–184. [CrossRef]
11. Chaudhary, P.P.; Gaci, N.; Borrel, G.; O'Toole, P.W.; Brugère, J.F. Molecular methods for studying methanogens of the human gastrointestinal tract: Current status and future directions. *Appl. Microbiol. Biotechnol.* **2015**, *99*, 5801–5815. [CrossRef] [PubMed]
12. Nakamura, N.; Lin, H.C.; McSweeney, C.S.; Mackie, R.I.; Gaskins, H.R. Mechanisms of Microbial Hydrogen Disposal in the Human Colon and Implications for Health and Disease. *Annu. Rev. Food Sci. Technol.* **2010**, *1*, 363–395. [CrossRef] [PubMed]
13. Sahakian, A.B.; Jee, S.R.; Pimentel, M. Methane and the gastrointestinal tract. *Dig. Dis. Sci.* **2010**, *55*, 2135–2143. [CrossRef] [PubMed]
14. Dridi, B.; Henry, M.; El Khéchine, A.; Raoult, D.; Drancourt, M. High prevalence of Methanobrevibacter smithii and Methanosphaera stadtmanae detected in the human gut using an improved DNA detection protocol. *PLoS ONE* **2009**, *4*, 1–6. [CrossRef]
15. Miller, T.L.; Wolin, M.J.; De Macario, E.C.; Macario, A.J.L. Isolation of Methanobrevibacter smithii from human feces. *Appl. Environ. Microbiol.* **1982**, *43*, 227–232. [CrossRef] [PubMed]
16. Ghavami, S.B.; Rostami, E.; Sephay, A.A.; Shahrokh, S.; Balaii, H.; Aghdaei, H.A.; Zali, M.R. Alterations of the human gut Methanobrevibacter smithii as a biomarker for inflammatory bowel diseases. *Microb. Pathog.* **2018**, *117*, 285–289. [CrossRef]
17. Eisenga, M.F.; Gomes-Neto, A.W.; van Londen, M.; Ziengs, A.L.; Douwes, R.M.; Stam, S.P.; Osté, M.C.J.; Knobbe, T.J.; Hessels, N.R.; Buunk, A.M.; et al. Rationale and design of TransplantLines: A prospective cohort study and biobank of solid organ transplant recipients. *BMJ Open* **2018**, *8*, e024502. [CrossRef]
18. Gavin, J.R.; Alberti, K.G.M.M.; Davidson, M.B.; DeFronzo, R.A.; Drash, A.; Gabbe, S.G.; Genuth, S.; Harris, M.I.; Kahn, R.; Keen, H.; et al. Report of the expert committee on the diagnosis and classification of diabetes mellitus. *Diabetes Care* **2003**, *26*, 5–20.
19. De Lacy Costello, B.P.J.; Ledochowski, M.; Ratcliffe, N.M. The importance of methane breath testing: A review. *J. Breath Res.* **2013**, *7*, 024001. [CrossRef]
20. Levitt, M.D.; Hirsh, P.; Fetzer, C.A.; Sheahan, M.; Levine, A.S. H2 excretion after ingestion of complex carbohydrates. *Gastroenterology* **1987**, *92*, 383–389. [CrossRef]
21. Yu, Z.; Morrison, M. Improved extraction of PCR-quality community DNA from digesta and fecal samples. *Biotechniques* **2004**, *36*, 808–812. [CrossRef] [PubMed]
22. De Goffau, M.C.; Luopajärvi, K.; Knip, M.; Ilonen, J.; Ruohtula, T.; Härkönen, T.; Orivuori, L.; Hakala, S.; Welling, G.W.; Harmsen, H.J. Fecal Microbiota Composition Differs Between Children With b-Cell Autoimmunity and Those Without. *Diabetes* **2013**, *62*, 1238–1244. [CrossRef] [PubMed]
23. Johnston, C.; Ufnar, J.A.; Griffith, J.F.; Gooch, J.A.; Stewart, J.R. A real-time qPCR assay for the detection of the nifH gene of Methanobrevibacter smithii, a potential indicator of sewage pollution. *J. Appl. Microbiol.* **2010**, *109*, 1946–1956. [CrossRef] [PubMed]
24. Samuel, B.S.; Hansen, E.E.; Manchester, J.K.; Coutinho, P.M.; Henrissat, B.; Fulton, R.; Latreille, P.; Kim, K.; Wilson, R.K.; Gordon, J.I. Genomic and metabolic adaptations of Methanobrevibacter smithii to the human gut. *Proc. Natl. Acad. Sci. USA* **2007**, *104*, 10643–10648. [CrossRef]
25. Levitt, M.D.; Furne, J.K.; Kuskowski, M.; Ruddy, J. Stability of human methanogenic flora over 35 years and a review of insights obtained from breath methane measurements. *Clin. Gastroenterol. Hepatol.* **2006**, *4*, 123–129. [CrossRef]
26. Cloarec, D.; Bornet, F.; Gouilloud, S.; Barry, J.L.; Salim, B.; Galmiche, J.P. Breath hydrogen response to lactulose in healthy subjects: Relationship to methane producing status. *Gut* **1990**, *31*, 300–304. [CrossRef]
27. Christl, S.U.; Gibson, G.R.; Cummings, J.H. Role of dietary sulphate in the regulation of methanogenesis in the human large intestine. *Gut* **1992**, *33*, 1234–1238. [CrossRef]
28. Gibson, G.R.; Cummings, J.H.; Macfarlane, G.T.; Allison, C.; Segal, I.; Vorster, H.H.; Walker, A.R. Alternative pathways for hydrogen disposal during fermentation in the human colon. *Gut* **1990**, *31*, 679–683. [CrossRef]
29. Smith, N.W.; Shorten, P.R.; Altermann, E.H.; Roy, N.C.; McNabb, W.C. Hydrogen cross-feeders of the human gastrointestinal tract. *Gut Microbes* **2019**, *10*, 270–288. [CrossRef]

30. Roediger, W.E.W.; Duncan, A.; Kapaniris, O.; Millard, S. Reducing sulfur compounds of the colon impair colonocyte nutrition: Implications for ulcerative colitis. *Gastroenterology* **1993**, *104*, 802–809. [CrossRef]
31. Leonel, A.J.; Alvarez-Leite, J.I. Butyrate: Implications for intestinal function. *Curr. Opin. Clin. Nutr. Metab. Care* **2012**, *15*, 474–479. [CrossRef] [PubMed]
32. Perman, J.A.; Modler, S. Glycoproteins as Substrates for Colonic Bacterial Flora. *Gastroenterology* **1982**, *83*, 388–393. [CrossRef]
33. Gibson, G.R.; Cummings, J.H.; Macfarlane, G.T. Use of a three-stage continuous culture system to study the effect of mucin on dissimilatory sulfate reduction and methanogenesis by mixed populations of human gut bacteria. *Appl. Environ. Microbiol.* **1988**, *54*, 2750–2755. [CrossRef] [PubMed]
34. Eutamene, H.; Beaufrand, C.; Harkat, C.; Theodorou, V. The role of mucoprotectants in the management of gastrointestinal disorders. *Expert Rev. Gastroenterol. Hepatol.* **2018**, *12*, 83–90. [CrossRef]
35. Miller, T.L.; Wolin, M.J. Enumeration of Methanobrevibacter smithii in human feces. *Arch. Microbiol.* **1982**, *131*, 14–18. [CrossRef]
36. Miller, T.L.; Wolin, M.J. Methanosphaera stadtmaniae gen. nov., sp. nov.: A species that forms methane by reducing methanol with hydrogen. *Arch. Microbiol.* **1985**, *141*, 116–122. [CrossRef]
37. Miller, T.L.; Wolin, M.J. Oxidation of Hydrogen and Reduction of Methanol to methane.pdf. *J. Bacteriol.* **1983**, *153*, 1051–1055. [CrossRef]
38. Lecours, P.B.; Marsolais, D.; Cormier, Y.; Berberi, M.; Haché, C.; Bourdages, R.; Duchaine, C. Increased prevalence of methanosphaera stadtmanae in inflammatory bowel diseases. *PLoS ONE* **2014**, *9*, 1–7. [CrossRef]
39. Bang, C.; Weidenbach, K.; Gutsmann, T.; Heine, H.; Schmitz, R.A. The intestinal archaea Methanosphaera stadtmanae and Methanobrevibacter smithii activate human dendritic cells. *PLoS ONE* **2014**, *9*, 1–9. [CrossRef]
40. Chaudhary, P.P.; Conway, P.L.; Schlundt, J. Methanogens in humans: Potentially beneficial or harmful for health. *Appl. Microbiol. Biotechnol.* **2018**, *102*, 3095–3104. [CrossRef]
41. Scanlan, P.D.; Shanahan, F.; Marchesi, J.R. Human methanogen diversity and incidence in healthy and diseased colonic groups using mcrA gene analysis. *BMC Microbiol.* **2008**, *8*, 1–8. [CrossRef] [PubMed]
42. Triantafyllou, K.; Chang, C.; Pimentel, M. Methanogens, methane and gastrointestinal motility. *J. Neurogastroenterol. Motil.* **2014**, *20*, 31–40. [CrossRef] [PubMed]
43. Vakili, S.T.T.; Taher, M.; Ebrahimi Daryani, N. Update on the management of ulcerative colitis. *Acta Med Iran.* **2012**, *50*, 363–372.
44. Deepak, P.; Bruining, D.H. Update on the Medical Management of Crohn' s Disease. *Curr. Gastroenterol. Rep.* **2015**, *17*, 1–10. [CrossRef] [PubMed]
45. Jia, Y.; Li, Z.; Liu, C.; Zhang, J. Methane Medicine: A Rising Star Gas with Powerful Anti-Inflammation, Antioxidant, and Antiapoptosis Properties. *Oxid. Med. Cell. Longev.* **2018**, *2018*, 1912746. [CrossRef] [PubMed]
46. Nafar, M.; Sahraei, Z.; Salamzadeh, J.; Samavat, S.; Vaziri, N.D. Oxidative stress in kidney transplantation causes, consequences, and potential treatment. *Iran. J. Kidney Dis.* **2011**, *5*, 357–372. [PubMed]
47. Boros, M.; Ghyczy, M.; Irces, D.; Varga, G.; Tokés, T.; Kupai, K.; Torday, C.; Kaszaki, J. The anti-inflammatory effects of methane. *Crit. Care Med.* **2012**, *40*, 1269–1278. [CrossRef]
48. Chen, O.; Ye, Z.; Cao, Z.; Manaenko, A.; Ning, K.; Zhai, X.; Zhang, R.; Zhang, T.; Chen, X.; Liu, W.; et al. Methane attenuates myocardial ischemia injury in rats through anti-oxidative, anti-apoptotic and anti-inflammatory actions. *Free Radic. Biol. Med.* **2016**, *90*, 1–11. [CrossRef]
49. Wolf, P.G.; Biswas, A.; Morales, S.E.; Greening, C.; Gaskins, H.R. H2 metabolism is widespread and diverse among human colonic microbes. *Gut Microbes* **2016**, *7*, 235–245. [CrossRef]
50. Christl, S.U.; Murgatroyd, P.R.; Gibson, S.R.; Cummings, J.H. Production, metabolism, and excretion of hydrogen in the large intestine. *Gastroenteroology* **1992**, *102*, 1269–1277. [CrossRef]
51. Santos-Marcos, J.A.; Rangel-Zuñiga, O.A.; Jimenez-Lucena, R.; Quintana-Navarro, G.M.; Garcia-Carpintero, S.; Malagon, M.M.; Landa, B.B.; Tena-Sempere, M.; Perez-Martinez, P.; Lopez-Miranda, J.; et al. Influence of gender and menopausal status on gut microbiota. *Maturitas* **2018**, *116*, 43–53. [CrossRef] [PubMed]

13

Management of Immunosuppression in Kidney Transplant Recipients who Develop Malignancy

Danwen Yang [1], Natanong Thamcharoen [2,*] and Francesca Cardarelli [1]

[1] Division of Nephrology, Beth Israel Deaconess Medical Center and Harvard Medical School, Boston, MA 02215, USA; yangdanwen@gmail.com (D.Y.); fcardare@bidmc.harvard.edu (F.C.)

[2] Section of Palliative Care, Division of General Medicine and Division of Nephrology, Beth Israel Deaconess Medical Center and Harvard Medical School, Boston, MA 02215, USA

* Correspondence: natthamcharoen@gmail.com

Abstract: The risk of cancer increases after transplantation. However, the consensus on immunosuppression (IS) adjustment after diagnosis of malignancy is lacking. Our study aims to assess the impact of IS adjustment on mortality of post-kidney transplant patients and allograft outcomes. We retrospectively reviewed the data in our center of 110 subjects. Our results showed IS dose adjustment was not statistically associated with mortality risk (HR 1.94, 95%CI 0.85–4.41, $p = 0.12$), and chemotherapy was the only factor that was significantly related to mortality (HR 2.3, 95%CI 1.21–4.35, $p = 0.01$). IS reduction was not statistically associated with worsening graft function (OR 3.8, 95%CI 0.77–18.71, $p = 0.10$), nor with graft survival (SHR 4.46, 95%CI 0.58–34.48, $p = 0.15$) after variables adjustment. Creatinine at cancer diagnosis and history of rejection were both negatively associated with graft survival (SHR 1.72, 95%CI 1.28–2.30, $p < 0.01$ and SHR 3.44, 95%CI 1.25–9.49, $p = 0.02$). Reduction of both mycophenolate and calcineurin inhibitors was associated with worsening graft function and lower graft survival in subgroup analysis (OR 6.14, 95%CI 1.14–33.15, $p = 0.04$; HR 17.97, 95%CI 1.81–178.78, $p = 0.01$). In summary, cancer causes high mortality and morbidity in kidney transplant recipients; the importance of cancer screening should be emphasized.

Keywords: malignancy; cancer; kidney transplant; immunosuppression; graft failure; survival

1. Introduction

The number of solid organ transplants has increased in the past decade, with 21,167 kidney transplants performed in the United States in 2018. Multiple studies have shown that there is an increased risk of malignancy in transplant recipients [1]. The overall cancer incidence rate is 90 per 1000 patients at 10 years after transplant, which is twice as high as in the general population, while the dialysis population has a 1.35 standardized cancer incident ratio compared to the general population [2]. Nonmelanoma skin cancer is even more frequent, with an incidence rate 14 times higher in transplant recipients compared to the general population.

The burden of malignancy in kidney transplant patients is very high, and the mortality risk in kidney transplant recipients diagnosed with cancer is also greater than nontransplant patients. The median survival of kidney transplant patients with cancer is significantly lower than kidney transplant patients without cancer (2.1 years vs. 8.3 years). Malignancy is currently the second most common cause of death in kidney transplant patients after cardiovascular disease [3].

Despite the surging incidence of cancer in kidney transplant recipients, there is very limited data of how immunosuppression (IS) should be managed after malignancy diagnosis. In current practice, the consensus is that IS dose should be decreased in renal transplant patients with newly diagnosed malignancy, since there is evidence supporting that IS is associated with an increased risk of malignancy and can promote tumor growth [4]. However, specific recommendations regarding how to adjust

IS after diagnosis of malignancy in kidney transplant patients are lacking, and management varies depending on institutions, and even by provider in the same practice. The regimen adjustment ranges from no dose reduction, dose reduction, or cessation of one or more immunosuppressive medications, to class switch. The aim of our study was to assess the impact of changes of IS on patient survival and graft function by retrospectively reviewing data on patients who were diagnosed with malignancy after kidney transplantation in our center.

2. Methods

This is a retrospective data analysis, in which we identified subjects by manual search of medical records of patients who had kidney transplantations and cancer diagnosis from January 1990 to December 2018 at Beth Israel Deaconess Medical Center, Boston, MA, USA. Data on immunosuppressive regimen, creatinine at cancer diagnosis and one year after diagnosis were extracted from medical records. Time from transplant to cancer diagnosis, patient and graft survival data were calculated from actual dates. Study data were collected and managed using REDCap (Research Electronic Data Capture) electronic data capture tools hosted at Harvard Catalyst—Beth Israel Deaconess Medical Center [5]. Data were collected by chart review following HIPAA guidelines. Institutional Review Board approval was obtained for data collection and analysis, with a waiver for individual consent.

We included all adult patients (18 years or older) who were diagnosed with malignancy after renal transplantation, as seen in Figure 1. Nonmelanoma skin cancer patients who did not require chemotherapy or radiation for cancer treatment were excluded from the analysis. The primary outcome in this study was patient survival. Secondary outcome included graft failure (defined as renal replacement therapy requirement) and worsening renal function (defined as glomerular filtration rate (GFR) reduction of more than 30% or developed graft failure at one year after cancer diagnosis). The mortality and graft function information were obtained from medical records. Our primary variable of interest was dose reduction defined by any types of IS dose reduction. Variables considered to have potential confounding effect were included in the multivariable models, specifically we included demographics of the subjects (i.e., age, race, gender), creatinine at cancer diagnosis, history of rejection, cancer type, donor type, history of chemotherapy, and history of radiation therapy. Races were divided into black and nonblack, which includes Asian, Hispanic, and others. Cancer types were differentiated as solid organ malignancy and hematologic malignancy. Missing data and loss to follow-up were excluded from the analysis. For survival analysis, loss to follow-up cases were censored.

We stratified the population based on whether individuals had IS dose reduction. Means and standard deviations were used to summarize continuous variables with normal distribution. Median (interquartile range) was used for skewed continuous variables. Categorical variables were summarized as percentage. We used t-test to assess the differences in continuous variables that were normally distributed. We tested the difference in categorical variables with Fisher's exact test. Wilcoxon rank sum test was used to test skewed continuous variables. We used logistic regression to assess variables for worsening graft function at one year after cancer diagnosis. For graft failure outcome, competing risk survival analysis (Fine and Gray model) was used to assess cumulative graft failure incidence, and the covariable effect on graft failure was reported as subdistribution hazard ratio. Death without graft failure was considered as a competing outcome. The Cox proportional hazards model was used to assess risk factors for mortality, and the data was censored by last follow-up date. Patient survival was analyzed using the Kaplan–Meier method with significance tested using the log-rank test.

For subgroup analysis, patients were divided into groups according to type of IS reduction (mycophenolate mofetil (MMF), calcineurin inhibitor (CNI), and reduction of both MMF and CNI). We compared each group to the group without any IS changes to assess the risk of worsening graft function and graft failure between these groups. Propensity score adjustment was utilized for subgroup analysis given the small number of subjects in each group. Propensity score of each subject was calculated based on significant factors derived from initial analysis of worsening graft function and graft failure.

Then, we performed regression analysis for worsening graft function outcome and Cox regression model for graft failure outcome. Propensity score was applied to the model for adjustment.

All multivariable models ware built based on clinical risk factors and statistically significant variables from univariable analyses. $p < 0.05$ was considered to be significant. The data collected were analyzed using the Stata software version 15.0 (Stata Corp., College Station, TX, USA).

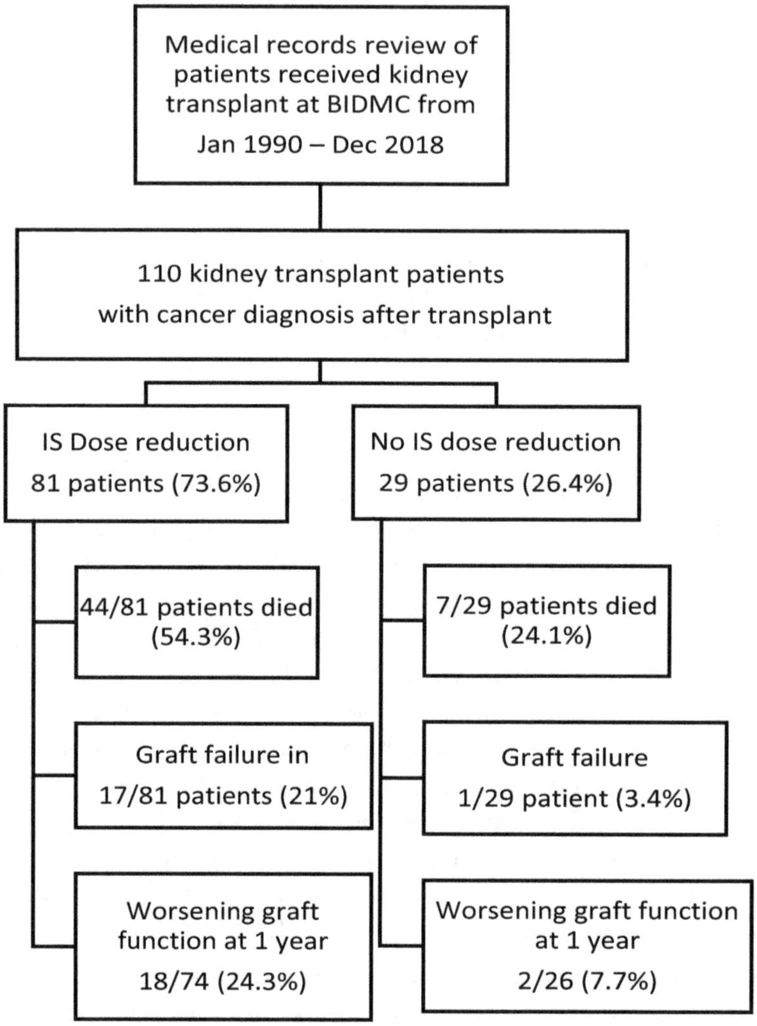

Figure 1. Summary of the study.

3. Results

3.1. Baseline Characteristics of the Study Population

One hundred and ten subjects who underwent kidney transplantation and developed malignancy were included in our analysis, as seen in Figure 1. Patients' demographics are shown in Table 1.

The mean age at cancer diagnosis was 60.2 years. Male gender contributed to 65.5% of subjects. The ethnicities of subjects were 77.3% non-Hispanic White, and 11.8% non-Hispanic Black. Our study population underwent transplantation during 1971–2018 (1971–1999 in 24 patients and 2000–2019 in 86 patients). Of the study population, 73.6% underwent IS regimen changes (dose reduction or class switch), 26.4% patients had no changes in their IS regimen. Among patients with IS reduction, 26 patients had reduction of both mycophenolate mofetil (MMF) and calcineurin inhibitor (CNI), 19 patients had reduction of CNI only, while 25 patients had reduction of MMF only.

The IS regimen of our patient population is presented in Figure 2. Degree of dose reduction for each IS was showed as median of percent reduced from precancer diagnosis dose in Table 2.

Table 1. Baseline characteristic of subjects (N = 110).

Characteristics	Dose Reduction (N = 81)	No Dose Reduction (N = 29)	*p* Value
Sex			
Male	55 (67.9%)	17 (58.6%)	0.37
Race			
White	61(75.3%)	24 (82.8%)	0.17
Black	8 (9.9%)	5 (17.2%)	
Asian	6 (7.4%)	0	
Hispanic	6 (7.4%)	0	
Age at cancer diagnosis	60.1 (11.2)	60.2 (9.1)	0.87
Primary disease			
Diabetes	28 (34.6%)	7 (24.1%)	0.33
Glomerulonephritis	15 (18.5%)	8 (27.6%)	
PKD	7 (8.6%)	3 (10.3%)	
Reflux	1 (1.2%)	2 (6.9%)	
Other	30 (37.0%)	9 (30.0%)	
Transplant type			
Deceased donor	41 (50.6%)	16 (55.2%)	0.77
Living unrelated donor	24 (29.6%)	9 (31.0%)	
Living related donor	16 (19.8%)	4 (13.8%)	
Mean creatinine at cancer diagnosis (mg/dL)	1.65 (1.44–1.87)	1.49 (1.27–1.70)	0.39
Type of cancer			
Hematological cancer	19 (23.5%)	4 (13.8%)	0.27
Solid organ cancer	62 (76.5%)	25 (86.2%)	
History of chemotherapy	48 (59.3%)	8 (27.6%)	<0.01
History of radiation	27 (33.3%)	11 (37.9%)	0.66
History of rejection	14 (17.3%)	5 (18.5%)	0.22

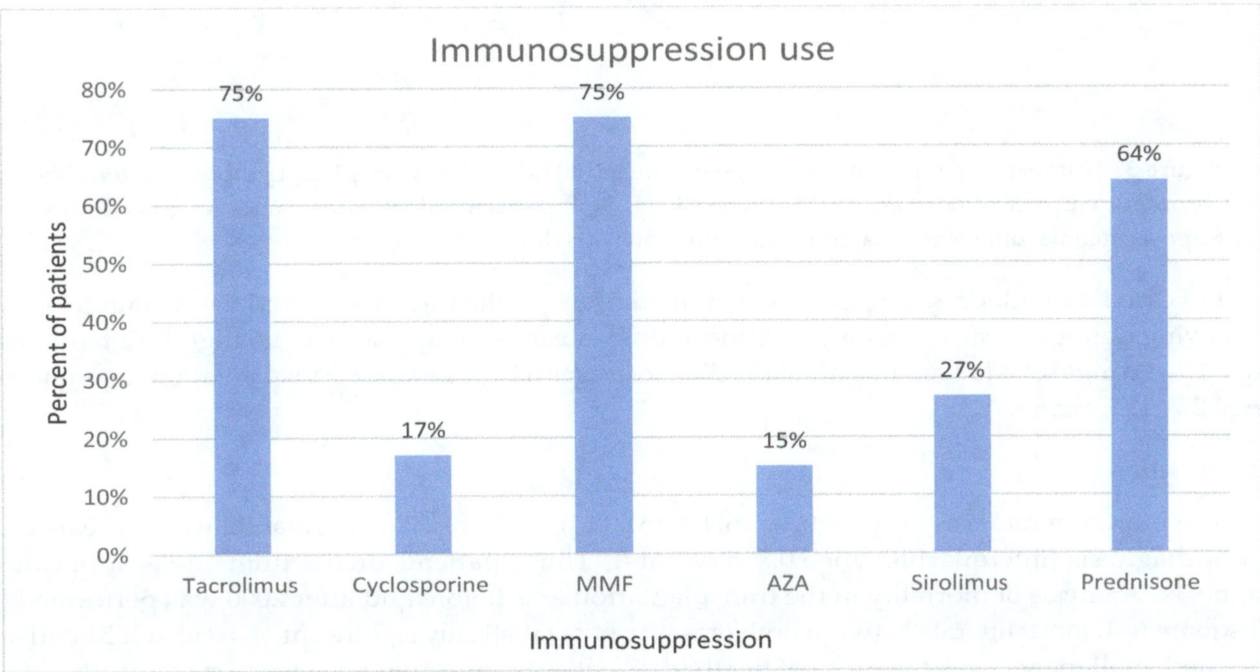

Figure 2. Types of immunosuppression (IS) used by subjects in the study. MMF = mycophenolate mofetil, AZA = azathioprine.

Table 2. Median percent dose reduction of each immunosuppression (100% = completely discontinuation of immunosuppression).

Immunosuppression	Median Percent Dose Reduction (IQR)
Tacrolimus	60% (29.17%–100%)
Cyclosporine	100% (100%–100%)
Mycophenolate mofetil (MMF) or mycophenolic acid	50% (50%–100%)

Medians of percent dose reduction were 60% for tacrolimus, 100% (completely discontinued) for cyclosporine, and MMF or mycophenolic acid. Solid organ malignancies represented 79.1% of the cases; the remainders were hematological cancers. Number of subjects for each type of malignancy are shown in Figure 3.

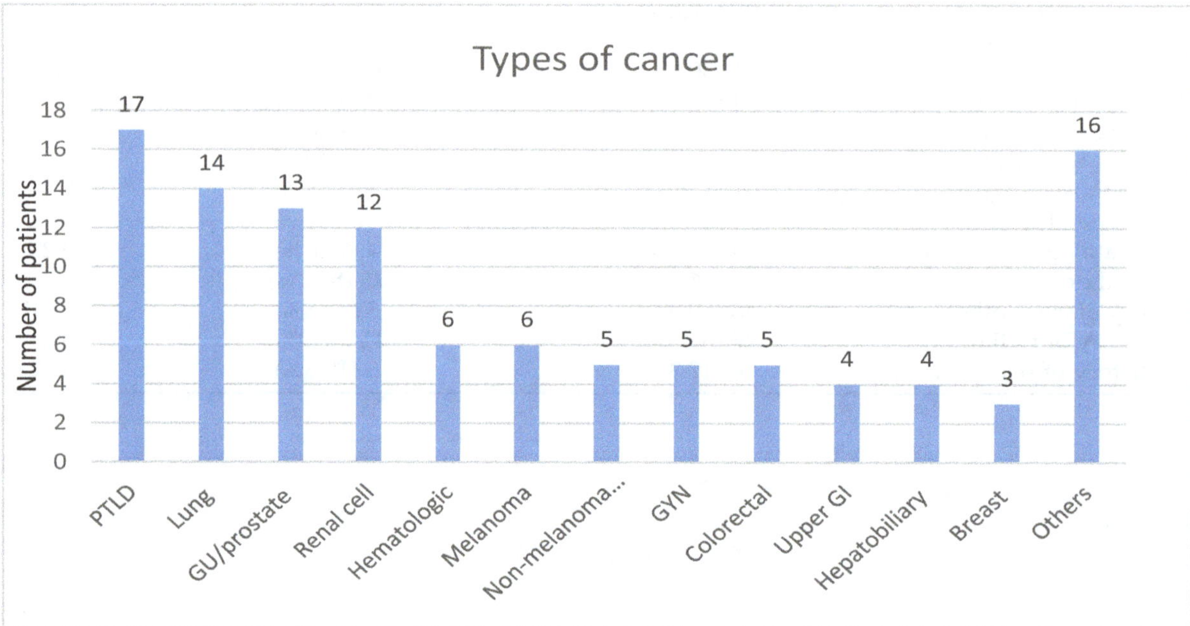

Figure 3. Number of patients in each type of cancer; PTLD = Post-transplant Lymphoproliferative Disorders, GU = Genitourinary, GYN = gynecology, GI = gastrointestinal. Other cancers are head/neck, Kaposi sarcoma, other sarcoma, brain, and unknown origin.

Deceased donor kidney transplant constituted 51.8% of the transplants, and the remainders were from living donors. Mean baseline creatinine at time of cancer diagnosis was 1.6 mg/dL (interquartile range 1.1–1.8 mg/dL). Median time of cancer diagnosis was 6.76 years after transplantation (interquartile range 2.7–11.7 years).

3.2. Mortality

The mortality rate was very high, at 46.4 % (51/110), with median survival time of 1.8 years after cancer diagnosis (interquartile range 0.7–5.6 years). Thirty patients died within one year of cancer diagnosis. Analysis of mortality in the transplantation eras before and after 2000 was performed by chi-square test, mortality rate between both eras was not statistically significant, $p = 0.65$. Of 51 patients who died, malignancy was the cause of death in 27 patients. Infection was the cause of death in four patients. Eighteen patients had no cause of death recorded. Other causes of death were cardiovascular disease and unknown cause. Kaplan–Meier curve and log-rank test revealed that IS dose reduction significantly increased mortality, $p = 0.01$, as seen in Figure 4.

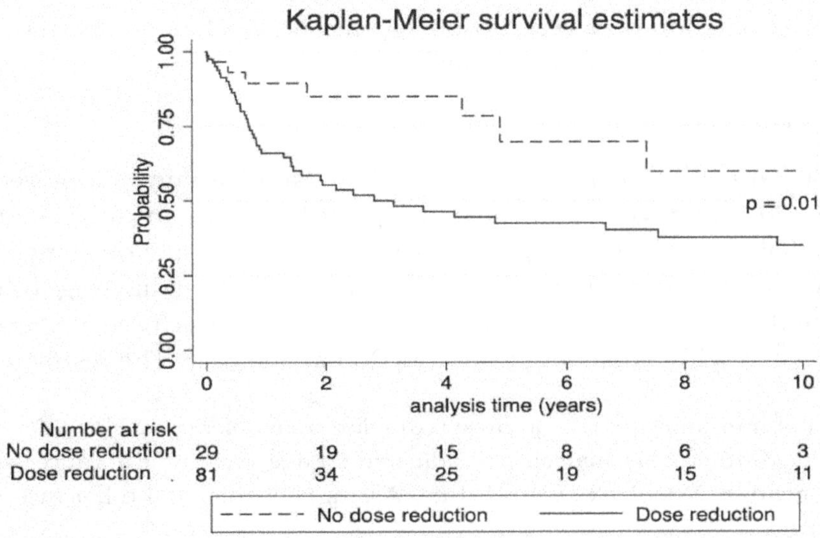

Figure 4. Kaplan–Meier curve and log-rank test of IS dose management and mortality risk.

We performed univariate Cox regression analysis to assess relationship of each variable to mortality, as shown in Table 3. According to our univariate regression analysis model, older age, male gender, IS dose reduction, and chemotherapy were associated with higher mortality. However, in the multivariate model, only chemotherapy remained significant (HR 2.3, 95%CI 1.21–4.35, $p = 0.01$). When we excluded patients who died within six months of cancer diagnosis, the results did not change.

Table 3. Effect of immunosuppression dose reduction on patients' mortality. Multivariable analysis was adjusted for age, IS dose reduction, chemotherapy history, and gender. Nonblack race = White, Asian, Hispanic, and other races. * = Statistically significant, $p < 0.05$.

Variables	Univariate Model		Multivariable Model	
	Hazard Ratio (95%CI)	***p*-Value**	**Hazard Ratio (95%CI)**	***p*-Value**
Age at cancer diagnosis	1.04 (1.02–1.07)	<0.01 *	1.02(0.99–1.05)	0.13
IS dose reduction	2.68 (1.21–6.00)	0.02 *	1.94 (0.85–4.41)	0.12
Chemotherapy	3.08 (1.69–5.61)	<0.01 *	2.30 (1.21–4.35)	0.01 *
Male	2.44 (1.24–4.77)	0.01 *	1.97 (0.98–3.99)	0.06
History of rejection	0.78 (0.37–1.67)	0.53		
Cr at cancer diagnosis	1.06 (0.80–1.42)	0.68		
Black Race +	0.36 (0.11–1.17)	0.09		
Solid organ cancer	1.24 (0.58–2.65)	0.57		
Radiation therapy	1.59 (0.91–2.79)	0.10		
Deceased donor	1.62 (0.92–2.84)	0.09		

We also checked the interaction between chemotherapy and dose reduction; the p value of 0.36, indicates no strong interaction between those two variables. The spearman correlation coefficient between chemotherapy and dose reduction was 0.28.

3.3. Worsening Graft Function

There were 100 patients who had post-cancer diagnosis creatinine at one year available. Twenty percent of patients (20/100) developed worsening graft function. In univariate logistic regression, creatinine at cancer diagnosis and female gender were associated with worsening renal function. Those variables remained significant in the multivariable analysis after adjusting for creatinine at cancer diagnosis, IS dose reduction, age, and gender. Interestingly, cancer type, chemotherapy, and donor type were not associated with worsening graft function at one year. The result is shown in Table 4.

Table 4. Impact of immunosuppression dose reduction on worsening GFR > 30% at one year after cancer diagnosis. Multivariable analysis was adjusted for age, creatinine at cancer diagnosis, IS dose reduction, and gender. Nonblack race = White, Asian, Hispanic, and other race. * = Statistically significant, $p < 0.05$.

Variables	Univariable Model		Multivariable Model	
	Odds Ratio (95%CI)	***p*-Value**	**Odds Ratio (95%CI)**	***p*-Value**
Age at cancer diagnosis	0.99 (0.94–1.03)	0.59	1.02 (0.97–1.08)	0.48
Cr at cancer diagnosis	2.37 (1.28–4.40)	<0.01 *	2.67 (1.35–5.28)	<0.01 *
IS dose reduction	3.86 (0.83–17.94)	0.09	3.80 (0.77–18.71)	0.10
Male	0.43 (0.16–1.16)	0.01 *	0.22 (0.06–0.77)	0.02 *
Black Race +	0.33 (0.04–2.72)	0.30		
Solid organ cancer	0.54 (0.18–1.63)	0.27		
Chemotherapy	2.05 (0.74–5.68)	0.17		
Radiation therapy	0.47 (0.13–1.36)	0.15		
Deceased donor	1.11 (0.41–2.96)	0.84		

It is important to note that the direction and magnitude of the estimates for IS dose reduction suggest a potentially strong effect on worsening graft function and mortality outcome, but our study did not have enough power to detect this, given the small number of patients.

3.4. Graft Failure

In our study, the graft failure rate was 16.4% (18/110). Median graft survival after cancer diagnosis in patients with graft failure was 2.97 years (interquartile range 0.56–4.22 years). Causes of graft failure were acute kidney injury in five patients, "chronic allograft nephropathy" in five patients, and acute rejection in five patients. BK nephropathy, multiple myeloma, and unknown cause contributed to the remaining patients.

As shown in Table 5, in competing risk survival model, creatinine at cancer diagnosis, history of rejection and hematologic cancer were associated with increased risk of graft failure in univariable analysis. After adjusting for age at cancer diagnosis, creatinine at cancer diagnosis, IS dose reduction, malignancy type, and history of rejection, our result showed that creatinine at cancer diagnosis and history of rejection have remained statistically significant with SHR 1.72, 95% CI 1.28–2.30, $p < 0.01$ and SHR 3.44, 95% CI 1.25–9.49, $p = 0.02$, respectively.

Table 5. Impact of immunosuppression dose reduction on graft survival. Multivariable analysis was adjusted for age, creatinine at cancer diagnosis, history of rejection, IS dose reduction, and cancer type. Nonblack race = White, Asian, Hispanic, and other races. * = Statistically significant, $p < 0.05$.

Variables	Univariable Model		Multivariable Model	
	SHR (95%CI)	*p*-Value	SHR (95%CI)	*p*-Value
Age at cancer diagnosis	0.97 (0.93–1.01)	0.16	0.99 (0.94–1.03)	0.62
Cr at cancer diagnosis	1.83 (1.45–2.30)	<0.01 *	1.72 (1.28–2.30)	<0.01 *
History of rejection	3.63 (1.45–9.08)	0.01 *	3.44 (1.25–9.49)	0.02 *
IS dose reduction	6.19 (0.82–46.73)	0.08	4.46 (0.58–34.48)	0.15
Solid organ cancer	0.35 (0.13–0.95)	0.04 *	0.48 (0.16–1.42)	0.18
Black Race +	0.91 (0.23–3.61)	0.90		
Male	0.67 (0.27–1.66)	0.39		
Chemotherapy	1.39 (0.56–3.46)	0.48		
Radiation therapy	0.93 (0.36–2.44)	0.89		
Deceased donor	0.80 (0.32–1.98)	0.62		

IS was reduced in all the patients who had graft failure, except for one patient who did not have his IS adjusted, as he was only on low dose tacrolimus monotherapy due to BK viremia. PTLD diagnosis contributed to five out of 18 cases of graft failure.

3.5. *Subgroup Analysis*

3.5.1. Worsening Graft Function

We performed subgroup analysis in patients who had IS reduction, defined by reduction of CNI (19 patients), reduction of MMF (25 patients), and reduction of both (29 patients), compared to 29 patients who had no IS change at all to analyze their impact on worsening graft function at one year. After adjusting for gender, age at cancer diagnosis, creatinine at cancer diagnosis using propensity score, reduction of two types of IS was a significant factor for worsening graft function at one year in logistic regression, OR 6.14, 95% CI 1.14–33.15, $p = 0.04$, as seen in Table 6.

Table 6. Impact of each type of IS reduction compared to no dose reduction on worsening GFR > 30% at one year after cancer diagnosis Adjusted for gender, age at cancer diagnosis, and creatinine at cancer diagnosis. * = Statistically significant, $p < 0.05$.

Immunosuppression Reduction (N)	OR (95% CI)	*p*-Value
CNI Reduction (19/29)	1.31 (0.16–10.59)	0.80
MMF Reduction (25/29)	5.28 (0.86–32.55)	0.07
Reduction of all IS (26/29)	6.14 (1.14–33.15)	0.04 *

3.5.2. Graft Failure

Subgroup analysis was also performed to assess the impact of different IS reduction regimens on graft failure. The patient groups are the same as subgroup analysis in worsening graft function. In the Cox model adjusted for age at cancer diagnosis, creatinine at cancer diagnosis, history of rejection, and cancer type using propensity score, reduction of both CNI and MMF was associated with graft failure, HR 17.97, 95%CI 1.81–178.78, $p = 0.01$, as seen in Table 7.

Table 7. Impact of each type of IS reduction compared to no dose reduction on graft survival. Adjusted for age at cancer diagnosis, creatinine at cancer diagnosis, history of rejection and cancer type. * = Statistically significant, $p < 0.05$.

Immunosuppression Reduction	HR (95%CI)	*p*-Value
CNI Reduction (19/29)	6.52 (0.46–92.70)	0.17
MMF/myfortic Reduction (25/29)	0.66(0.04–11.14)	0.77
Reduction of all IS (26/29)	17.97 (1.81–178.78)	0.01 *

4. Discussion

Although there is increasing evidence of high morbidity and mortality of kidney transplant patients diagnosed with malignancy, specific recommendation on how to adjust IS is lacking. A randomized trial comparing low cyclosporine dose to regular dose found no difference in graft survival or function, although the low-dose regimen was associated with fewer malignant disorders and more frequent rejections [6]. Another randomized controlled trial in 489 kidney transplant patients with 20-year follow-up showed that azathioprine and cyclosporine-based regimens were associated with similar overall long-term cancer risks. In addition, gender, previous antithymocyte globulin (ATG) exposure, and graft failure showed no association with development of malignancy, excluding skin cell carcinoma [7]. One retrospective observational study in heart transplant patients showed that everolimus treatment was associated with lower malignancy risk than MMF [8]. Previous studies showed that sirolimus was associated with reduction in the risk of malignancy and nonmelanoma skin cancer in kidney transplant recipients; however, it was associated with increased mortality risk [9].

KDIGO guidelines published in 2010 recommend considering a reduction of IS for kidney transplant recipients with malignancy (2C recommendation). Important factors to consider (not graded) include the stage of cancer at diagnosis, malignancies which are likely to be exacerbated by IS, available therapies, and whether IS interferes with ability to administer standard chemotherapy [10]. The likelihood of cancer being exacerbated by IS can be assessed using standardized incidence ratio (SIR), which compares the malignancy risk in kidney transplant patients to that in the general population. Cancers with SIR > 3, such as Kaposi's sarcoma, PTLD, and ano-genital cancer, are mostly associated with viral infections, e.g., Human Herpesvirus 8 (HHV8), Epstein–Barr virus (EBV), human papillomavirus (HPV). It has been shown that the incidence of Kaposi's sarcoma, non-Hodgkin's lymphoma, HPV related ano-genital cancer, and melanoma were significantly elevated in patients with functioning transplant graft, but not after transplant failure, when patients were back on dialysis, suggesting that IS has significant effect on these types of cancer. As a consequence, IS adjustment should be strongly considered in these types of malignancy [11,12].

Our study showed that mortality rate in kidney transplant patients with diagnosis of malignancy was high (46.4%), with median survival time of 1.8 years after cancer diagnosis (interquartile range 0.7–5.6 years). Mortality rate was not significantly different between patients who had transplantation before and after year 2000. Interestingly, in our study, malignancy was the main cause of death in subjects whose cause of death was recorded, while the leading cause of death in kidney transplant recipients in general is cardiovascular disease. This data suggests that malignancy contributes to major of mortality in kidney transplant recipients with cancer diagnosis. In addition, more than half of deceased subjects died within two years of their cancer diagnosis, possibly reflecting advanced cancer at presentation and/or aggressive disease in transplant patients. Our data emphasizes that the appropriate cancer screening could reduce mortality and its importance should be particularly stressed in transplant recipients.

The possible causes of increased mortality risk in this population have been attributed to reduction of immune surveillance in the setting of IS and limited use of certain chemotherapy regimens due to reduced renal function. Notably, kidney transplant recipients and patients with HIV share a similar pattern of increased risk of cancer. Consequently, the increased risk of malignancy after kidney transplantation is thought to be caused by viral infection along with chronic IS use [2].

The significant variable between dose reduction and no reduction groups was whether patients required chemotherapy, suggesting that physicians are more inclined to reduce IS when the cancer is more advanced. The type of cancer (hematologic or solid organ malignancy) did not appear to affect the decision of changing the IS. According to Kaplan–Meier analysis, mortality was significantly higher in the dose reduction group, which is likely confounded by the fact that patients with more advanced stage malignancy tended to have their IS adjusted. Our result is comparable to a previous study in a different center [13]. For multivariate analysis, our study demonstrated that chemotherapy is the only variable associated with mortality, which could be similarly explained by the severity of disease.

As expected, patients with baseline poor kidney function had higher risk of graft failure. The degree of IS dose reduction was significant in majority of patients (IS dose was reduced by at least 50% to completely stopped) putting patients at higher risk of acute allograft rejection. Interestingly, our data showed a novel and important factor in subgroup analysis, reduction of both CNI and MMF put patients at higher risk of graft failure. As a consequence, we recommend that providers should carefully weigh the risks and benefits before drastically changing IS in transplant recipients after cancer diagnosis. A multidisciplinary approach is necessary, focusing on the individual patient's wishes and goals in terms of survival, quality of life, and factor in the possibility of graft failure and return to dialysis. Patients with renal allograft failure returning to dialysis seem to have inferior quality of life and higher rate of depression compared to wait-listed transplant naive patients [14].

Based on our cohort, patients with PTLD had the highest mortality (seven out of 17 patients). Graft failure incidence in patients diagnosed with PTLD was also the highest compared to any other malignancy, as five out of 18 patients who had graft failure were diagnosed with PTLD.

Our study has many limitations. First, it is an uncontrolled retrospective study; therefore, the direct and independent effect of IS changes on mortality could not be clearly determined. Second, our database is from a single center, which has a relatively small number of subjects and heterogeneous cancer types, which might contribute a major confounder. Third, despite adjusting for chemotherapy and radiation therapy, cancer staging was not included in our analysis due to lack of record and heterogeneity of cancer diagnosis. While some chemotherapy regimens could have been a cause graft failure, we did not include this data in our analysis. Lastly, we disregarded the effect of sirolimus and steroid adjustment since both drugs are not part of the standard immunosuppressive regimen at our transplant center.

5. Conclusions

Our study shows no difference in mortality and graft survival outcomes between reduction and no reduction of IS in kidney transplant recipients diagnosed with cancer. However, it is important to note that the direction and magnitude of the estimates for IS dose reduction suggest a potentially strong effect on worsening graft function and mortality outcome, but a lacking power, caused by the small group of subjects, prevented us to detect the differences. The mortality rate in this population is high and malignancy is usually aggressive; therefore, kidney transplant patients would benefit from early detection of disease by routine cancer screening. The data from our study reveals a novel finding: the risk of graft failure appears remarkably higher after adjusting two immunosuppressive medications. Most importantly, providers should have an extensive discussion with patients regarding the risk and benefit of IS adjustment, chances of prolonging survival from cancer treatment, and worsening quality of life in case patients develop kidney allograft failure requiring dialysis. As a future direction, a prospective study might be the key to define the temporal effect of IS adjustment on patient's survival, malignancy, and allograft outcomes in kidney transplant recipients.

Author Contributions: All authors had full access to all of the data in the study and take responsibility for the integrity of the data and the accuracy of the data analysis. Conceptualization, Supervision, F.C.; Methodology, Data Curation, Data Analysis, Draft Preparation, D.Y. and N.T. D.Y. and N.T. equally have contributed to this manuscript as first authors.

Acknowledgments: We acknowledge the statistic consultation from Harvard Catalyst. REDCap is a secure, web-based application designed to support data capture for research studies, providing (1) an intuitive interface for validated data entry; (2) audit trails for tracking data manipulation and export procedures; (3) automated export procedures for seamless data downloads to common statistical packages; and (4) procedures for importing data from external sources.

References

1. Collett, D.; Mumford, L.; Banner, N.R.; Neuberger, J.; Watson, C. Comparison of the incidence of malignancy in recipients of different types of organ: A UK registry audit. *Am. J. Transpl.* **2010**, *10*, 1889–1896. [CrossRef] [PubMed]
2. Chapman, J.R.; Webster, A.C.; Wong, G. Cancer in the transplant recipient. *Cold Spring Harb. Perspect. Med.* **2013**, *3*, 1–15. [CrossRef] [PubMed]
3. Au, E.; Wong, G.; Chapman, J.R. Cancer in kidney transplant recipients. *Nat. Rev. Nephrol.* **2018**, *14*, 508–520. [CrossRef] [PubMed]
4. Dantal, J.; Soulillou, J.-P. Immunosuppressive Drugs and the Risk of Cancer after Organ Transplantation. *N. Engl. J. Med.* **2005**, *352*, 1371–1373. [CrossRef] [PubMed]
5. Harris, P.A.; Taylor, R.; Thielke, R.; Payne, J.; Gonzalez, N.; Conde, J.G. Research electronic data capture (REDCap)-A metadata-driven methodology and workflow process for providing translational research informatics support. *J. Biomed. Inform.* **2009**, *42*, 377–381. [CrossRef] [PubMed]
6. Dantal, J.; Hourmant, M.; Cantarovich, D.; Giral, M.; Blancho, G.; Dreno, B.; Soulillou, J.P. Effect of long-term immunosuppression in kidney-graft recipients on cancer incidence: Randomised comparison of two cyclosporin regimens. *Lancet* **1998**, *351*, 623–628. [CrossRef]
7. Gallagher, M.P.; Kelly, P.J.; Jardine, M.; Perkovic, V.; Cass, A.; Craig, J.C.; Eris, J.; Webster, A.C. Long-Term Cancer Risk of Immunosuppressive Regimens after Kidney Transplantation. *J. Am. Soc. Nephrol.* **2010**, *21*, 852–858. [CrossRef] [PubMed]
8. Wang, Y.J.; Chi, N.H.; Chou, N.K.; Huang, S.C.; Wang, C.H.; Wu, I.H.; Yu, H.Y.; Chen, Y.S.; Tsao, C.I.; Shun, C.T.; et al. Malignancy after Heart Transplantation under Everolimus Versus Mycophenolate Mofetil Immunosuppression. *Transplant. Proc.* **2016**, *48*, 969–973. [CrossRef] [PubMed]
9. Knoll, G.A.; Kokolo, M.B.; Mallick, R.; Beck, A.; Buenaventura, C.D.; Ducharme, R.; Barsoum, R.; Bernasconi, C.; Blydt-Hansen, T.D.; Ekberg, H.; et al. Effect of sirolimus on malignancy and survival after kidney transplantation: Systematic review and meta-analysis of individual patient data. *BMJ* **2014**, *349*, g6679. [CrossRef] [PubMed]
10. Chapman, J.R. The KDIGO clinical practice guidelines for the care of kidney transplant recipients. *Transplantation* **2010**, *89*, 644–645. [CrossRef] [PubMed]
11. Van Leeuwen, M.T.; Webster, A.C.; McCredie, M.R.; Stewart, J.H.; McDonald, S.P.; Amin, J.; Kaldor, J.M.; Chapman, J.R.; Vajdic, C.M.; Grulich, A.E. Effect of reduced immunosuppression after kidney transplant failure on risk of cancer: Population based retrospective cohort study. *BMJ* **2010**, *340*, c570. [CrossRef] [PubMed]
12. Yanik, E.L.; Clarke, C.A.; Snyder, J.J.; Pfeiffer, R.M.; Engels, E.A. Variation in Cancer Incidence among Patients with ESRD during Kidney Function and Nonfunction Intervals. *J. Am. Soc. Nephrol.* **2016**, *27*, 1495–1504. [CrossRef] [PubMed]

13. Hope, C.M.; Krige, A.J.; Barratt, A.; Carroll, R.P. Reductions in immunosuppression after haematological or solid organ cancer diagnosis in kidney transplant recipients. *Transpl. Int.* **2015**, *28*, 1332–1335. [CrossRef] [PubMed]
14. Perl, J.; Zhang, J.; Gillespie, B.; Wikström, B.; Fort, J.; Hasegawa, T.; Fuller, D.S.; Pisoni, R.L.; Robinson, B.M.; Tentori, F. Reduced survival and quality of life following return to dialysis after transplant failure: The Dialysis Outcomes and Practice Patterns Study. *Nephrol. Dial. Transplant.* **2012**, *27*, 4464–4472. [CrossRef] [PubMed]

14

Changes in Office Blood Pressure Control, Augmentation Index and Liver Steatosis in Kidney Transplant Patients after Successful Hepatitis C Infection Treatment with Direct Antiviral Agents

Aureliusz Kolonko [1,*], Joanna Musialik [1], Jerzy Chudek [2], Magdalena Bartmańska [1], Natalia Słabiak-Błaż [1], Agata Kujawa-Szewieczek [1], Piotr Kuczera [1], Katarzyna Kwiecień-Furmańczuk [1] and Andrzej Więcek [1]

1 Department of Nephrology, Transplantation and Internal Medicine, Medical University of Silesia, Francuska 20/24, 40-027 Katowice, Poland; jmusialik@sum.edu.pl (J.M.); bartmanska.m@gmail.com (M.B.); nataliablaz@gazeta.pl (N.S.-B.); agata.szewieczek@gmail.com (A.K.-S.); p.m.kuczera@gmail.com (P.K.); kapril@go2.pl (K.K.-F.); awiecek@spskm.katowice.pl (A.W.)

2 Department of Internal Medicine and Oncological Chemotherapy, Medical University of Silesia, Reymonta 8, 40-035 Katowice, Poland; chj@poczta.fm

* Correspondence: uryniusz@wp.pl

Abstract: Hepatitis C virus (HCV) infection in kidney transplant recipients (KTRs) can be successfully treated with direct antiviral agents (DAA). The aim of our study was to analyze different measures of vascular function during and after the DAA treatment. As we have observed the improvement of blood pressure (BP) control in some individuals, we have conducted an analysis of potential explanatory mechanisms behind this finding. Twenty-eight adult KTRs were prospectively evaluated before and 15 months after start of DAA therapy. Attended office BP (OBP), augmentation index (AIx), pulse wave velocity (PWV), flow-mediated dilation (FMD), liver stiffness measurement (LSM), and liver steatosis assessment (controlled attenuation parameter (CAP)) were measured. In half of the patients, improvement of OBP control (decline of systolic BP by at least 20 mmHg or reduction of the number of antihypertensive drugs used) and parallel central aortic pressure parameters, including AIx, was observed. There was a significant decrease in CAP mean values (241 ± 54 vs. 209 ± 30 dB/m, $p < 0.05$) only in patients with OBP control improvement. Half of our KTRs cohort after successful HCV eradication noted clinically important improvement of both OBP control and central aortic pressure parameters, including AIx. The concomitant decrease of liver steatosis was observed only in the subgroup of patients with improvement of blood pressure control.

Keywords: blood pressure; eradication; interferon-free regimen; hepatitis C infection; kidney transplant

1. Introduction

Arterial hypertension is highly prevalent in kidney transplant recipients (KTRs) as a consequence of common pretransplant hypertension and as an additional effect of immunosuppressive medications [1,2]. It has been shown that blood pressure (BP) control is suboptimal (systolic BP > 140 mmHg) in 50% of KTRs [3–5]. In addition, higher BP values were associated with reduced graft and patient survival [5]. Notably, cardiovascular disease is the primary cause of mortality among kidney transplant recipients, mostly due to long-term consequences of chronic kidney disease (CKD) [6]. CKD-related systemic inflammation, calcium-phosphate abnormalities, and oxidative stress promote endothelial dysfunction, vascular calcification, and accelerated atherosclerosis in addition to the traditional risk factors [7,8]. Vascular injury caused by the uremic milieu results in an increased arterial stiffness and reduced flow-mediated dilation (FMD) [9,10].

Chronic hepatitis C virus (HCV) infection has been shown to independently worsen posttransplant survival [11]. HCV infection is a risk factor for increased aortic stiffness and cardiovascular events in dialysis patients [12], whereas advanced HCV-derived liver fibrosis is associated with increased endothelial dysfunction, independently of common cardiovascular risk factors [13]. On the other hand, patients with chronic HCV infection also demonstrate impaired autonomic nervous system function [14]. All the above disturbances caused by coexisting HCV infection may partially worsen blood pressure control in KTRs.

A few years ago a breakthrough in the treatment of chronic hepatitis C occurred. The previous interferon-based therapy, which was contraindicated for kidney transplanted patients due to increased risk of organ rejection, was replaced by new, direct acting antiviral (DAA) drug regimens. In our observation, the effectiveness of this therapy, based on sofosbuvir, reached 100% [15]. We hypothesized that the successful eradication of HCV infection may directly or indirectly improve the endothelial function. In the present study, patients were prospectively evaluated regarding different measures of their vascular function, including endothelial function, arterial stiffness measurement, and blood pressure control. Concurrently, we assessed the liver stiffness and steatosis before and after the DAA treatment. As we observed the improvement of blood pressure control in some individuals, we conducted an analysis of potential explanatory mechanisms behind this finding.

2. Material and Methods

2.1. *Study Group*

The study protocol was accepted by the Bioethics Committee of the Medical University of Silesia in Katowice (KNW/0022/KB1/119/16) and all participants provided written informed consent. The study was conducted in accordance with the Declaration of Helsinki. We prospectively studied all eligible adult kidney transplant recipients (KTRs) who completed treatment with DAA therapy due to HCV infection and completed both baseline and follow-up examination at least 12 months after the start of DAA therapy.

2.2. *Clinical, Anthropometric, and Laboratory Measurements*

Body weight and height were measured following standard procedures and body mass index (BMI) was then calculated (kg/m^2). Body surface area (BSA) was calculated according to the DuBois formula and was expressed in m^2.

Kidney graft function was measured by the estimated glomerular filtration rate (eGFR), which was calculated according to the abbreviated Modification of Diet in Renal Disease formula.

HOMA-IR (Homeostatic model assessment of insulin resistance) was calculated to assess insulin resistance.

HCV RNA was measured with COBAS® AmpliScreen HCV v.1.0, with lower limit of detection of 15 IU/mL (Roche Diagnostics, USA). HCV genotyping and viral load was performed with Linear Array Genotyping Test and COBAS®TaqMan® Quantitative test v.1.0, with lower limit of detection of 21 IU/mL (TaqMan; Roche Diagnostics, Branchburg, NJ, USA).

Concentrations of blood glycated hemoglobin (HbA_{1C}), serum creatinine, total cholesterol, triglycerides, and total bilirubin concentrations, as well as aspartate aminotransferase (AST), alanine aminotransferase (ALT), and gamma glutamyl transpeptidase (GGT) activity were routinely measured during standard outpatient visits. Additional blood samples were withdrawn in a closed system into tubes containing citrate and ethylenediaminetetraacetic acid (EDTA) for nonroutine analyses. The tubes were allowed to stand for 2 h at room temperature, then centrifuged (15 min, 3000 rpm), and finally plasma aliquots were preserved at −70 °C.

The plasma concentrations of high-sensitivity C-reactive protein (hsCRP) were assessed with the use of an enzyme-linked immunosorbent assay (ELISA) (Immundiagnostic AG, Bensheim, Germany), with the limit of quantification (LoQ) of 0.09 mg/L, intra-assay variation <6%, and inter-assay variation <11.6%. Plasma concentrations of interleukin-6 (IL-6) were assessed with an ELISA (R&D Systems, Minneapolis, MN, USA) with a LoQ of 0.7 pg/mL, intra-assay variation <4.2%, and inter-assay variation <6.4%. Plasma concentrations of fibroblast growth factor 21 (FGF-21) were assessed with an ELISA (Biovendor, Brno, Czech Republic) with a LoQ of 7 pg/mL, intra-assay variation <2.0%, and inter-assay variation <3.3%. Plasma concentrations of C-peptide and insulin were measured using a Cobas E411 analyzer with intermediate precision <5.0% and <2.8%, respectively.

Each study examination consisted of the measurement of office BP and central arterial pressure parameters. Echocardiography, pulse wave velocity (PWV), FMD, liver stiffness measurement (LSM), and liver steatosis assessment (controlled attenuation parameter (CAP)) were also performed at the same time points.

Attended office blood pressure measurements (OBP) were performed three times in the sitting position after more than a 5-min rest in the sitting position on the arm without arterio-venous fistula at the beginning of the study. Patients with systolic BP values ≥140 mmHg and/or diastolic BP values ≥90 mmHg or those who received antihypertensive medication were diagnosed as hypertensive. For the present post hoc analysis, the OBP control improvement was defined as the decline of attended office systolic pressure by at least 20 mmHg without pharmacotherapeutic changes or the reduction of antihypertensive treatment due to the BP decline during the follow-up period. The cut-off value (20 mmHg) was established based on doubled maximum measurement error of 10 mmHg [16,17]. Patients were divided into two study subgroups based on the BP control improvement during the follow-up period.

2.3. *Echocardiography*

Echocardiographic measurements were performed using Toshiba Xario 100 Diagnostic Ultrasound System (Toshiba, Toshiba Medical System Corporation, Tochigi 324-8550, Japan). M-mode and two-dimensional measurements were performed as recommended by the American Society of Echocardiography [18], including left ventricular end-diastolic and end-systolic diameters, intraventricular septum, and posterior wall end-diastolic thickness. Left ventricular mass (LVM) was calculated according to the Devereux formula [19]. LVM was indexed for BSA (LVMI).

2.4. *Brachial Artery Flow-Mediated Dilation*

FMD was measured in the morning, after 10 min of lying in a quiet dimmed room using the Toshiba Xario 100. During the examination, the patients rested in a seated position with their forearms and backs supported. A manual sphygmomanometer cuff was placed on the arm without arteriovenous fistula and the diameter (lumen) of the brachial artery was measured with a linear transducer. The cuff was then inflated at approximately 50 mmHg above the current systolic pressure for 5 min [20]. After the deflation of the cuff, the serial measurements during diastole were recorded and the widest dilation of the brachial artery was used for FMD calculation: $FMD\% = (A - B)/B \times 100\%$, where A is the diameter of the artery during reactive hyperemia, and B is the initial diameter of the artery.

Non-endothelial dependent vasodilation (NMD) was assessed after at least a 15-min rest from the FMD acquisition. Similarly to FMD measurements, vessel diameters were assessed before and after sublingual nitroglycerin (400 μg) application (Nitromint (glyceroli trinitras), Proterapia, Poland). Of importance, as we observed unexpected reduction of NMD values in some patients, we repeated all NMD measurements using a double dose of nitroglycerin, i.e., 800 μg, after approximately 6 months from the previous follow-up series.

2.5. Central Aortic Pressure and Arterial Stiffness Measurement

Pulse waveform analysis was performed with the commercially available SphygmoCor 2000 (AtCor Medical, Sydney, Australia). Peripheral pressure waveforms were recorded from the radial artery using applanation tonometry. After the acquisition of at least 20 sequential waveforms, a validated generalized transfer function was used to generate the corresponding central aortic pressure waveform. Central blood pressure measurements, including central aortic systolic and diastolic blood pressure, central pulse pressure, and augmentation index were performed. Augmentation index was then normalized according to the heart rate (AIx@75). Only high-quality recordings, defined as an in-device quality index greater than 80% and visually acceptable curves by the investigator, were included in the analysis. The entire pulse wave analysis was performed in the sitting position under standardized conditions in the morning hours, after at least 15 min of rest in the supine position.

Arterial stiffness was also assessed using SphygmoCor 2000 placed over the carotid and femoral arteries. Pressure signals were calibrated using brachial BP and PWV was calculated as the time of the pulse wave between the diagnosed points (distance (m)/time (s)).

2.6. Liver Elastography

The controlled attenuation parameter (CAP) and liver stiffness measurement (LSM) were performed using transient elastography with a M-probe (FibroScan 502 Touch, Echosense, Paris, France). The operator was a technician certified by Echosense and unaware of patient status. The measurements were performed using a 3.5-MHz standard probe on the right hepatic lobe through the intercostal spaces with the patient lying in a supine position. As recommended by the manufacturer, 10 successful measurements were performed for each patient and only those with a success rate of at least 60% and an interquartile range/median value of less than 0.3 were considered reliable. The final CAP and liver stiffness were expressed in dB/m and kPa, respectively [21,22].

2.7. Data and Statistical Analysis

Statistical analyses were performed using the STATISTICA 13.0 PL for Windows software package (StatSoft Poland, Cracow, Poland). The values were presented as mean values with 95% confidence interval (CI) (for variables with normal distribution), medians with Q25-Q75 quartile values (for variables with not normal distribution), or frequencies. Comparisons between groups were done by using the Student t-test for quantitative variables or the χ^2 test for qualitative variables. Variables with not normal distribution were compared using the Mann–Whitney U test. The comparison of baseline and follow-up values was performed using the Student t-test, or the Wilcoxon test for variables with not normal distribution. Correlation coefficients were calculated using the Pearson test. Due to its not normal distribution, FGF-21 data were logarithmized before the correlation analyses. In all statistical tests, 'p' values below 0.05 were considered as statistically significant.

3. Results

3.1. Study Group

Out of all 73 KTRs with the presence of anti-HCV antibodies, HCV-RNA was detected in 40 patients. These patients were qualified to further HCV genotyping and viral load. Out of them, 8 patients had started DAA therapy without baseline examination planned for the present study and were not included in the final analysis. The other 32 patients were treated with the DAA anti-HCV protocol, including 8 with a 6-month regimen and 24 patients with a 3-month regimen based on sofosbuvir. The DAA regimen was shortened in the later enrolled patients as the treatment recommendations were updated during the study period. Out of this group, 4 KTRs were excluded: 2 of them were normotensive prior to HCV treatment and 2 others did not finalize the study protocol (Figure 1). Hence, the final study group consisted of 28 hypertensive patients who completed DAA therapy and both baseline and follow-up examinations. In all study patients, the diagnosis of HCV infection was established prior to kidney transplantation. In all patients, HCV viremia was not detectable after the first month of treatment and they all reached sustained virologic response at 48 weeks from DAA treatment start (SVR48) time point. The clinical characteristics of the study patients are presented in Table 1.

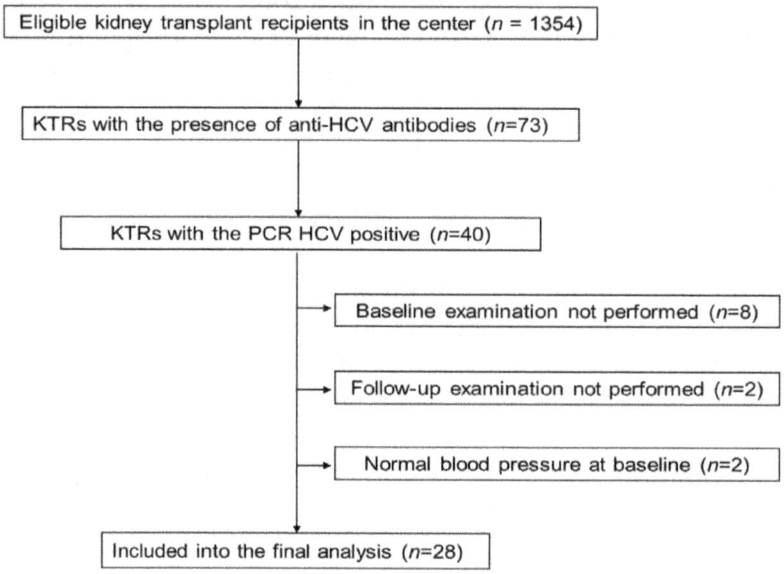

Figure 1. Study flow chart. KTRs, kidney transplant recipients; HCV, hepatitis C virus; PCR, polymerase chain reaction.

Table 1. Characteristics of direct antiviral agents-treated kidney transplant recipients stratified to subgroups based on blood pressure control improvement in the follow-up period.

	OBP Control Improvement $n = 14$	No OBP Control Improvement $n = 14$	p
Age at the start of DAA therapy (years, means and 95%CI)	49.8 (42.8–56.8)	48.5 (42.2–54.9)	0.78
Sex (M/F)	8/6	11/3	0.23
Baseline BMI (kg/m^2, means and 95%CI)	24.9 (22.8–26.9)	24.0 (22.3–25.7)	0.48
Follow-up BMI (kg/m^2, means and 95%CI)	25.6 (23.5–27.6) ##	24.4 (22.6–26.3)	0.40
Baseline eGFR (mL/min/1.73 m^2, means and 95%CI)	58.1 (45.1–71.2)	54.2 (36.3–72.1)	0.51
Follow-up eGFR (mL/min/1.73 m^2, means and 95%CI)	54.6 (39.4–69.8)	51.7 (35.0–68.5)	0.51
Diabetes (n (%))	4 (28.6)	4 (28.6)	1.0
Duration of HCV infection (years, means and 95%CI)	11.0 (6.9–15.1)	16.4 (12.6–20.1)	<0.05
Dialysis vintage (months, median and IQR)	30 (18–59)	42 (20–83)	0.37
Time after KTx (months, means and 95%CI)	121 (56–186)	125 (80–169)	0.92
Calcineurin inhibitor (CyA/Tc) (n)	8/6	7/7	0.70
Baseline HCV viremia (IU/mL, median and IQR)	340,258 (29,882–1,149,502)	78,631 (14,847–330,000)	0.40

$p < 0.01$ versus baseline. CI, confidence interval; IQR, interquartile range; OBP, attended office blood pressure; DAA, direct antiviral drug therapy; BMI, body mass index; eGFR, estimated glomerular filtration rate; KTx, kidney transplantation; CyA, cyclosporine A; Tc, tacrolimus.

3.2. Study Subgroups Based on Blood Pressure Control

In the follow-up period, half of the patients showed an improvement of OBP control (subgroup 1). Patients with OBP improvement had initially higher systolic BP (SBP) ($p = 0.02$), but similar diastolic BP (DBP) (Table 2). In addition, they received more antihypertensive medications (mean: 2.5 vs. 1.9 drugs) before the start of DAA therapy; however, this difference was not statistically significant. The observed overall SBP (Δ −20.4, 95% CI, −26.2 to −14.6 mmHg) and DBP (Δ −12.5, 95% CI, −16.5 to −8.5 mmHg) decline in subgroup 1 was obtained despite the reduction in the number of antihypertensive drugs in 9 subjects. We also observed mild reduction in SBP (Δ −5.2, 95 % CI, −9.7 to −0.8 mmHg) and DBP (Δ −4.6, 95% CI, −9.6 to 0.3 mmHg) in the second subgroup.

At baseline, the antihypertensive treatment was used in all patients: Beta-blockers in 67.9%, calcium channel blockers in 25%, angiotensin-converting enzyme inhibitor or angiotensin receptor blocker in 32.1%, alpha-blocker in 25%, and diuretics in 32.1% of study participants. The structure of antihypertensive medication classes was similar in both study subgroups (data not shown).

Both study subgroups did not differ in respect to age, gender, BMI, pretransplant dialysis vintage, time after kidney transplantation, and the occurrence of diabetes (Table 1). The time from diagnosis of HCV infection to DAA treatment was significantly longer in the subgroup 2 (Table 1), however, the percentage of patients with HCV infection lasting more than 13.7 years (mean value in the whole group) did not differ between study subgroups ($p = 0.13$). Out of whole group, only 4 patients were previously treated with interferon-based anti-HCV regimens. There were no differences in regards to baseline values of serum lipid concentrations, fasting glucose and insulin concentrations, glycated hemoglobin, and HOMA-IR values between subgroups (Supplementary Table S1).

Also, the HCV genotypes were similar in both subgroups, including 11 patients with genotype 1b in each group. The percentage of patients with advanced fibrosis, defined based on a METAVIR score >2, was comparable (28.6 vs. 38.5%, $p = 0.59$). The mean time between baseline and follow-up study examinations was also similar (15.0 ± 1.4 vs. 15.9 ± 2.1 months, $p = 0.22$).

Both study subgroups were similar in respect to calcineurin inhibitor (CNI) structure (Table 1). There were no CNI-type conversions during the whole study period. At baseline, median cyclosporine (CyA) doses were comparable (100 (100–125) mg in subgroup 1 vs. 125 (100–150) mg in subgroup 2, $p = 0.60$), whereas median tacrolimus (Tc) doses were significantly greater in subgroup 2 (4.0 (2.5–6.0) mg vs. 1.0 (1.0–2.0) mg in subgroup 1, $p < 0.05$). Notably, median CyA (97 (70–128) vs. 125 (100–146) ng/mL, respectively; $p = 0.30$) and Tc (7.1 (6.1–7.4) vs. 8.4 (6.7–8.7) ng/mL, respectively; $p = 0.22$) blood trough concentrations were similar. During and after DAA treatment, the improved liver function resulted in the reduction of calcineurin inhibitor (cyclosporine or tacrolimus) blood trough concentrations as compared with baseline values, which were similar in both study subgroups (−21.4 (−37.2 to −5.7) vs. −11.3 (−33.5 to 10.9)%, respectively; $p = 0.42$) and required individual dose adjustments in 61% of patients ($n = 17$) as soon as after one month of therapy. The consecutive CNI dose adjustments were made at physician discretion and were guided by the drug blood concentration, to prevent the CyA level decreasing below 70 ng/mL or Tc level decreasing below 5 ng/mL. Overall, the median CNI dose changes in both study subgroups were similar (13.4 (interquartile range (IQR) 0–25) vs. 25 (0–75)%, respectively; $p = 0.26$). Also, the absolute median dose changes of CyA (0 (0–75) vs. 25 (12.5–25) mg, respectively; $p = 0.73$) and Tc (0.5 (0.5–1.0) vs. 0 (−1.5–0.5) mg, respectively; $p = 0.26$) were similar.

Table 2. Office BP measurements and antihypertensive treatment before and after successful DAA therapy, divided into two subgroups based on changes in OBP control after treatment.

	OBP Control Improvement (n = 14)			p	**No OBP Control Improvement** (n = 14)			p
	Baseline	**Follow-up**	**Δ**		**Baseline**	**Follow-up**	**Δ**	
SBP (mmHg, mean and 95% CI)	145.5 (138.3–152.7)	125.1 (116.3–133.8)	−20.4 (−26.2–−14.6)	<0.001	135.6 (130.4–140.1)	130.4 (125.1–135.6)	−5.2 (−9.7–−0.8)	<0.05
DBP (mmHg, mean and 95% CI)	84.3 (78.8–89.8)	71.8 (67.0–76.6)	−12.5 (−16.5–−8.5)	<0.01	86.9 (83.6–90.1)	82.2 (79.3–85.1)	−4.6 (−9.6–0.3)	0.07
PP (mmHg, mean and 95% CI)	61.2 (52.7–69.7)	53.3 (43.2–63.3)	−7.9 (−14.1–−1.8)	<0.05	48.7 (43.8–53.6)	48.1 (42.1–54.2)	−0.6 (−5.3 – 4.2)	0.86
Number of antihypertensive drugs (mean and 95% CI)	2.5 (1.3–3.7)	1.9 (0.8–2.9)	−0.6 (−1.0- −0.3)	<0.05	1.9 (1.4–2.5)	2.2 (1.5–3.0)	0.3 (0.0–0.6)	<0.07

CI, confidence interval; OBP, attended office blood pressure; DAA, direct antiviral drug therapy; SBP, systolic blood pressure; DBP, diastolic blood pressure; PP, pulse pressure.

3.3. Liver Function Tests and Liver Morphologic Assessments

At baseline, there was a numerical difference in HCV viremia between subgroups (Table 1), but neither HCV viremia nor baseline liver function tests differed significantly. In both subgroups, there was a significant reduction in aminotransferases and GGT activities after DAA treatment (Supplemental Materials Table S2). Liver elastography measurements were performed with a success rate near 100% (only 3 out of 28 patients needed 11 total measurements to obtain 10 valid results). Baseline liver stiffness measurements did not differ between subgroups and remained unchanged thereafter. On the contrary, CAP values only declined significantly in subgroup 1 (Supplementary Materials Table S2 and Figure 2).

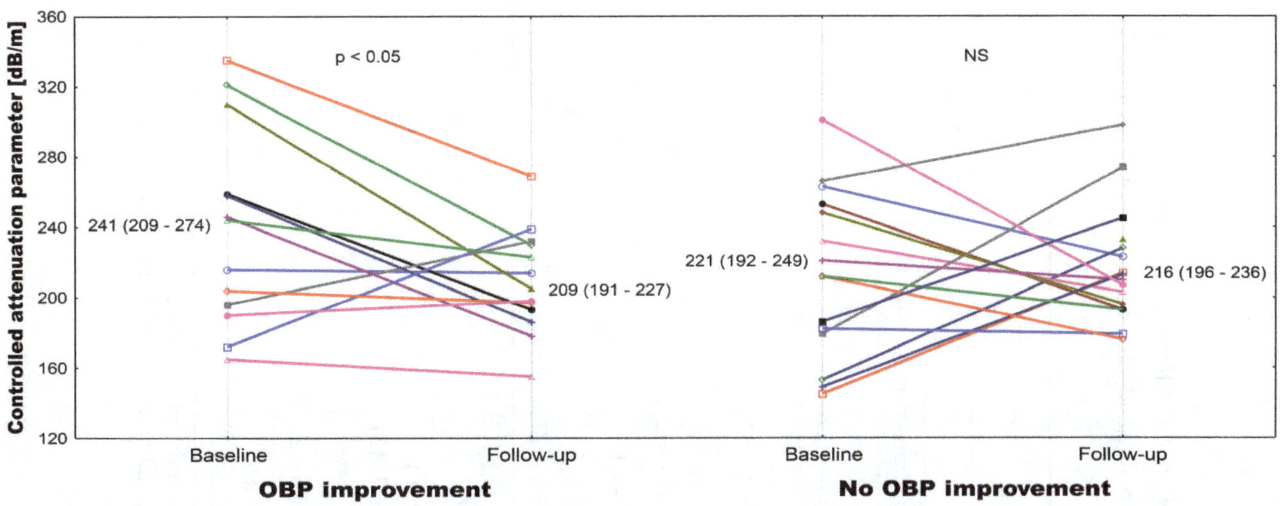

Figure 2. Individual plot of the controlled attenuation parameter at baseline and after the follow-up in patients with and without attended office blood pressure control improvement.

3.4. Central Blood Pressure Parameters

Both baseline and follow-up values of central aortic systolic pressure and central aortic pulse pressure correlated with corresponding values of OBP (baseline $r = 0.669$, $p < 0.001$, follow-up $r = 0.557$, $p < 0.01$ for SBP; and baseline $r = 0.730$, $p < 0.001$, follow-up $r = 0.502$, $p < 0.01$ for pulse pressure, respectively). There were also significant correlations between baseline augmentation index values standardized to heart rate (AIx@75) and both baseline and follow-up values of office SBP and pulse pressure (baseline $r = 0.660$, $p < 0.001$ and $r = 0.562$, $p < 0.01$, respectively; follow-up $r = 0.484$, $p < 0.01$ and $r = 0.545$, $p < 0.01$, respectively) (Table 3).

Parallel to OBP, we observed a 15.4% decline in aortic systolic pressure, a 12.1% decline in aortic diastolic pressure, and a 21.7% decline in aortic pulse pressure in subgroup 1 after successful DAA treatment (Table 3). Of note, AIx@75 values decreased significantly only in subgroup 1. On the contrary, only a mild decline of systolic aortic pressure (7.2%) was observed in subgroup 2. There was a positive correlation between the percentage change in CAP values and both the change in central aortic systolic pressure ($r = 0.438$, $p < 0.05$) and the change in AIx@75 ($r = 0.446$, $p < 0.05$). Of note, both baseline ($r = 0.479$, $p < 0.05$) and follow-up ($r = 0.431$, $p < 0.05$) CAP results correlated with corresponding BMI values.

Table 3. The central blood pressure parameters and the measurements of arterial stiffness (pulse wave velocity (PWV)) and endothelial function (flow-mediated dilation, (FMD) and nitroglycerine-mediated dilation (NMD)) measured before and after successful DAA treatment in kidney transplant recipients in both study subgroups, based on changes in OBP control after treatment.

	OBP Control Improvement (n = 14)			p	**No OBP Control Improvement (n = 14)**			p
	Baseline	**Follow-up**	**Δ**		**Baseline**	**Follow-up**	**Δ**	
Central blood pressure measurement								
AoSys (mmHg, mean and 95%CI)	136 (124–148)	114 (104–124)	−21.8 (−30.1–−13.5)	<0.01	131 (121–141)	120 (114–127)	−10.6 (−19.4–−1.9)	0.06
AoDia (mmHg, mean and 95%CI)	89 (81–96)	77 71–83)	−11.6 (−19.2–−4.1)	<0.05	87 (81–92)	82 (76–87)	−5.0 (−12.8–−2.8)	0.19
AoPP (mmHg, mean and 95%CI)	47 (38–57)	37 (29–46)	−10.1 (−14.1–−6.2)	0.09	44 (37–51)	39 (33–44)	−5.6 (−12.3–1.1)	0.19
AIx@75 (%, median and IQR)	20.5 (8.6–25.1)	16.9 (2.0–20.2)	−4.4 (−13.4–−1.1)	<0.05	15.5 (10.6–21.1)	16.5 (8.2–21.8)	0.0 (−8.2–7.8)	0.85
Arterial wall assessments								
PWV (m/s, mean and 95%CI)	8.5 (7.4–9.7)	8.7 (7.5–9.8)	0.1 (−0.7–0.9)	0.65	8.3 (7.1–9.5)	8.0 (6.9–9.2)	−0.3 (−1.4–0.8)	0.55
FMD (%,median and IQR)	9.2 (8.1–12.5)	9.3 (4.9–17.9)	2.1 (−6.5–3.3)	0.88	9.9 (7.5–15.0)	9.6 (5.6–12.2)	−1.6 (−2.8–0.6)	0.36
NMD (%,mean and 95%CI)	12.9 (10.3–15.6)	11.1 (8.4–13.8)	−1.8 (−5.5–1.8)	0.30	11.8 (9.9–13.7)	6.3 (3.7–8.9)	−5.5 (−9.1–−2.0)	<0.001
NMD with double dose (%,mean and 95%CI)	12.9 (10.3–15.6)	13.4 (10.3–16.6)	0.5 (−2.2–3.2)	0.80	11.8 (9.9–13.7)	10.5 (5.7–15.3)	−1.3 (−6.0–3.5)	0.59

CI, confidence interval; IQR, interquartile range; OBP, office blood pressure; AoSys, aortic systolic pressure; AoDia, aortic diastolic pressure; AoPP, aortic pulse pressure; AIx75, aortic augmentation index normalized to heart rate of 75/min; PWV, pulse wave velocity; FMD, flow-mediated dilation; NMD, nitroglycerin-mediated dilation. For all comparisons of baseline values between two study subgroups, p values were >0.05.

3.5. Arterial Structural and Functional Measurements

At baseline and in the follow-up period, PWV values were similar in both subgroups (Table 3). FMD values were stable in both subgroups, while NMD measured using the standard (400 μg) dose of nitroglycerin did not change in subgroup 1, but showed a significant reduction in subgroup 2 (Table 3). However, in an additional repeated NMD measurement with a double dose of nitroglycerin there was no significant NMD change compared with baseline values in both study subgroups.

3.6. Cardiac Parameters

At baseline, both mean LVM (210 (169–250) vs. 211 (173–250) g, $p = 0.84$)) and mean LVMI (113 (94–131) vs. 114 (95–133) g/m^2, $p = 0.98$) were comparable in subgroups 1 and 2, respectively. Similarly, there were no differences in the follow-up LVM and LVMI values (0.70 and 0.87, respectively), and their absolute changes during the study period did not differ significantly (LVM 7.9 (−23.5 to 39.2) vs. −0.3 (−44.4 to 43.8), $p = 0.57$; LVMI 3.3 (−13.4 to 19.9) vs. −1.3 (−23.2 to 20.6) g/m^2, $p = 0.70$).

3.7. Inflammatory Markers

The baseline median of CRP concentration was slightly higher in subgroup 1 (1.7 (IQR 1.1–2.4) vs. 0.9 (0.4–1.4) mg/L in subgroup 2, with borderline significance ($p = 0.07$)). At follow-up assessment, there was a borderline increase of median hsCRP in subgroup 2 (3.6 (0.5–6.7), $p = 0.06$), whereas no difference was noted in subgroup 1 (1.8 (1.5–3.0), $p = 0.33$). There were no significant differences in IL-6 concentration median values, both at baseline (2.7 (2.2–3.2) vs. 2.2 (1.8–2.5) pg/mL, $p = 0.23$) and at the follow-up examination (2.7 (1.7–4.1) vs. 2.6 (1.7–5.7) pg/mL, $p = 0.76$). Levels did not change significantly during the study period.

3.8. Fibroblast Growth Factor 21 Levels

Median values of FGF-21 measured at follow-up increased significantly in subgroup 1 (411 (204–706) vs. 215 (120–535) pg/mL at baseline, $p < 0.01$), while they remained unchanged in subgroup 2 (189 (147–481) vs. 226 (116–267) pg/mL at baseline, $p = 0.22$). The baseline number of antihypertensive drugs was borderline associated with log values of baseline FGF-21 ($r = 0.375$, $p = 0.05$) and significantly associated with follow-up values of FGF-21 ($r = 0.467$, $p < 0.05$). However, the log values of both baseline and follow-up FGF-21 did not correlate with baseline SBP or DBP values, whereas they correlated significantly with baseline central systolic aortic pressure ($r = 0.388$, $p < 0.05$, and $r = 0.434$, $p < 0.05$, for baseline and follow-up FGF-21 log values, respectively) and borderline with central diastolic aortic pressure ($r = 0.357$, $p < 0.05$, and $r = 0.385$, $p < 0.05$, respectively). Moreover, the log values of follow-up FGF-21 negatively correlated with the change of central systolic and diastolic aortic pressures ($r = -0.361$ and $r = -0.367$, respectively) with both p values = 0.06.

4. Discussion

In the present study, we demonstrated the clinically important improvement of blood pressure control, defined as the decline of attended office systolic pressure by at least 20 mmHg without pharmacotherapeutic changes or the reduction of antihypertensive treatment due to the BP decline, in half of our cohort of HCV-infected stable kidney transplant recipients after successful HCV eradication with sofosbuvir-based DAA therapy. In this subgroup of patients, we observed the reduction of systolic BP values despite the de-escalation of antihypertensive treatment in 9 out of 14 subjects. Moreover, we also documented the parallel decline of central aortic pressure parameters, obtained with the Sphygmo-Cor device, including augmentation index, in patients with improved BP control. Finally, we noted the corresponding decrease of liver steatosis, measured by the controlled attenuation parameter, in this subgroup of patients, which may suggest the potential underlying mechanism of beneficial vascular changes.

We are aware that nowadays a majority of dialysis patients with previously diagnosed HCV infection have already been successfully treated with DAA regimen even before they get a kidney transplant. Nevertheless, the confirmation of relatively moderate BP control improvement in patients being currently on dialysis would be much more difficult due to procedural-related fluctuations in volemia. Thus, the present study findings may help to elucidate or confirm some mechanisms linking the HCV infection with BP control in CKD patients.

There are several possible pathomechanisms linking the chronic HCV infection with elevated blood pressure and increased cardiovascular risk, including increased arterial stiffness [23], endothelial dysfunction [13], and the direct effect of liver steatosis on BP regulation [24]. The virus plays an etiological and pathogenic role in the development of vasculitis and renal involvement with subsequent elevated BP and cardiovascular events. Notably, in the present study, the time from HCV diagnosis to DAA treatment was significantly shorter in the subgroup with improved BP control thereafter, which may confirm that the longer duration of HCV infection determines the degree of irreversible vascular damage and, therefore, influences the net effect of HCV eradication on BP control. Recently, an increased augmentation index following viral eradication with DAA therapy was found in patients with advanced fibrosis (≥9.5 kPa) [25]. Of note, in patients with non-advanced fibrosis, the authors observed a stable augmentation index and significantly lower values of both office and central systolic pressure at the SVR12 time point [25]. In contrast, we observed a significant decrease of the normalized augmentation index in a subgroup with BP improvement, whereas any change in arterial stiffness, measured by pulse wave velocity, was found in our cohort, independently of BP changes after DAA treatment.

When considering the possible changes of endothelial function after successful HCV eradication with DAA, the reduction of endothelium-derived adhesion molecule levels at the SVR12 time point was confirmed by two small studies [26,27], but the improvement of FMD values was observed only in one group [26], and Davis et al. did not find changes in bedside microvascular reactivity, measured by peripheral arterial tonometry [27]. Of note, both studies were performed in individuals with normal renal function. In our cohort, we observed stable FMD values and significantly lower NMD values after DAA treatment; however, a repeated measurement with a double dose of nitroglycerin did not confirm the preceding finding. As we previously reported, the significant decrease of calcineurin inhibitor levels shortly after successful HCV eradication in this group [15], we may speculate that this effect was caused by an improved liver metabolic efficiency, which limited the biologic effect of a standard nitroglycerin dose used originally. Furthermore, the calcineurin inhibitor co-medication may also influence the endothelial function in our group [28], though the proportion of cyclosporine A- and tacrolimus-treated patients was similar in both study subgroups.

It is important to notice that both analyzed subgroups did not differ at baseline in terms of demographics, co-morbidity, or kidney graft function. Also, arterial stiffness and endothelial function measures, as well as liver function tests and liver stiffness measurements, were comparable. There were significantly higher baseline office systolic blood pressure and pulse pressure values, but not central blood pressure parameters, in subgroup 1. The posttreatment follow-up evaluation, along with the substantial BP control improvement, revealed a significant decrease of CAP values in these patients. Notably, in patients without known cause of chronic liver disease, increased CAP was shown to be a good indicator of fatty liver disease with metabolic abnormalities that manifest even before a sonographic fatty change appears [29].

In HCV-infected patients, an intrahepatic viral load directly enhances the liver steatosis [30], especially in the setting of multiple metabolic abnormalities (expansion of visceral adipose tissue, insulin resistance, reversible hypocholesterolemia, arterial hypertension, and hyperuricemia). On the other hand, in patients with non-alcoholic fatty liver disease (NAFLD), steatosis grade was the most important factor for endothelial dysfunction [31]. Furthermore, lower FMD values were shown in pediatric NAFLD patients, in whom systolic and diastolic blood pressures were significantly higher than in healthy controls, but also higher than obese children with normal livers [32]. Even more importantly, fatty liver was shown to be associated with 24-h systolic blood pressure and daytime diastolic blood pressure measurements [24]. Recently, Wang et al. demonstrated that NAFLD is independently associated with hypertension and blood pressure category [33]. In this study, the CAP value was the predictor of diastolic, but not systolic BP in stepwise analysis for the whole study group, not only in NAFLD participants [33]. Of note, CAP alone was not sufficient for predicting hypertension in this study.

It is well known that in the population of KTRs, the measures of vascular damage are conditioned by many factors, including the duration of chronic kidney disease, pretransplant dialysis vintage, concomitant immunosuppressive regimen, and non-optimal kidney graft function. Thus, the possibility for marked improvement of vascular elasticity and distensibility after the successful HCV treatment is much lower than in the general population. Nonetheless, overall results of our investigation may indirectly confirm the notable role of decreasing liver steatosis in the BP control improvement in the study group.

Finally, FGF-21 levels are reported to increase in acute liver injury, but decrease in chronic hepatitis B patients [34], especially those with advanced fibrosis [35]. We analyzed FGF-21 concentrations before and after the successful treatment of chronic HCV infection. Its levels significantly increased only in patients with initially more advanced steatosis as shown by CAP and improved BP control after DAA therapy and HCV elimination. The concomitant decrease of liver steatosis after DAA therapy observed in our study is in line with previously published papers [36,37] and may play a significant role in improved BP control.

The main limitation of our analyzed cohort was its small size, which limited multivariate analysis of factors independently associated with the BP control improvement. Therefore, our preliminary data should be investigated in a larger multicenter cohort. However, we included all eligible KTRs with the sustained elimination of chronic HCV infection. Of note, the structure of DAA regimen in our patients was uniform: All were treated with a sofosbuvir-based therapy. Another limitation was the method of OBP measurement used in this study, specifically the lack of unattended BP measurement, which eliminated the potential bias related to the 'white coat' effect. In addition, we did not perform the 24-h ambulatory blood pressure monitoring; however, we observed the central blood pressure values and found a strong association with OBP results. Lastly, we would like to acknowledge the lack of monitoring of the adherence to antihypertensive medication in our study.

5. Conclusions

In conclusion, we observed the clinically important improvement of both office blood pressure control and central aortic pressure parameters, including augmentation index, in half of our cohort of HCV-infected stable kidney transplant recipients after successful HCV eradication with a sofosbuvir-based DAA therapy. The concomitant decrease of liver steatosis, measured by the controlled attenuation parameter, was only observed in this subgroup of patients, which may suggest the potential underlying mechanism of beneficial hemodynamic changes. Further investigation would elucidate the pathomechanism of the observed improvement of blood pressure control, however, the increased availability of DAA therapy already resulted in pretransplant eradication of HCV infection in a majority of currently dialysis patients. We believe that patients receiving DAA therapy in the pretransplant period will benefit even more. Nevertheless, the confirmation of relatively moderate BP improvement in dialysis patients would be much more difficult due to procedural-related fluctuations in volemia.

Author Contributions: Conceptualization and methodology, A.K. and J.M.; formal analysis, A.K. and J.C.; investigation, M.B., N.S.-B., A.K.-S., and P.K.; data curation, A.K. and K.K.-F.; writing—original draft preparation, A.K., J.M., and J.C.; writing—review and editing, A.W.; supervision, A.K. and A.W.; funding acquisition, A.K. All authors have read and agreed to the published version of the manuscript.

References

1. Divac, N.; Naumovic, R.; Stojanovic, R.; Prostran, M. The role of immunosuppressive medications in the pathogenesis of hypertension and efficacy of antihypertensive agents in kidney transplant recipients. *Curr. Med. Chem.* **2015**, *23*, 1941–1952. [CrossRef]
2. Wadei, H.M.; Textor, S.C. Hypertension in the kidney transplant recipients. *Transplant. Rev.* **2010**, *24*, 105–120. [CrossRef]
3. Arias, M.; Fernández-Fresnedo, G.; Gago, M.; Rodrigo, E.; Gómez-Alamillo, C.; Toyos, C.; Allende, N. Clinical characteristics of resistant hypertension in renal transplant recipients. *Nephrol. Dial. Transplant.* **2012**, *27* (Suppl. 4), 36–38. [CrossRef]
4. Azancot, M.A.; Ramos, N.; Moreso, F.J.; Ibernon, M.; Espinel, E.; Torres, I.B.; Fort, J.; Seron, D. Hypertension in chronic kidney disease: The influence of renal transplantation. *Transplantation* **2014**, *98*, 537–542. [CrossRef] [PubMed]
5. Opelz, G.; Wujciak, T.; Ritz, E. Association of chronic kidney graft failure with recipient blood pressure. *Kidney Int.* **1998**, *53*, 217–222. [CrossRef] [PubMed]
6. Sarnak, M.J.; Levey, A.S.; Schoolwerth, A.C.; Coresh, J.; Culleton, B.; Hamm, L.L.; McCullough, P.A.; Kasiske, B.L.; Kelepouris, E.; Klag, M.J.; et al. Kidney disease as a risk factor for development of cardiovascular disease: A statement from the American Heart Association Councils on Kidney in Cardiovascular Disease, High Blood Pressure Research, Clinical Cardiology, and Epidemiology and Prevention. *Circulation* **2002**, *108*, 154–169.
7. Stenvinkel, P.; Carrero, J.J.; Axelsson, J.; Lindholm, B.; Heimburger, O.; Massy, Z. Emerging biomarkers for evaluating cardiovascular risk in the chronic kidney disease patient: How do new pieces fit into the uremic puzzle? *Clin. J. Am. Soc. Nephrol.* **2008**, *3*, 505–521. [CrossRef]
8. Hogas, S.M.; Voroneanu, L.; Serban, D.N.; Segall, L.; Hogas, M.M.; Serban, I.L.; Covic, A. Methods and potential biomarkers for the evaluation of endothelial dysfunction in chronic kidney disease: A critical approach. *J. Am. Soc. Hypertens.* **2010**, *4*, 116–127. [CrossRef]
9. Wang, M.C.; Tsai, W.C.; Chen, J.Y.; Huang, J.J. Stepwise increase in arterial stiffness corresponding with the stages of chronic kidney disease. *Am. J. Kidney Dis.* **2005**, *45*, 494–501. [CrossRef]
10. Recio-Mayoral, A.; Banerjee, D.; Streather, C.; Kaski, J.C. Endothelial dysfunction, inflammation and atherosclerosis in chronic kidney disease—A cross-sectional study of predialysis, dialysis and kidney-transplantation patients. *Atherosclerosis* **2011**, *216*, 446–451. [CrossRef]
11. Pedroso, S.; Martins, L.; Fonseca, I.; Dias, L.; Henriques, A.C.; Sarmento, A.M.; Cabrita, A. Impact of hepatitis C virus on renal transplantation: Association with poor survival. *Transplant. Proc.* **2006**, *38*, 1890–1894. [CrossRef] [PubMed]
12. Oyake, N.; Shimada, T.; Murakami, Y.; Ishibashi, Y.; Satoh, H.; Suzuki, K.; Matsumory, A.; Oda, T. Hepatitis C virus infection as a risk factor for increased aortic stiffness and cardiovascular events in dialysis patients. *J. Nephrol.* **2008**, *21*, 345–353. [PubMed]
13. Barone, M.; Viggiani, M.T.; Amoruso, A.; Schiraldi, S.; Zito, A.; Devito, F.; Cortese, F.; Gesualdo, M.; Brunetti, N.; Di Leo, A.; et al. Endothelial dysfunction correlates with liver fibrosis in chronic HCV infection. *Gastroenterol. Res. Pract.* **2015**, *2015*, 682174. [CrossRef] [PubMed]
14. Osztovits, J.; Horváth, T.; Abonyi, M.; Tóth, T.; Visnyei, Z.; Bekö, G.; Csák, T.; Lakatos, P.L.; Littvay, L.; Fehér, J.; et al. Chronic hepatits C virus infection associated with autonomic dysfunction. *Liver Int.* **2009**, *29*, 1473–1478. [CrossRef] [PubMed]
15. Musialik, J.; Kolonko, A.; Kwiecień, K.; Owczarek, A.J.; Więcek, A. Effectiveness and safety of sofosbuvir-based therapy against hepatitis C infection after successful kidney transplantation. *Transpl. Infect. Dis.* **2019**, *21*, e13090. [CrossRef] [PubMed]

16. Babbs, C.F. The origin of Korotkoff sounds and the accuracy of auscultatory blood pressure measurements. *J. Am. Soc. Hypertens.* **2015**, *9*, 935–950. [CrossRef] [PubMed]
17. Padwal, R.; Jalali, A.; McLean, D.; Anwar, S.; Smith, K.; Raggi, P.; Ringrose, J.S. Accuracy of oscillometric blood pressure algorithms in healthy adults and in adults with cardiovascular risk factors. *Blood Press. Monit.* **2019**, *24*, 33–37. [CrossRef]
18. Lang, R.M.; Bierig, M.; Devereux, R.B.; Flaschkampf, F.A.; Foster, E.; Pellikka, P.A.; Picard, M.H.; Roman, M.J.; Seward, J.; Shanewise, J.S.; et al. Recommendations for Chamber Quantification: A report from the American Society of Echocardiography's Guidelines and Standards Committee and the Chamber Quantification Writing group. *J. Am. Soc. Echocardiogr.* **2005**, *18*, 1440–1463. [CrossRef]
19. Devereux, R.B.; Reichek, N. Echocardiographic determination of left ventricular mass in man. Anatomic validation of the method. *Circulation* **1977**, *55*, 613–618. [CrossRef]
20. Thijssen, D.H.J.; Bruno, R.M.; van Mil, A.C.C.M.; Holder, S.M.; Faita, F.; Greyling, A.; Zock, P.L.; Taddei, S.; Deanfield, J.E.; Luscher, T.; et al. Expert consensus and evidence-based recommendations for the assessment of flow-mediated dilation in humans. *Eur. Heart J.* **2019**, *40*, 2534–2547. [CrossRef]
21. Jun, B.G.; Park, W.Y.; Park, E.J.; Jang, J.Y.; Jeong, S.W.; Lee, S.H.; Kim, S.G.; Cha, S.W.; Kim, Y.S.; Cho, Y.D.; et al. A prospective comparative assessment of the accuracy of the FibroScan in evaluating liver steatosis. *PLoS ONE* **2017**, *12*, e01827784. [CrossRef] [PubMed]
22. Sandrin, L.; Fourquet, B.; Hasquenoph, J.M.; Yon, S.; Fournier, C.; Mal, F.; Christidis, C.; Ziol, M.; Poulet, B.; Kazemi, F.; et al. Transient elastography: A new noninvasive method for assessment of hepatic fibrosis. *Ultrasound Med. Biol.* **2003**, *29*, 1705–1713. [CrossRef] [PubMed]
23. Chou, C.-H.; Ho, C.-S.; Tsai, W.-C.; Wang, M.-C.; Tsai, Y.-S.; Chen, J.-Y. Effects of chronic hepatitis C infection on arterial stiffness. *J. Am. Soc. Hypertens.* **2017**, *11*, 716–723. [CrossRef] [PubMed]
24. Vasunta, R.-L.; Kesaniemi, Y.A.; Ylitalo, A.S.; Ukkola, O.H. High ambulatory blood pressure values associated with non-alcoholic fatty liver in middle-aged adults. *J. Hypert.* **2012**, *30*, 2015–2019. [CrossRef] [PubMed]
25. Cheng, P.-N.; Chen, J.-Y.; Chiu, Y.-C.; Chiu, H.-C.; Tsai, L.-M. Augmenting central arterial stiffness following eradication of HCV by direct acting antivirals in advanced fibrosis patients. *Sci. Rep.* **2019**, *9*, 1426. [CrossRef] [PubMed]
26. Schmidt, F.P.; Zimmermann, T.; Wenz, T.; Schnorbus, B.; Ostad, M.A.; Feist, C.; Grambihler, A.; Schattenberg, J.M.; Sprinzl, M.F.; Münzel, T.; et al. Interferon- and ribavirin-free therapy with new direct acting antivirals (DAA) for chronic hepatitis C improves vascular endothelial function. *Int. J. Cardiol.* **2018**, *271*, 296–300. [CrossRef]
27. Davis, J.S.; Young, M.; Lennox, S.; Jones, T.; Piera, K.; Pickles, R.; Oakley, S. The effect of curing hepatitis C with direct-acting antiviral treatment on endothelial function. *Antivir. Ther.* **2018**, *23*, 687–694. [CrossRef]
28. Akoglu, H.; Seringec, N.; Yildirim, T.; Yilmaz, R.; Okutucu, S.; Turkmen, E.; Evranos, B.; Kaya, E.B.; Dikmenoglu, N.; Arici, M.; et al. Relationship between hemorheology and endothelial dysfunction in renal transplant patients receiving calcineurin inhibitors. *J. Nephrol.* **2013**, *26*, 931–940. [CrossRef]
29. Kwak, M.S.; Chung, G.E.; Yang, J.I.; Yim, J.Y.; Chung, S.J.; Jung, S.Y.; Kim, J.S. Clinical implications of controlled attenuation parameter in a health check-up cohort. *Liver Int.* **2017**, *38*, 915–923. [CrossRef]
30. Ramalho, F. Hepatitis C virus infection and liver steatosis. *Antivir. Res.* **2003**, *60*, 125–127. [CrossRef]
31. Sapmaz, F.; Uzman, M.; Basyigit, S.; Ozkan, S.; Yavuz, B.; Yeniova, A.; Kefeli, A.; Asilturk, Z.; Nazligül, Y. Steatosis grade is the most important risk factor for development of endothelial dysfunction in NAFLD. *Medicine* **2016**, *95*, e3280. [CrossRef] [PubMed]
32. Pacifico, L.; Anania, C.; Martino, F.; Cantisani, V.; Pascone, R.; Marcantonio, A.; Chiesa, C. Functional and morphological vascular changes in pediatric nonalcoholic fatty liver disease. *Hepatology* **2010**, *52*, 1643–1651. [CrossRef] [PubMed]
33. Wang, Y.; Zeng, Y.; Lin, C.; Chen, Z. Hypertension and non-alcoholic fatty liver disease proven by transient elastography. *Hepatol. Res.* **2016**, *46*, 1304–1310. [CrossRef] [PubMed]
34. Wu, L.; Pan, Q.; Wu, G.; Qian, L.; Zhang, J.; Zhang, L.; Fang, Q.; Zang, G.; Wang, Y.; Lau, G.; et al. Diverse changes of circulating fibroblast growth factor 21 levels in hepatitis B virus-related diseases. *Sci. Rep.* **2017**, *7*, 16482. [CrossRef] [PubMed]
35. Iwasa, M.; Mifuji-Moroka, R.; Kobayashi, Y.; Takei, Y.; D'Alessandro-Gabazza, C.; Gabazza, E.C. Comment on serum FGF21 and RBP4 levels in patients with chronic hepatits C. *Scand. J. Gastroent.* **2012**, *48*, 252–253. [CrossRef] [PubMed]

36. Tada, T.; Kumada, T.; Toyoda, H.; Sone, Y.; Takeshima, K.; Ogawa, S.; Goto, T.; Wakahata, A.; Nakashima, M.; Nakamuta, M.; et al. Viral eradication reduces both liver stiffness and steatosis in patients with chronic hepatitis C virus infection who received direct-acting anti-viral therapy. *Aliment. Pharmacol. Ther.* **2018**, *7*, 1012–1022. [CrossRef]

37. Kobayashi, N.; Iijima, H.; Tada, T.; Kumada, T.; Yoshida, M.; Aoki, T.; Nishimura, T.; Nakano, C.; Takata, R.; Yoh, K.; et al. Changes in liver stiffness and steatosis among patients with hepatitis C virus infection who received direct-acting antiviral therapy and achieved sustained virological response. *Eur. J. Gastroenterol. Hepatol.* **2018**, *5*, 546–551. [CrossRef]

15

Living Donor Kidney Transplantation Improves Graft and Recipient Survival in Patients with Multiple Kidney Transplants

Maria Irene Bellini *, Aisling E Courtney and Jennifer A McCaughan

Regional Nephrology and Transplant Unit, Belfast City Hospital, 51 Lisburn Road, Belfast BT9 7AB, UK; aisling.courtney@belfasttrust.hscni.net (A.E.C.); jennifer.mccaughan@belfasttrust.hscni.net (J.A.M.)
* Correspondence: mariairene.bellini@nhs.net

Abstract: Background: Failed kidney transplant recipients benefit from a new graft as the general incident dialysis population, although additional challenges in the management of these patients are often limiting the long-term outcomes. Previously failed grafts, a long history of comorbidities, side effects of long-term immunosuppression and previous surgical interventions are common characteristics in the repeated kidney transplantation population, leading to significant complex immunological and technical aspects and often compromising the short- and long-term results. Although recipients' factors are acknowledged to represent one of the main determinants for graft and patient survival, there is increasing interest in expanding the donor's pool safely, particularly for high-risk candidates. The role of living kidney donation in this peculiar context of repeated kidney transplantation has not been assessed thoroughly. The aim of the present study is to analyse the effects of a high-quality graft, such as the one retrieved from living kidney donors, in the repeated kidney transplant population context. Methods: Retrospective analysis of the outcomes of the repeated kidney transplant population at our institution from 1968 to 2019. Data were extracted from a prospectively maintained database and stratified according to the number of transplants: 1st, 2nd or 3rd+. The main outcomes were graft and patient survivals, recorded from time of transplant to graft failure (return to dialysis) and censored at patient death with a functioning graft. Duration of renal replacement therapy was expressed as cumulative time per month. A multivariate analysis considering death-censored graft survival, decade of transplantation, recipient age, donor age, living donor, transplant number, ischaemic time, time on renal replacement therapy prior to transplant and HLA mismatch at HLA-A, -B and -DR was conducted. In the multivariate analysis of recipient survival, diabetic nephropathy as primary renal disease was also included. Results: A total of 2395 kidney transplant recipients were analysed: 2062 (83.8%) with the 1st kidney transplant, 279 (11.3%) with the 2nd graft, 46 (2.2%) with the 3rd+. Mean age of 1st kidney transplant recipients was 43.6 ± 16.3 years, versus 39.9 ± 14.4 for 2nd and 41.4 ± 11.5 for 3rd+ ($p < 0.001$). Aside from being younger, repeated kidney transplant patients were also more often males ($p = 0.006$), with a longer time spent on renal replacement therapy ($p < 0.0001$) and a higher degree of sensitisation, expressed as calculated reaction frequency ($p < 0.001$). There was also an association between multiple kidney transplants and better HLA match at transplantation ($p < 0.0001$). A difference in death-censored graft survival by number of transplants was seen, with a median graft survival of 328 months for recipients of the 1st transplant, 209 months for the 2nd and 150 months for the 3rd+ ($p = 0.038$). The same difference was seen in deceased donor kidneys ($p = 0.048$), but not in grafts from living donors ($p = 0.2$). Patient survival was comparable between the three groups ($p = 0.59$). Conclusions: In the attempt to expand the organ donor pool, particular attention should be reserved to high complex recipients, such as the repeated kidney transplant population. In this peculiar context, the quality of the donor has been shown to represent a main determinant for graft survival—in fact, kidney retrieved from living donors provide comparable outcomes to those from single-graft recipients.

Keywords: living donation; repeated kidney transplantation; graft survival; prolonged ischaemic time; patient survival; pre-emptive transplantation

1. Introduction

The proportion of end-stage renal disease (ESRD) patients with a failed kidney transplant is increasing each year [1,2]; 25% of patients on the US kidney transplant waiting list have a failed transplant [3] and in the Eurotransplant area, the number of patients being re-waitlisted after returning to dialysis steadily ranges between 17.9% and 18.9% [4].

Morbidity and mortality for patients with a failed kidney transplant on dialysis is high; there is a two- to three-fold risk of death compared to patients with a functioning graft and a median recipient survival after graft failure of three years [3,5]. This increased mortality [6] relates to higher rates of cardiovascular, neoplastic and infective events, in which the burden of immunosuppressive therapy is no longer counterbalanced by the benefits of a working kidney transplant [7]. The single modifiable factor which has the greatest impact on recipient survival in this group is the time to re-transplantation [6]; however, the suboptimal outcome of repeated kidney re-transplantation has generated increasing debate regarding the overall management and resource allocation within this subgroup. Nevertheless, previous reports have shown that there is a significative survival benefit after repeat deceased donor kidney transplantation over remaining on the waiting list, due to significative improvement in better immunological screening, crossmatching, HLA matching, post-operative management and immunosuppression protocols [8], although the overall outcome remains impaired by an inferior survival compared to first kidney transplant recipients [9].

Yet, other fundamental outcome drivers, for example the impact of a high-quality living donor graft, have not been fully investigated in the peculiar context of repeated kidney transplantation.

One of the primary advantages in fact of receiving a kidney from a living donor is that the organ is generally healthier and more resistant to the occurrence and extension of the subsequent ischaemic reperfusion injury. To become eligible, living donors undergo full screening of their kidney function, tissue and immunological compatibility with the recipient and a comprehensive overall physical health check. This is in contrast with grafts retrieved from deceased donors, where already the stress and the damage related to the death of the individual determine a systemic storm summing up to the usual longer time in cold storage to allow retrieval and transfer between different teams and hospitals. All together, these factors can temporarily reduce and potentially compromise the organ function irreversibly [10].

The incidence of delayed graft function in kidneys from deceased donors varies, but is overall as high as 30%; it might also take weeks before the recipient is fully dialysis independent [11,12], thus the recipients are more exposed and vulnerable in the post-operative period. Conversely, kidneys from living donors tend to function immediately, reducing the risk of hospitalisation and renal replacement therapy after transplant to less than 4% [13] and setting in this way the recipient for the best short- and long-term outcome.

Why is it so important an immediate graft function? As stated above, the more complex the procedure, the higher the likelihood of the prolonged ischaemic insult and the resultant impact on challenging recipients. Previously failed grafts, a long history of comorbidities, side effects of long-term immunosuppression and previous surgical interventions are common characteristics in the repeated kidney transplant population, leading to significant immunological and technical challenges.

Intuitively, it might initially seem sensible to withdraw immunosuppression in patients after graft failure to reduce the risk of cardiovascular, neoplastic and infective complications. However, for those who are fit for a subsequent transplant, this commonly results in a high degree of sensitisation to HLA, namely the production of donor-specific HLA antibodies (DSA) and other panel-reactive antibodies (PRAs) [14]. This reduces access to compatible donors and may result in an extremely prolonged wait for transplantation, with the associated morbidity and mortality [15]. This increased waiting time might also have a worse synergistic effect with the often extended ischemic time, due to the technical challenges associated with re-transplantation, namely adhesions from previous surgery, difficulties accessing the iliac vasculature or earlier manipulation of the bladder to establish the ureterovesical anastomosis [16].

The aim of this study is to analyse the experience of repeated kidney transplantation in our institution over 50 years, with a focus on outcomes in recipients of first, second and third/fourth kidney transplants and factors which impact these outcomes.

2. Methods

All recipients of kidney transplants in Northern Ireland between 1968 and 2019 were included in the analysis. Recipients were identified using a prospectively maintained database which records data on all transplant recipients. Recipients were followed up until death or 1 September 2019. The clinical and research activities being reported are consistent with the principles of the Declaration of Helsinki and comply with the Declaration of Istanbul. Approval for this study was granted by the Regional Ethics Committee (12/NI/1078).

Death-censored graft survival was measured from time of transplant to graft failure (return to dialysis) and censored when a patient died with a functioning graft. Duration of renal replacement therapy was expressed as cumulative time per month. Recipient survival was measured from transplantation to death. Pre-transplant sensitisation levels were expressed as a calculated reaction frequency (cRF), which is calculated as the proportion of the last 10,000 UK, blood group-identical, deceased donors to which the patient has DSAs. Recipients were considered highly sensitized if they had a cRF greater than 85%.

Immunosuppression: No routine induction was used in any era. Maintenance regimen was on prednisolone and azathioprine before 1989; from 1989 to 1998, cyclosporine was introduced and patients commenced on triple therapy; in 1998, mycophenolate mofetil replaced azathioprine in the triple-therapy regimen; and from 2000, tacrolimus replaced cyclosporine. Overall, the majority of patients were maintained on two agents in the long term, with 25% on the calcineurin inhibitor-free regimen.

Living donors: Numbers of living donors performed varied according to the decade considered: 3.3% from 1968 to 1977; 9.8% from 1978 to 1987; 4% from 1988 to 1997; 10.6% from 1998 to 2007 and 55.3% from 2008 to 2017.

Statistical Analysis

Continuous variables are presented as the mean ± standard deviation. Analysis of variance and *t* test were used to compare continuous variables between groups. For nominal or non-parametric variables, the Pearson χ^2 test was performed. Kaplan–Meier and Cox regression analyses were applied for survival analysis. In a multivariate analysis for death-censored graft survival, factors previously associated in our population were included: decade of transplantation, recipient age, donor age, living donor, transplant number, ischaemic time, time on renal replacement therapy prior to transplant and HLA mismatch at HLA-A, -B and -DR. In the multivariate analysis of recipient survival, diabetic nephropathy as primary renal disease was also included. Confidence interval was set to 95%, and p was considered significant at less than 0.05. Analysis was performed using SPSS (IBM SPSS Statistics for Windows, Version 20.0; IBM Corp, Armonk, NY, USA).

3. Results

A total of 2395 kidney transplant recipients were included: 2062 (83.8%) received a 1st kidney transplant, 279 (11.3%) received a 2nd kidney transplant, 46 (1.9%) received a 3rd kidney transplant and 8 (0.3%) received a 4th kidney transplant. The outcomes of the 3rd and 4th kidney transplants were grouped together (3rd+).

Table 1 summarises donor and recipient characteristics. Recipients of 3rd+ kidney transplants were significantly more likely to receive a living donor kidney ($p < 0.0001$).

Table 1. Demographics of kidney transplants performed in Northern Ireland in the period 1968–2019.

	1st Transplant $n = 2062$	2nd Transplant $n = 279$	3rd+ Transplant $n = 54$	p Value
Recipient				
Recipient age (mean+SD, years)	43.6 ± 16.3	39.9 ± 14.4	41.4 ± 11.5	0.001
Recipient sex (male)	1244 (60%)	187 (67%)	38 (73%)	0.006
Renal replacement therapy duration (mean+SD, months)	22.5 ± 26.6	124.7 ± 95.8	207.3 ± 106.8	<0.0001
Calculated reaction frequency (cRF) (mean+SD, %)	15.3 ± 29.7	54.1 ± 40.3	75.7 ± 34.5	<0.0001
Donor				
Donor age (mean+SD, years)	49.7 ± 9	39.4 ± 16.1	43.5 ± 16	0.166
Donor sex (male)	1159 (56%)	152 (54%)	28 (54%)	0.171
Living donor	549 (26%)	82 (29%)	22 (42%)	<0.0001
Transplant				
Pre-emptive transplantation	308 (14.9%)	22 (7.9%)	3 (5.6%)	<0.0001
HLA-A, -B, -DR mismatch (mean+SD, number)	2.4 ± 1.3	2 ± 1.4	1.4 ± 1.4	<0.0001
Ischaemic time (mean+SD, hours)	17.5 + 18	16.6 + 16.5	13 + 9.9	0.197

Donor age, donor sex and cold ischaemic time did not statistically differ between the groups.

In total, 99% of recipients were White. Recipients of repeated kidney transplants were more likely to be male ($p = 0.006$) and were younger ($p < 0.001$): mean age of 1st KTRs was 43.6 ± 16.3 years, versus 39.9 ± 14.4 for 2nd and 41.4 ± 11.5 for 3rd+ KTRs. Furthermore, these patients were also significantly more sensitised, with an increasing cRF from 15% (1st transplant) to 54% (2nd transplant), to 76% (3rd+ transplant) ($p < 0.0001$). As a consequence, there was also an association between multiple kidney transplants and better HLA match at transplantation ($p < 0.0001$). The pre-emptive rate was significantly lower in recipients of multiple transplants ($p < 0.0001$).

3.1. *Surgical Information*

All kidney transplants were performed extraperitoneally and graft nephrectomy was only performed in four cases: one in relation to uncontrolled antibody mediated rejection with systemic involvement, one following a catastrophic bleed, one simultaneously to the implant and one to create space for a potential 4th graft. The final patient had had multiple gynaecology procedures and the peritoneal content would not have been easily mobilised to allow graft implantation.

Only one major bleeding event occurred that required graft nephrectomy (2nd implant), but the recipient underwent successful implantation of a 3rd graft three years later. Urological complications were not recorded.

3.2. *Death-Censored Graft and Recipient Survival*

Figure 1 shows death-censored graft survival, with a median of 328 months for 1st kidney transplant recipients (KTRs) in blue, 209 months for 2nd KTRs in green and 150 months for 3rd+ KTRs in red ($p = 0.04$).

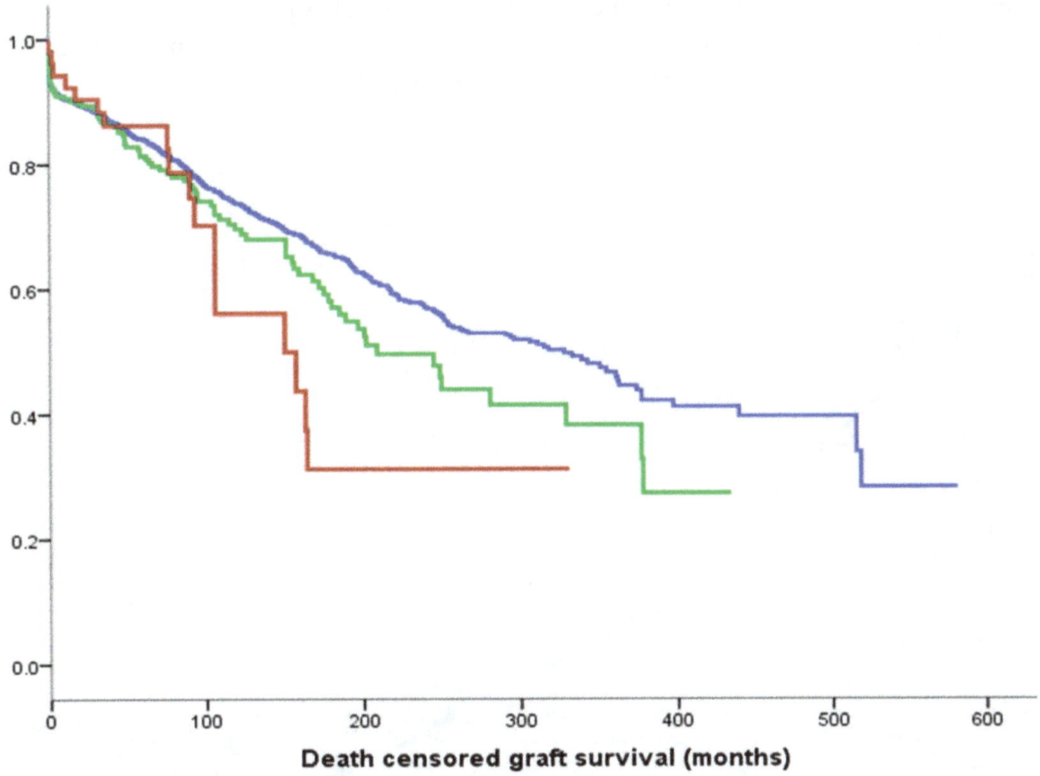

Figure 1. Median death-censored graft survival: 328 months for 1st graft (blue line), 209 months for 2nd (green line) and 150 months for 3rd+ (red line). ($p = 0.04$).

Death-censored graft survival remained significantly different between the three groups in the case of deceased donor transplants (Figure 2a), but there was no significant difference in death-censored graft survival between the groups in living donor transplantation (Figure 2b).

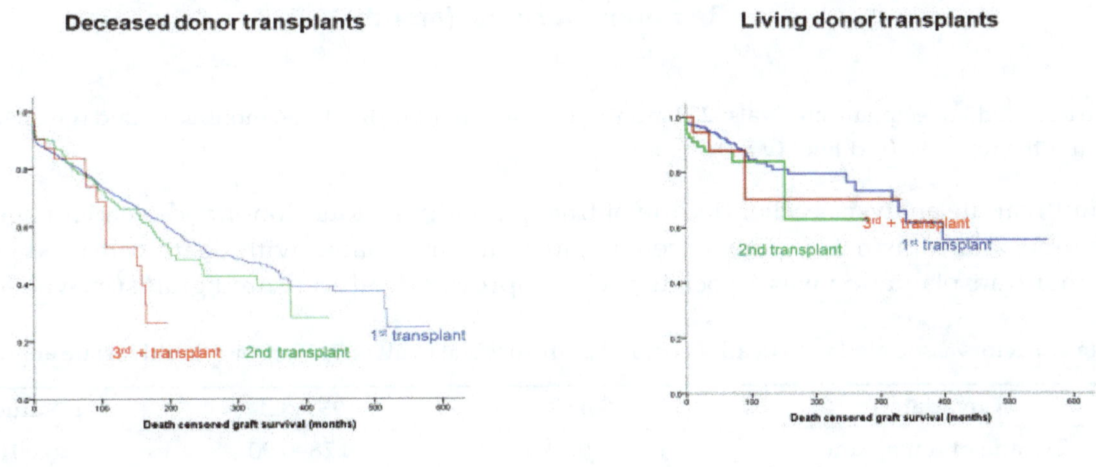

Figure 2a p = 0.048

Figure 2b p = 0.2

Figure 2. Difference in death-censored graft survival is seen in deceased donor transplants (**a**) but not in kidneys retrieved from living donors (**b**). Prolonged ischaemia is significantly detrimental to long-term survival in deceased donor grafts and 3rd and 4th transplants are associated with prolonged ischaemic times. These are marginal patients with difficult vasculature—marginal kidneys do less well in this context while good kidneys cope fine. Blue line: recipients of 1st kidney transplant; green line: recipients of 2nd kidney transplant; red line: recipients of 3rd kidney transplant.

Recipient survival was comparable between the three groups ($p = 0.59$), with a median of 234 months for 1st KTRs in blue, 256 months for 2nd KTRs in green and 298 months for 3rd+ KTRs in red (Figure 3). The 10 year recipient survival for all groups exceeded 70%.

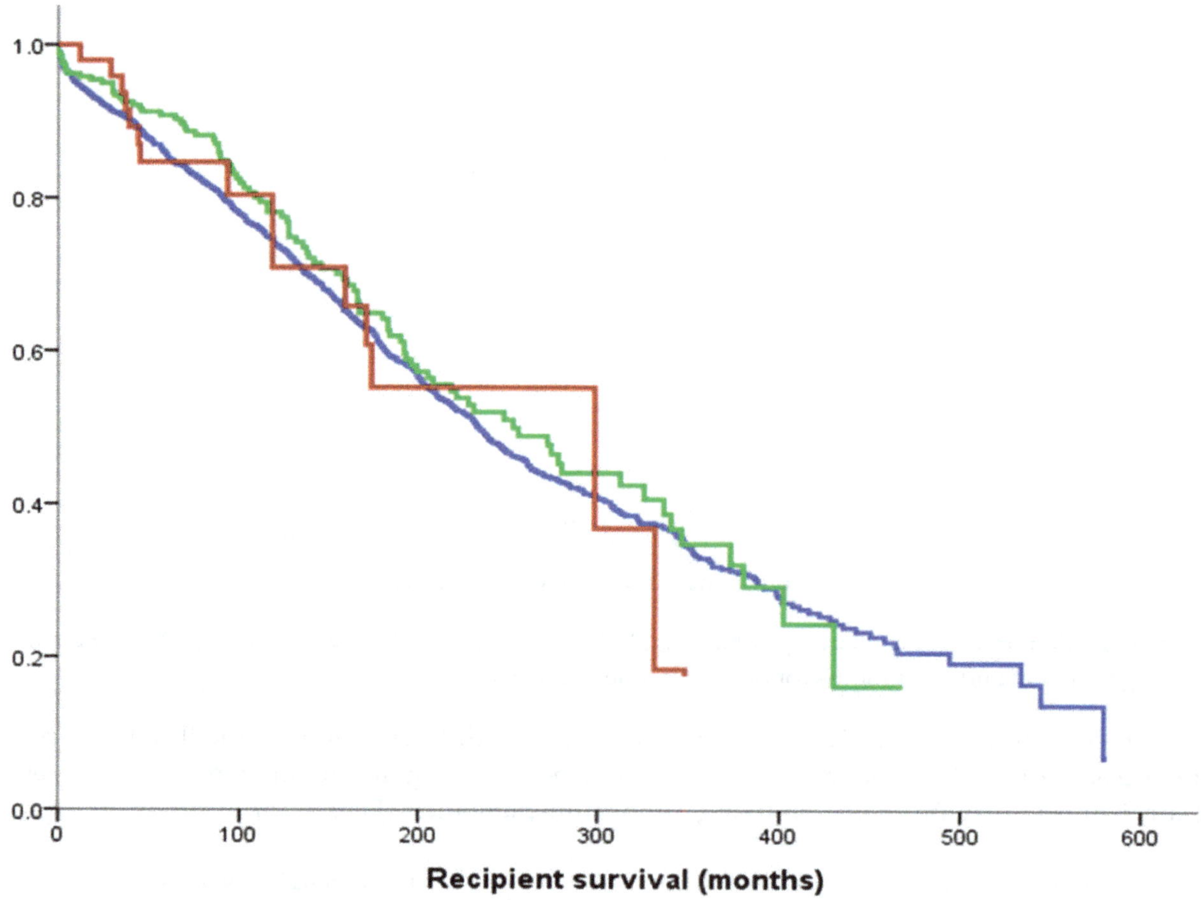

Figure 3. Median recipient survivals: 234 months for 1st graft (blue line); 256 months for 2nd (green line); 298 months for 3rd+ (red line) ($p = 0.59$).

In multivariate analysis, earlier decade of transplantation, older donor and recipient age, longer ischemic time, and transplant number were significantly associated with death-censored graft loss. Living donor transplantation was associated with improved death-censored graft survival (Table 2).

Table 2. Factors associated with death-censored graft survival in all recipients on a multivariate analysis.

Covariate	HR	95% CI	*p* Value
Decade of transplant	0.84	0.78–0.90	<0.001
Recipient age (per decade)	0.90	0.86–0.96	<0.001
Living donor	0.61	0.45–0.83	0.002
Donor age (per decade)	1.14	1.08–1.20	<0.001
Transplant number	1.23	1.03–1.48	0.02
Ischaemic time (per 6h)	1.09	1.01–1.17	0.02

Time on RRT and HLA mismatch at HLA-A, - B and -DR were not significant and dropped out of model.

For recipients of 3rd+ transplants, the association with a living donor is the only factor associated with death-censored graft survival (Table 3).

Table 3. Multivariate analysis for death-censored graft survival in 3rd+ recipients.

Covariate	HR	95% CI	p Value
Decade of transplant	0.98	0.49–1.96	0.9
Recipient age (per decade)	0.85	0.51–1.39	0.5
Living donor	0.10	0.01–0.89	0.04
Donor age (per decade)	0.76	0.63–1.40	0.8
Ischaemic time (per 6h)	0.57	0.30–1.10	0.08

Despite small numbers, a living donor transplant was associated with a 90% reduction in death-censored graft loss.

In multivariate analysis for recipient survival, significant factors were decade of transplant, recipient age, recipient primary disease of diabetic nephropathy, duration of RRT pre-transplant, living donor, donor age and ischaemic time (Table 4).

Table 4. Multivariate analysis for recipient survival in all transplants.

Covariate	HR	95% CI	p Value
Decade of transplant	0.60	0.56–0.65	<0.001
Recipient age (per decade)	1.7	1.6–1.8	<0.001
Recipient primary disease diabetic nephropathy	2.8	2.3–3.5	<0.001
RRT pre-transplant (per month)	1.002	1.00–1.004	0.02
Living donor	0.75	0.56–1.00	0.05
Donor age (per decade)	1.07	1.02–1.1	0.03
Ischaemic time (per 6h)	1.1	1.04–1.2	0.002

HLA mismatch at HLA-A, -B and -DR and transplant number were not significant and dropped out of model.

4. Discussion

This study investigated the outcomes of repeated kidney transplantation at our institution and demonstrated excellent graft and recipient outcomes (Figures 1 and 3), despite a significantly more sensitised population and a longer vintage of ESRD. There was also an association between multiple kidney transplants and better HLA match at transplantation ($p < 0.0001$); this is unsurprising, as more highly sensitised patients require better matched kidneys. Our results are in contrast to a recent European multicentre analysis reporting that mortality and graft loss after 3rd+ KTRs were higher as compared to 1st KTRs, despite receiving grafts with more favourable HLA matches [17]. More in detail, Assfalg et al. analysed the outcomes of 1464 patients from 42 centres in the Eurotransplant area who received a third or fourth kidney transplant in the period 1996–2010, confirming a younger age compared to first transplant recipients, a more frequently favourable HLA match, but a higher rate of graft loss, death with functioning graft and primary non-function. Their conclusion was, therefore, to set an upper limit for the number of sequential transplantations in order to consider also the prospect of success of transplantation. In our study, it was confirmed that there is a significant difference in death-censored graft survival by number of transplants, as shown in Figure 1, with a median graft survival of 328 months for 1st KTRs, 209 months for 2nd KTRs and 150 months for 3rd+ KTRs, but the death-censored graft survival remained significantly different in the case of deceased donor transplants (Figure 2a), but not after living donor transplantation (Figure 2b). This suggests that living donor transplantation confers a significant benefit in the context of repeated kidney transplantation and challenges the assumption that repeated transplant recipients as well as any other special group of patients should be a priori denied access to transplantation [18]. Important modifiable factors, such as the quality of the implanted graft or the time at which the operation is performed, could significantly affect the overall outcome and this should be taken into consideration when planning such a complex procedure and before fixing an arbitrary cut off number to waitlist transplant candidates.

In this regard, an extensive patient work up with multidisciplinary input is highly recommended to maximise the chances of successful waitlisting for the candidate, to be followed by a successful repeated kidney transplantation. Further, in our study, in fact, 3rd+ KTRs are overall better matched compared to 1st or 2nd KTRs ($p < 0.001$), reflecting the broad immunological work up. Yet, despite a similar finding to the study from Dabare et al. [19], where patient survival did not differ significantly by transplant number even considering third or fourth KTRs and, therefore, confirming the survival benefit for this population over remaining on dialysis, we disagree with the authors' conclusion. In our present analysis, we observed a significant decline in graft survival only in the case of deceased donor grafts, with a progressive worsening survival curve in parallel with the progressive increase in repeated kidney transplant number (Figure 2a). The conclusion that regardless of the donor type, there is an inferior graft survival for the repeated kidney transplant population is not confirmed instead for grafts retrieved from living donors (Figure 2b). Therefore, the authors' suggestion to use HLA-incompatible living donors and extended criteria deceased donors in the peculiar context of the repeated kidney transplant population is not justifiable from our experience.

Prolonged ischaemic time is significantly detrimental to long-term survival for deceased donor grafts [20], with preservation strategies being key for suboptimal and extended criteria deceased donor organs [12]. Often 3rd and 4th kidney transplants are associated with prolonged ischaemic times due to increasing technical complexity: KTRs of 3rd and 4th transplants may have difficult vasculature that often requires additional surgical time. The deceased donor kidney performs less well in this context, while better-quality living donor kidneys can tolerate the insult. In our centre, where there is a high rate of living donor transplantation, there is for this reason an even higher proportion of organs retrieved from living donors in the case of 3rd+ KTRs (Table 1). To overcome living donor shortage, broad educational campaigns aiming to educate and inform the general population [21] and particularly via social media, have demonstrated an increase in donation rates [22]. With the current organ donor shortage and more patients dying on the waiting list, living donor kidney donation seems, therefore, to satisfy and significantly contribute to expand the donor pool for the general population, and more specifically for those who might not survive a long waiting list time or a major operation, like in the case of the repeated kidney transplantation subgroup. In addition, every living donor transplant that occurs removes one person from the transplant waiting list, shortening the waiting list for a deceased donor transplant, too.

With increasing evidence of how the preservation time and modality significantly impact organs retrieved from marginal donors [10] and with an even increasing debate in how to safely implement the donor pool, without compromising recipient outcomes, until a general consensus on how to best treat and preserve deceased donor grafts [23], an effort to find alternative ways of influencing patient and graft survivals should be canvassed in the ethical attempt to provide the best renal replacement therapy to those who need it.

Another important advantage offered by living donation is that an elective operation allows diligent planning and the presence of additional surgical expertise for complex cases [24]. This might also contribute to better outcomes, independently from the quality of the donor [19], with a standardised elective procedure taking place at an optimal time and that, despite being a major operation, has a minor impact [25] on the recovery of the healthy donor, who usually can plan ahead for time off work, for family care for and for a full recovery.

With deceased donor transplantation, the surgery often takes place out of hours; additionally, emergency procedures usually carry out extra unanticipated risks [26], along with the impossibility to schedule the time and avoid the waitlist consequences and deterioration on the general health status of the candidate, who might even be transplanted after several years, because of the complex immunological status. Inevitably, the elderly and sickest candidates might, therefore, be more susceptible to the vicious cycle of repeated kidney transplantation, becoming not transplantable, with a significant drop out from the list, or a detrimental transplant outcome. In our opinion, this is, therefore, why living donor kidney donation is so fundamental to expand the donor pool: removing successfully a difficult transplant candidate from the transplant waiting list and ensuring that the next person on the list will not have to wait as long for a deceased donor transplant.

The preferred surgical approach in the case of repeated kidney transplantation at our centre is extraperitoneal to avoid ileus and expedite an enhanced recovery [27]. In the case of native polycystic kidney disease, further space for transplantation might become a challenge, and therefore the affected patients are more likely to undergo native nephrectomy before the planned transplant, as they are already vintage patients [28]. In our series, 13 patients (23.6% of the total population) underwent bilateral native nephrectomy.

Differently from native nephrectomy, kidney transplantectomy was rarely performed in the case of a failed graft. The British Transplant Society guidelines [29] suggest limited indications for graft nephrectomy: localised symptoms that are resistant to medical therapy, to create space for re-transplantation, to enable complete withdrawal of immunosuppression and where there is risk of graft rupture or graft malignancy. This caution with regard to graft nephrectomy is partly due to its immunological effect [30], as nephrectomy and the cessation of immunosuppression can precipitate the development of HLA antibodies (DSAs and PRAs), which limits access to re-transplantation. In our series, only four graft nephrectomies were recorded: because of antibody mediated rejection with systemic involvement, because of a bleeding catastrophe after the transplant and to create space for a potential further kidney transplant. The limited number of graft nephrectomy at our institution is in contrast with other centres' experiences, estimated at approximately 40% from a Turkish report [31] and up to 75% in a UK single-centre experience from 2009 [32]. We tend to avoid, as a general principle, an additional operation, unless not strictly required, in consideration of the controversy affecting the immunological recipient status and the likelihood of finding a suitable match, with antibody absorption from the graft itself. [30,32]. As previously stated, in fact the graft nephrectomy would imply the cessation of the immunosuppression, giving rise to antibody production due to the persistence of donor antigen-presenting cells after the transplantectomy. Furthermore, with the evidence that HLA matching plays a fundamental role in the context of repeated kidney transplantation, from the present study and another large registry analysis [17], we think that a synergistic approach to optimise the recipient condition and general immunological status would better satisfy increased complexity at the moment of transplantation in the eventuality that a prolonged surgical time would be required to find a suitable implantation site. Once again, we emphasize the importance of a high-quality graft, like the one retrieved from a living donor, to better resist a prolonged ischaemic insult.

Finally, given the increased morbidity in patients with failed kidney transplants, special attention should be paid to the attainment of cardiovascular and other infective or malignant events [33], the main cause of death in the long term and also in particular for the repeated KTRs. In our centre, we acknowledge this extra care and, notably, recipient survival did not differ between the groups.

5. Limitations

The main limitation of this study is the retrospective data assessment from a single institution, subjected to selection bias by the nature of the study itself, with a change in the immunosuppression and overall management of kidney transplant recipients over time. There is also an immortal bias due to younger age and higher fitness of the recipients of repeated kidney transplantation, possibly leading to comparable patient survival between the subgroups. Nevertheless, the comprehensive assessment from the same institution over a period of more than 50 years shed light on the context of the failing kidney transplant population, for which the best treatment and donor selection remains unclear in terms of long-term outcomes.

6. Conclusions

In conclusion, a living donor kidney has the greatest impact on improving graft and recipient survival in patients with multiple kidney transplants. We recommend early work up of recipients with failing grafts to achieve pre-emptive transplantation and minimise time on dialysis, and early pursuit of a living donor option for these individuals.

In our view, it is fundamental to consider that not only recipients' factors but also donors' characteristics are strongly related to short- and long-term results after kidney transplantation and that the higher the risk represented by the recipient, as in the case of the repeated kidney transplant population, the more likely stress and damage in the immediate and longer follow up will occur, therefore potentially irreversibly compromising the graft.

Living donor kidneys represent an undervalued resource significantly impacting the transplant outcome for higher-risk candidates, where a standard donor is instead more likely to be affected by the recipient status.

Author Contributions: M.I.B.: study conception; writing the original manuscript and revision; data analysis; A.E.C.: study conception; data collection; manuscript revision; J.A.M.: study conception, data collection and analysis; manuscript revision. All authors have read and agreed to the published version of the manuscript.

Abbreviations

Abbr.	Original Word
DSA	Donor-specific antibody
ESRD	End-stage renal disease
KTR	Kidney transplant recipient
PRA	Panel-reactive antibody
RRT	Renal replacement therapy (cumulative time)

References

1. *U.S. Renal Data System, USRDS 2009 Annual Data Report: Atlas of Chronic Kidney Disease and End-Stage Renal Disease in the United States*; National Institutes of Health, National Institute of Diabetes and Digestive and Kidney Diseases: Bethesda, MD, USA, 2009.
2. *U.S. Renal Data System, USRDS 2010 Annual Data Report: Atlas of Chronic Kidney Disease and End-Stage Renal Disease in the United States*; National Institutes of Health, National Institute of Diabetes and Digestive and Kidney Diseases: Bethesda, MD, USA, 2010.
3. Kaplan, B.; Meier-Kriesche, H.U. Death after graft loss: An important late study endpoint in kidney transplantation. *Am. J. Transplant.* **2002**, *2*, 970–974. [CrossRef] [PubMed]
4. Mehrabi, S.; Sohn, S.; Li, D.; Pankratz, J.J.; Therneau, T.; Sauver, J.L.S.; Liu, H.; Palakal, M. Temporal pattern and association discovery of diagnosis codes using deep learning. In Proceedings of the 2015 International Conference on Healthcare Informatics, Richardson, TX, USA, 21–23 October 2015; pp. 408–416.
5. Fernandez Fresnedo, G.; Ruiz, J.C.; Gomez Alamillo, C.; de Francisco, A.L.; Arias, M. Survival after dialysis initiation: A comparison of transplant patients after graft loss versus nontransplant patients. *Transplant. Proc.* **2008**, *40*, 2889–2890. [CrossRef]
6. McCaughan, J.A.; Patterson, C.C.; Maxwell, A.P.; Courtney, A.E. Factors influencing survival after kidney transplant failure. *Transplant. Res.* **2014**, *3*, 18. [CrossRef] [PubMed]
7. Knoll, G.; Muirhead, N.; Trpeski, L.; Zhu, N.; Badovinac, K. Patient survival following renal transplant failure in Canada. *Am. J. Transplant.* **2005**, *5*, 1719–1724. [CrossRef] [PubMed]
8. Coupel, S.; Giral-Classe, M.; Karam, G.; Morcet, J.F.; Dantal, J.; Cantarovich, D.; Blancho, G.; Bignon, J.D.; Daguin, P.; Soulillou, J.P.; et al. Ten-year survival of second kidney transplants: Impact of immunologic factors and renal function at 12 months. *Kidney Int.* **2003**, *64*, 674–680. [CrossRef]

9. Redfield, R.R.; Gupta, M.; Rodriguez, E.; Wood, A.; Abt, P.L.; Levine, M.H. Graft and patient survival outcomes of a third kidney transplant. *Transplantation* **2015**, *99*, 416–423. [CrossRef]
10. Bellini, M.I.; Nozdrin, M.; Yiu, J.; Papalois, V. Machine perfusion for abdominal organ preservation: A systematic review of kidney and liver human grafts. *J. Clin. Med.* **2019**, *8*, 1221. [CrossRef]
11. Perico, N.; Cattaneo, D.; Sayegh, M.H.; Remuzzi, G. Delayed graft function in kidney transplantation. *Lancet* **2004**, *364*, 1814–1827. [CrossRef]
12. Bellini, M.I.; Charalampidis, S.; Herbert, P.E.; Bonatsos, V.; Crane, J.; Muthusamy, A.; Dor, F.; Papalois, V. Cold pulsatile machine perfusion versus static cold storage in kidney transplantation: A single centre experience. *BioMed. Res. Int.* **2019**, *2019*, 7435248. [CrossRef]
13. Redfield, R.R.; Scalea, J.R.; Zens, T.J.; Muth, B.; Kaufman, D.B.; Djamali, A.; Astor, B.C.; Mohamed, M. Predictors and outcomes of delayed graft function after living-donor kidney transplantation. *Transpl. Int.* **2016**, *29*, 81–87. [CrossRef]
14. Lucisano, G.; Brookes, P.; Santos-Nunez, E.; Firmin, N.; Gunby, N.; Hassan, S.; Gueret-Wardle, A.; Herbert, P.; Papalois, V.; Willicombe, M.; et al. Allosensitization after transplant failure: The role of graft nephrectomy and immunosuppression—A retrospective study. *Transpl. Int.* **2019**, *32*, 949–959. [CrossRef]
15. McCaughan, J.A.; Courtney, A.E. Successful kidney transplantation in highly sensitized, ultra-long-term dialysis patients. *Transpl. Int.* **2017**, *30*, 844–846. [CrossRef]
16. Ooms, L.S.; Roodnat, J.I.; Dor, F.J.; Tran, T.C.; Kimenai, H.J.; Ijzermans, J.N.; Terkivatan, T. Kidney retransplantation in the ipsilateral iliac fossa: A surgical challenge. *Am. J. Transplant.* **2015**, *15*, 2947–2954. [CrossRef]
17. Assfalg, V.; Selig, K.; Tolksdorf, J.; van Meel, M.; de Vries, E.; Ramsoebhag, A.M.; Rahmel, A.; Renders, L.; Novotny, A.; Matevossian, E.; et al. Repeated kidney re-transplantation-the Eurotransplant experience: A retrospective multicenter outcome analysis. *Transpl. Int.* **2020**. [CrossRef] [PubMed]
18. Morath, C.; Süsal, C. Three is not enough. *Transpl. Int.* **2020**, *33*, 612–614. [CrossRef] [PubMed]
19. Dabare, D.; Kassimatis, T.; Hodson, J.; Khurram, M.A.; Papadakis, G.; Rompianesi, G.; Shaw, O.; Karydis, N.; Callaghan, C.; Olsburgh, J.; et al. Outcomes in third and fourth kidney transplants based on the type of donor. *Transplantation* **2019**, *103*, 1494–1503. [CrossRef]
20. Aubert, O.; Kamar, N.; Vernerey, D.; Viglietti, D.; Martinez, F.; Duong-Van-Huyen, J.P.; Eladari, D.; Empana, J.P.; Rabant, M.; Verine, J.; et al. Long term outcomes of transplantation using kidneys from expanded criteria donors: Prospective, population based cohort study. *Br. Med. J.* **2015**, *351*, h3557. [CrossRef] [PubMed]
21. Bellini, M.I.; Charalampidis, S.; Stratigos, I.; Dor, F.; Papalois, V. The effect of Donors' demographic characteristics in renal function post-living kidney donation. Analysis of a UK single centre cohort. *J. Clin. Med.* **2019**, *8*, 883. [CrossRef]
22. Bellini, M.I.; Parisotto, C.; Dor, F.J.M.F.; Kessaris, N. Social Media Use Among Transplant Professionals in Europe: A Cross-Sectional Study From the European Society of Organ Transplantation. *Exp. Clin. Transpl.* **2020**, *18*, 169–176. [CrossRef]
23. Bellini, M.I.; D'Andrea, V. Organ preservation: Which temperature for which organ? *J. Int. Med. Res.* **2019**, *47*, 2323–2325. [CrossRef]
24. Chandak, P.; Byrne, N.; Coleman, A.; Karunanithy, N.; Carmichael, J.; Marks, S.D.; Stojanovic, J.; Kessaris, N.; Mamode, N. Patient-specific 3D printing: A novel technique for complex pediatric renal transplantation. *Ann. Surg.* **2019**, *269*, e18–e23. [CrossRef] [PubMed]
25. Bellini, M.; Wilson, R.S.; Veitch, P.; Brown, T.; Courtney, A.; Maxwell, A.P.; D'Andrea, V.; McDaid, J. Hyperamylasemia post living donor nephrectomy does not relate to pain. *Cureus* **2020**, *12*, e8217. [CrossRef] [PubMed]
26. The National Confidential Enquiry into Patient Outcome and Death. National Confidential Enquiry into Perioperative Outcome and Death. Who Operates when 1995/6? Available online: www.ncepod.org.uk/1995_6.html (accessed on 13 October 2019).
27. Mazzucchi, E.; Danilovic, A.; Antonopoulos, I.M.; Piovesan, A.C.; Nahas, W.C.; Lucon, A.M.; Srougi, M. Surgical aspects of third and subsequent renal transplants performed by the extraperitoneal access. *Transplantation* **2006**, *81*, 840–844. [CrossRef]
28. Bellini, M.I.; Charalmpidis, S.; Brookes, P.; Hill, P.; Dor, F.; Papalois, V. Bilateral nephrectomy for adult polycystic kidney disease does not affect the graft function of transplant patients and does not result in sensitisation. *BioMed. Res. Int.* **2019**, *2019*, 7423158. [CrossRef]

29. British Transplantation Society guidelines. Available online: https://bts.org.uk/wp-content/uploads/2016/09/13_BTS_Failing_Graft-1.pdf (accessed on 13 October 2019).
30. Lin, J.; Wang, R.; Xu, Y.; Chen, J. Impact of renal allograft nephrectomy on graft and patient survival following retransplantation: A systematic review and meta-analysis. *Nephrol. Dial. Transplant.* **2018**, *33*, 700–708. [CrossRef] [PubMed]
31. Yagmurdur, M.C.; Emiroğlu, R.; Ayvaz, I.; Sozen, H.; Karakayali, H.; Haberal, M. The effect of graft nephrectomy on long-term graft function and survival in kidney retransplantation. *Transplant. Proc.* **2005**, *37*, 2957–2961. [CrossRef] [PubMed]
32. Ahmad, N.; Ahmed, K.; Mamode, N. Does nephrectomy of failed allograft influence graft survival after re-transplantation? *Nephrol. Dial. Transplant.* **2009**, *24*, 639–642. [CrossRef]
33. McCaughan, J.A.; Courtney, A.E. The clinical course of kidney transplant recipients after 20 years of graft function. *Am. J. Transplant.* **2015**, *15*, 734–740. [CrossRef]

16

Inpatient Burden and Mortality of Goodpasture's Syndrome in the United States: Nationwide Inpatient Sample 2003–2014

Wisit Kaewput [1,*], Charat Thongprayoon [2], Boonphiphop Boonpheng [3], Patompong Ungprasert [4], Tarun Bathini [5], Api Chewcharat [2], Narat Srivali [6], Saraschandra Vallabhajosyula [7] and Wisit Cheungpasitporn [8]

1 Department of Military and Community Medicine, Phramongkutklao College of Medicine, Bangkok 10400, Thailand
2 Division of Nephrology, Department of Medicine, Mayo Clinic, Rochester, MN 55905, USA; charat.thongprayoon@gmail.com (C.T.); api.che@hotmail.com (A.C.)
3 Department of Medicine, David Geffen School of Medicine, University of California, Los Angeles, Los Angeles, CA 90095, USA; boonpipop.b@gmail.com
4 Clinical Epidemiology Unit, Department of Research and Development, Faculty of Medicine, Siriraj Hospital, Mahidol University, Bangkok, 10700, Thailand; p.ungprasert@gmail.com
5 Department of Internal Medicine, University of Arizona, Tucson, AZ 85721, USA; tarunjacobb@gmail.com
6 Department of Internal Medicine, St. Agnes Hospital, Baltimore, MD 21229, USA; nsrivali@gmail.com
7 Department of Cardiovascular Medicine, Mayo Clinic, Rochester, MN 55905, USA; Vallabhajosyula.Saraschandra@mayo.edu
8 Division of Nephrology, Department of Medicine, University of Mississippi Medical Center, Jackson, MS 39216, USA; wcheungpasitporn@gmail.com
* Correspondence: wisitnephro@gmail.com

Abstract: Background: Goodpasture's syndrome is a rare, life-threatening, small vessel vasculitis. Given its rarity, data on its inpatient burden and resource utilization are lacking. We conducted this study aiming to assess inpatient prevalence, mortality, and resource utilization of Goodpasture's syndrome in the United States. **Methods:** The 2003–2014 National Inpatient Sample was used to identify patients with a principal diagnosis of Goodpasture's syndrome. The inpatient prevalence, clinical characteristics, in-hospital treatment, end-organ failure, mortality, length of hospital stay, and hospitalization cost were studied. Multivariable logistic regression was performed to identify independent factors associated with in-hospital mortality. **Results:** A total of 964 patients were admitted in hospital with Goodpasture's syndrome as the principal diagnosis, accounting for an overall inpatient prevalence of Goodpasture's syndrome among hospitalized patients in the United States of 10.3 cases per 1,000,000 admissions. The mean age of patients was 54 ± 21 years, and 47% were female; 52% required renal replacement therapy, whereas 39% received plasmapheresis during hospitalization. Furthermore, 78% had end-organ failure, with renal failure and respiratory failure being the two most common end-organ failures. The in-hospital mortality rate was 7.7 per 100 admissions. The factors associated with increased in-hospital mortality were age older than 70 years, sepsis, the development of respiratory failure, circulatory failure, renal failure, and liver failure, whereas the factors associated with decreased in-hospital mortality were more recent year of hospitalization and the use of therapeutic plasmapheresis. The median length of hospital stay was 10 days. The median hospitalization cost was $75,831. **Conclusion:** The inpatient prevalence of Goodpasture's syndrome in the United States is 10.3 cases per 1,000,000 admissions. Hospitalization of patients with Goodpasture's syndrome was associated with high hospital inpatient utilization and costs.

Keywords: Goodpasture syndrome; anti-GBM disease; epidemiology; hospitalization; outcomes

1. Introduction

Goodpasture's syndrome (GS) is a rare, life-threatening, small vessel vasculitis that is mediated by circulating anti-glomerular basement membrane (anti-GBM) autoantibodies against the NC1 domain of the alpha 3 chain of type IV collagen, targeting capillaries of the kidneys and lungs [1–4]. It is considered as one of the organ-specific autoimmune diseases that typically presents as a rapidly progressive glomerulonephritis (RPGN), accompanied by alveolar hemorrhage with pathology characterized by crescentic glomerulonephritis with classic linear polyclonal immunoglobulin (Ig) G deposits on immunofluorescence staining of the GBM on analysis of kidney biopsy samples [1,2,5–7]. Without prompt diagnosis and treatment, patients with GS can develop organ failure, resulting in significant morbidities and mortality [1–3].

Among European and Asian populations, the incidence of GS is estimated to have a frequency of 0.5 to 1.8 cases per million population per year [1–3,8,9]. A recent study from Ireland reported a nationwide disease incidence of GS of 1.64 per million population per year [10]. While it is well known that patients with GS can have both pulmonary and renal involvement requiring a mechanical ventilator and renal replacement therapy [3,4], data on its inpatient burden and resource utilization are lacking.

Thus, we conducted this study using the 2003–2014 National Inpatient Sample (NIS) database to assess inpatient prevalence, mortality, and resource utilization of GS in the United States.

2. Materials and Methods

2.1. Data Source

The 2003–2014 NIS database was used to conduct this cohort study. The NIS is the publicly available, inpatient, all-payer database in the United States. This database was developed and maintained by the Healthcare Cost and Utilization Project (HCUP) under the sponsorship of the Agency for Healthcare Research and Quality (AHRQ). The dataset contains more than 7 million hospitalizations annually, which were obtained from a 20% stratified sample of over 4000 non-federal acute care hospitals in more than 40 states of the United States. A survey procedure using discharge weights provided by the HCUP-NIS database was used to generate national estimates for 95% of hospitalizations nationwide [11]. This dataset includes codes for principal and secondary diagnosis as well as codes for procedures performed during the hospitalization.

2.2. Study Population

All patients with a principal diagnosis of GS, based on the International Classification of Diseases, Ninth Revision, Clinical Modification (ICD-9 CM) diagnosis code of 446.21 for the hospitalization were included.

2.3. Variables and Outcome of Interest

Patient characteristics included age, sex, race, year of hospitalization, smoking, hemoptysis, and the presence of anti-neutrophil cytoplasmic antibody (ANCA)-associated vasculitis, which consisted of granulomatosis polyangiitis, microscopic polyangiitis, and sepsis. Treatments included respiratory support consisting of invasive mechanical ventilation and non-invasive ventilation, renal replacement therapy, therapeutic plasmapheresis, and blood transfusion. Patient outcomes included organ failure or dysfunction, which consisted of respiratory failure, circulatory failure, renal failure, liver failure, hematologic failure, metabolic failure, and neurologic failure, as well as in-hospital mortality. Resource utilization included length of hospital stay and hospitalization cost.

2.4. Statistical Analysis

Discharge-level weights published by the HCUP were used to estimate the total number of GS patients. Continuous variables were summarized as mean ± standard deviation for normally-distributed data, and median with interquartile range for skewed data. Categorical variables were summarized as count with percentage. The annual inpatient prevalence of GS in hospitalized patients in the United States from 2003 to 2014 was calculated. Independent factors associated with in-hospital mortality were identified using multivariable logistic regression with the forward stepwise selection method. A two-tailed p-value of less than 0.05 was considered statistically significant. All analyses were performed using JMP statistical software (version 10, SAS Institute, Cary, NC).

3. Results

3.1. Patient Characteristics and In-Hospital Treatment

Of 93,377,054 hospital admissions during the study period, 964 patients were admitted to hospital with GS as the principal diagnosis. The mean age of patients was 54 ± 21 years; 47% were female, 65% were Caucasian, and 9% had a co-diagnosis of ANCA-associated vasculitis. Of patients with GS, 19% needed invasive mechanical ventilation, 5% needed non-invasive ventilation support, and 52% required renal replacement therapy. Plasmapheresis was performed in 39% of patients. Table 1 shows clinical characteristics and in-hospital treatment of GS patients in this cohort.

Table 1. Clinical characteristics, treatments, outcomes, and resource utilization of Goodpasture's syndrome patients.

	All (*N* = 964)
Clinical characteristics	
Age (years)	54 ± 21
≤39	260 (27)
40–49	91 (9)
50–59	141 (15)
60–69	199 (21)
≥70	273 (28)
Male sex	456 (47)
Caucasian	622 (65)
Year of hospitalization	
2003–2006	281 (29)
2007–2010	357 (37)
2011–2014	326 (34)
Smoking	95 (10)
Hemoptysis	267 (28)
ANCA vasculitis	84 (9)
Granulomatosis with polyangiitis	54 (6)
Microscopic polyangiitis	30 (3)
Sepsis	62 (6)

Table 1. *Cont.*

	All (*N* = 964)
Treatments	
Respiratory support	216 (23)
Invasive mechanical ventilation	181 (19)
Non-invasive ventilation	49 (5)
Renal replacement therapy	499 (52)
Hemodialysis	494 (51)
Peritoneal dialysis	10 (1)
Therapeutic plasmapheresis	376 (39)
Blood transfusion	391 (41)
Outcomes	
Number of organ failure	
0	230 (24)
1	369 (38)
2	242 (25)
≥3	123 (13)
Respiratory failure	283 (29)
Circulatory failure/shock	53 (6)
Renal failure	597 (62)
Liver failure	10 (1)
Hematologic failure	127 (13)
Metabolic failure	159 (17)
Neurological failure	50 (5)
In-hospital death	74 (8)
Resource utilization	
Length of stay (days), median (IQR)	10 (5–18)
<5	215 (22)
5–9	229 (24)
10–14	188 (20)
≥15	332 (34)
Hospitalization cost ($), median (IQR)	75,831.5 (31,687.3–163,201.0)

3.2. Inpatient Prevalence of GS

Table 2 shows the annual distribution and inpatient prevalence of GS in hospitalized patients. The inpatient prevalence of GS ranged from 6.7 to 12.1 per 1,000,000 admissions between the years 2003 and 2014 in the United States with an overall inpatient prevalence of GS over 12 years of 10.3 cases per 1,000,000 admissions (Figure 1).

Table 2. The distribution and inpatient prevalence of Goodpasture's syndrome from 2003 to 2014.

Year	Total Number of Goodpasture's Syndrome Patients	Total Number of Admissions	Inpatient Prevalence (per 1,000,000 Admissions)
2003	72	7,977,728	9.0
2004	54	8,004,571	6.7
2005	66	7,995,048	8.3
2006	89	8,074,825	11.0
2007	97	8,043,415	12.1
2008	84	8,158,381	10.3
2009	85	7,810,762	10.9
2010	91	7,800,441	11.7
2011	92	8,023,590	11.5
2012	75	7,296,968	10.3
2013	86	7,119,563	12.1
2014	73	7,071,762	10.3
Total	964	93,377,054	10.3

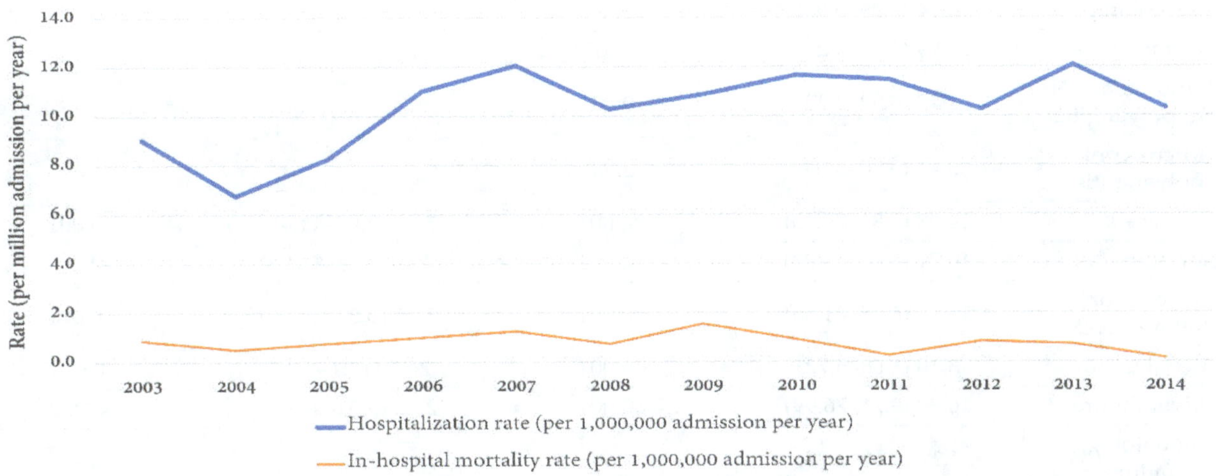

Figure 1. Rate of hospital admission and in-hospital mortality rate for Goodpasture's syndrome stratified by year.

3.3. *Organ Failure and In-Hospital Mortality*

Seventy-six percent of patients had at least one end-organ failure. Renal failure was the most common end-organ failure (62%), followed by respiratory failure (29%), metabolic failure (17%), hematologic failure (13%), circulatory failure (6%), neurological failure (5%), and liver failure (1%) (Table 1). The number of end-organ failures was significantly associated with increased in-hospital mortality with an adjusted OR of 2.19 (95% CI 0.45–10.58) for one end-organ failure, 7.60 (95% CI 1.67–34.56) for two end-organ failures, and 19.86 (95% CI 4.10–96.19) for ≥3 end-organ failures.

Of 964 patients with GS, 74 (8%) died in the hospital. In the multivariable logistic regression, age older than 70 years (OR 3.62; 95% CI 1.52–8.61 compared to age ≤ 39 years), sepsis (OR 5.38; 95% CI 2.53–11.45), respiratory failure (OR 7.41; 95% CI 3.85–14.26), circulatory failure (OR 7.85; 95% CI 3.37–18.26), renal failure (OR 2.55; 95% CI 1.21–5.37), and liver failure (OR 32.32; 95% CI 3.51–297.19) were associated with increased in-hospital mortality. In contrast, more recent year of hospitalization (OR 0.23; 95% CI 0.10–0.55 for year 2011–2014 compared to year 2003–2006) and the use of therapeutic plasmapheresis (OR 0.43; 95% CI 0.22–0.84) were associated with decreased in-hospital mortality (Table 3).

Table 3. Univariable and multivariable analysis assessing factors associated with in-hospital mortality in Goodpasture's syndrome patients.

Characteristics	Univariable Analysis		Multivariable Analysis	
	Crude OR (95% CI)	*P*-Value	Adjusted OR (95% CI)	*P*-Value
Age (years)				
≤39	1 (ref)		1 (ref)	
40–49	0.85 (0.23–3.17)	0.81	0.76 (0.17–3.35)	0.71
50–59	0.54 (0.15–2.01)	0.36	0.58 (0.13–2.52)	0.47
60–69	2.34 (1.05–5.22)	0.04	1.68 (0.62–4.54)	0.31
≥70	4.42 (2.16–9.02)	<0.001	3.62 (1.52–8.61)	<0.01
Male	1.34 (0.83–2.16)	0.23		
Caucasian	1.34 (0.83–2.17)	0.23		
Year of admission				
2003–2006	1 (ref)		1 (ref)	
2007–2010	1.11 (0.65–1.91)	0.70	0.92 (0.47–1.79)	0.80
2011–2014	0.46 (0.23–0.90)	0.02	0.23 (0.10–0.55)	0.001
Smoking	0.24 (0.06–0.99)	0.04		
Hemoptysis	1.99 (1.22–3.23)	<0.01		
Granulomatosis with polyangiitis	1.42 (0.59–3.43)	0.43		
Microscopic polyangiitis	0.41 (0.06–3.03)	0.38		
Sepsis	14.03 (7.85–25.10)	<0.001	5.38 (2.53–11.45)	<0.001
Respiratory failure	10.71 (6.04–19.02)	<0.001	7.41 (3.85–14.26)	<0.001
Circulatory failure/shock	11.72 (6.35–21.66)	<0.001	7.85 (3.37–18.26)	<0.001
Renal failure	3.10 (1.68–5.72)	<0.001	2.55 (1.21–5.37)	0.01
Liver failure	16.90 (3.71–76.99)	<0.001	32.32 (3.51–297.19)	<0.01
Hematologic failure	1.17 (0.60–2.28)	0.66		
Metabolic failure	1.32 (0.73–2.39)	0.36		
Neurological failure	3.32 (1.59–6.95)	0.001		
Invasive mechanical ventilation	11.26 (6.72–18.86)	<0.001		
Non-invasive ventilation	1.74 (0.71–4.23)	0.22		
Dialysis	1.40 (0.87–2.27)	0.17		
Therapeutic plasmapheresis	0.89 (0.54–1.46)	0.64	0.43 (0.22–0.84)	0.01
Blood transfusion	0.83 (0.51–1.36)	0.46		

3.4. Length of Hospital Stay and Hospitalization cost

The median length of hospital stay was 10 (IQR 5–18) days. The median hospitalization cost was $75,831 (IQR 31,687–163,201) (Table 1).

4. Discussion

To the best of our knowledge, our study is the first to evaluate inpatient prevalence, mortality, and resource utilization of GS in the United States. We demonstrated overall inpatient prevalence of GS among hospitalized patients in the United States of 10.3 cases per 1,000,000 admissions. The in-hospital mortality rate was 8%. The factors associated with increased in-hospital mortality were age older than 70 years, sepsis, the development of respiratory failure, circulatory failure, renal failure, and liver failure, whereas the factors associated with decreased in-hospital mortality were more recent year of hospitalization and the use of therapeutic plasmapheresis.

GS is often described to have an incidence of GS of 0.5 to 1.8 cases per million population per year in European and Asian populations, primarily based on single-center biopsy or serology-based series [1–3,8,9,12]. A recent nationwide study from Ireland identified all GS cases over a decade via reference immunology laboratories and a nationwide pathology database over an 11-year period, which reported a disease rate of 1.64 per million population per year [10]. In this study, we utilized the United States inpatient hospitalization data from the NIS database and demonstrated inpatient prevalence of GS among hospitalized patients in the United States of 10.3 cases per 1,000,000 admissions. Although hospitalization for GS is infrequent, we found that hospitalized patients with GS commonly had high rates of end-organ failure, including renal failure (62%) and respiratory failure (29%). While 19% of hospitalization for GS required invasive mechanical ventilation, 52% required renal replacement therapy. The median hospitalization cost for GS was as high as $75,831.

Our findings confirmed a bimodal age distribution of GS, with younger patients <39 years having a male predominance, whereas older patients >60 years old were more frequently female [2,12]. We also observed an increase in the inpatient prevalence of GS from 2004 to 2007, which subsequently stabilized (Figure 1). Although the reason remains unclear, we speculated that this is because of the increasing awareness and widespread availability of diagnostic tests around that time [4,13]. Previous studies have suggested that, in addition to genetic factors, environmental factors can also trigger the development of GS, such as cigarette smoking, inhaled hydrocarbons, or potential infectious triggers damaging the alveolar basement membrane and exposing type IV collagen epitopes [3,4,6,14–18]. Future studies are needed to assess if these factors play an important role in the trends of inpatient prevalence of GS in the United States.

Our study demonstrated that 52% of hospitalization for GS required dialysis, which was consistent with previous literature indicating that approximately half of patients with GS require hemodialysis [19]. There are limited data on how frequently artificial ventilation is required. Small series estimated that this occurred in 11% of patients with GS [20–23]. Our study demonstrated that 19% of hospitalizations for GS needed invasive mechanical ventilation, and 5% needed non-invasive ventilation support. GS is life-threatening, with irreversible kidney damage and respiratory failure. Aggressive therapy with modern treatment protocols with antibody removal by plasmapheresis, use of corticosteroids, and immunosuppressive agents, particularly cyclophosphamide, has dramatically improved patient outcomes compared to the past [4,18,24–26]. The 5-year survival rate exceeds 80% and fewer than 30% of patients require long-term dialysis [2]. In our study, we demonstrated that in-hospital mortality rate of GS in the United States between the years 2003 and 2014 was 8%. Although the data on medication were limited in the database, we found that recent year of hospitalization and the use of therapeutic plasmapheresis were associated with decreased in-hospital mortality among patients with GS. While the underlying explanations of decreased in-hospital mortality among patients with GS in the recent years of hospitalization remain unclear and require further investigations, this finding may potentially represent an improvement in patient care of GS in recent years of hospitalization.

There are several limitations of this study. Firstly, although the utilization of the NIS database allowed us to evaluate U.S. inpatient prevalence and burden of patients with GS, possible inaccuracies in ICD-9 CM coding may have confounded the results. Secondly, given the administrative nature of the dataset, the data on medication such as immunosuppression were limited in this study. Consequently, we could not assess the potential effects of immunosuppression, such as cyclophosphamide treatment on hospital outcomes of patients with GS. Thirdly, this was an analysis of an inpatient database in the United States. Sixty-five percent of patient populations with GS in NIS database were Caucasian, and this limits generalizability to the patient population in other countries. Fourthly, kidney biopsy, and laboratory data were lacking in the database. Previous studies have suggested that no patient with 100% glomerular crescents and dialysis dependence at presentation recovered kidney function, and so current guidelines do not recommend treatment in these cases [27,28]. Furthermore, studies have also demonstrated that those patients with higher serum creatinine (5.7 mg/dL or higher) and reduced proportion of normal glomeruli on kidney biopsy have poor renal outcomes [2,13]. Therefore, future studies are needed to assess the impacts of kidney biopsy findings on the treatment and outcomes during hospitalizations for GS.

5. Conclusions

In summary, we demonstrate overall inpatient prevalence among patients with GS between the years 2003 and 2014 in the United States, with 10.3 cases per 1,000,000 admissions. Although the in-hospital mortality rate was only 8%, hospitalization of patients with GS was associated with high hospital inpatient utilization and costs.

Author Contributions: Conceptualization, W.K., C.T., P.U., T.B., A.C., N.S., S.V., and W.C.; Data curation, WK and BB; Formal analysis, W.K.; Investigation, W.K., C.T., and W.C.; Methodology, W.K., C.T., S.V., and W.C.; Project administration, B.B., P.U., T.B., A.C., and N.S.; Resources, B.B.; Software, W.K.; Supervision, W.C.; Validation, W.K. and W.C.; Visualization, C.T. and T.B.; Writing—original draft, W.K.; Writing—review and editing, W.K., C.T., B.B., P.U., A.C., N.S., S.V., and W.C. All authors have read and agreed to the published version of the manuscript.

References

1. Gulati, K.; McAdoo, S.P. Anti-Glomerular Basement Membrane Disease. *Rheum. Dis. Clin. North. Am.* **2018**, *44*, 651–673. [CrossRef]
2. Greco, A.; Rizzo, M.I.; De Virgilio, A.; Gallo, A.; Fusconi, M.; Pagliuca, G.; Martellucci, S.; Turchetta, R.; Longo, L.; De Vincentiis, M. Goodpasture's syndrome: A clinical update. *Autoimmun. Rev.* **2015**, *14*, 246–253. [CrossRef] [PubMed]
3. McAdoo, S.P.; Pusey, C.D. Anti-Glomerular Basement Membrane Disease. *Clin. J. Am. Soc. Nephrol.* **2017**, *12*, 1162–1172. [CrossRef] [PubMed]
4. Henderson, S.R.; Salama, A.D. Diagnostic and management challenges in Goodpasture's (anti-glomerular basement membrane) disease. *Nephrol. Dial. Transplant.* **2018**, *33*, 196–202. [CrossRef] [PubMed]
5. Alchi, B.; Griffiths, M.; Sivalingam, M.; Jayne, D.; Farrington, K. Predictors of renal and patient outcomes in anti-GBM disease: Clinicopathologic analysis of a two-centre cohort. *Nephrol. Dial. Transplant.* **2015**, *30*, 814–821. [CrossRef]
6. Angioi, A.; Cheungpasitporn, W.; Sethi, S.; De Vriese, A.S.; Lepori, N.; Schwab, T.R.; Fervenza, F.C. Familial antiglomerular basement membrane disease in zero human leukocyte antigen mismatch siblings. *Clin. Nephrol.* **2017**, *88*, 277–283. [CrossRef]
7. Cheungpasitporn, W.; Zacharek, C.C.; Fervenza, F.C.; Cornell, L.D.; Sethi, S.; Herrera Hernandez, L.P.; Nasr, S.H.; Alexander, M.P. Rapidly progressive glomerulonephritis due to coexistent anti-glomerular basement membrane disease and fibrillary glomerulonephritis. *Clin. Kidney J.* **2016**, *9*, 97–101. [CrossRef]
8. Tang, W.; McDonald, S.P.; Hawley, C.M.; Badve, S.V.; Boudville, N.C.; Brown, F.G.; Clayton, P.A.; Campbell, S.B.; Zoysa, J.R.; Johnson, D.W. Anti-glomerular basement membrane antibody disease is an uncommon cause of end-stage renal disease. *Kidney Int.* **2013**, *83*, 503–510. [CrossRef]
9. Kluth, D.C.; Rees, A.J. Anti-Glomerular Basement Membrane Disease. *J. Am. Soc. Nephrol.* **1999**, *10*, 2446–2453.
10. Canney, M.; O'Hara, P.V.; McEvoy, C.M.; Medani, S.; Connaughton, D.M.; Abdalla, A.A.; Doyle, R.; Stack, A.G.; O'Seaghdha, C.M.; Clarkson, M.R.; et al. Spatial and Temporal Clustering of Anti-Glomerular Basement Membrane Disease. *Clin. J. Am. Soc. Nephrol.* **2016**, *11*, 1392–1399. [CrossRef]

11. Introduction to the HCUP Nationwide Inpatient Sample (NIS) 2009. Available online: http://www.hcup-us.ahrq.gov/db/nation/nis/NIS_2009_INTRODUCTION.pdf (accessed on 1 February 2020).
12. Savage, C.O.; Pusey, C.D.; Bowman, C.; Rees, A.J.; Lockwood, C.M. Antiglomerular basement membrane antibody mediated disease in the British Isles 1980-4. *Br. Med. J. (Clin. Res. Ed.).* **1986**, *292*, 301–304. [CrossRef]
13. Moroni, G.; Ponticelli, C. Rapidly progressive crescentic glomerulonephritis: Early treatment is a must. *Autoimmun. Rev.* **2014**, *13*, 723–729. [CrossRef]
14. Donaghy, M.; Rees, A.J. CIGARETTE SMOKING AND LUNG HAEMORRHAGE IN GLOMERULONEPHRITIS CAUSED BY AUTOANTIBODIES TO GLOMERULAR BASEMENT MEMBRANE. *Lancet.* **1983**, *2*, 1390–1393. [CrossRef]
15. Huart, A.; Josse, A.G.; Chauveau, D.; Korach, J.M.; Heshmati, F.; Bauvin, E.; Cointaul, O.; Kamar, N.; Ribes, D.; Pourrat, J.; et al. Outcomes of patients with Goodpasture syndrome: A nationwide cohort-based study from the French Society of Hemapheresis. *J. Autoimmun.* **2016**, *73*, 24–29. [CrossRef]
16. Taylor, D.M.; Yehia, M.; Simpson, I.J.; Thein, H.; Chang, Y.; De Zoysa, J.R. Anti-glomerular basement membrane disease in Auckland. *Int. Med. J.* **2012**, *42*, 672–676. [CrossRef]
17. Srivastava, A.; Rao, G.K.; Segal, P.E.; Shah, M.; Geetha, D. Characteristics and outcome of crescentic glomerulonephritis in patients with both antineutrophil cytoplasmic antibody and anti-glomerular basement membrane antibody. *Clin. Rheumatol.* **2013**, *32*, 1317–1322. [CrossRef]
18. Pusey, C.D. Anti-glomerular basement membrane disease. *Kidney Int.* **2003**, *64*, 1535–1550. [CrossRef]
19. Levy, J.B.; Turner, A.N.; Rees, A.J.; Pusey, C.D. Long-Term Outcome of Anti-Glomerular Basement Membrane Antibody Disease Treated with Plasma Exchange and Immunosuppression. *Ann. Intern. Med.* **2001**, *134*, 1033–1042. [CrossRef]
20. Lazor, R.; Bigay-Game, L.; Cottin, V.; Cadranel, J.; Decaux, O.; Fellrath, J.M.; Cordier, J.F. Alveolar Hemorrhage in Anti-Basement Membrane Antibody Disease: A Series of 28 cases. *Medicine.* **2007**, *86*, 181–193. [CrossRef]
21. Herbert, D.G.; Buscher, H.; Nair, P. Prolonged venovenous extracorporeal membrane oxygenation without anticoagulation: A case of Goodpasture syndrome-related pulmonary haemorrhage. *Crit. Care Resusc.* **2014**, *16*, 69–72.
22. Balke, L.; Both, M.; Arlt, A.; Rosenberg, M.; Bewig, B. Severe Adult Respiratory Distress Syndrome from Goodpasture syndrome. Survival Using Extracorporeal Membrane Oxygenation. *Am. J. Respir. Crit. Care Med.* **2015**, *191*, 228–229. [CrossRef]
23. Legras, A.; Mordant, P.; Brechot, N.; Bel, A.; Boussaud, V.; Guillemain, R.; Cholley, B.; Gibault, L.; Le Pimpec-Barthes, F.; Combes, A. Prolonged extracorporeal membrane oxygenation and lung transplantation for isolated pulmonary anti-GBM (Goodpasture) disease. *Intensive Care Med.* **2015**, *41*, 1866–1868. [CrossRef]
24. Shah, M.K.; Hugghins, S.Y. Characteristics and outcomes of patients with Goodpasture's syndrome. *South. Med. J.* **2002**, *95*, 1411–1418. [CrossRef]
25. Johnson, J.P.; Moore, J., Jr.; Austin, H.A., 3rd; Balow, J.E.; Antonovych, T.T.; Wilson, C.B. Therapy of anti-glomerular basement membrane antibody disease: Analysis of prognostic significance of clinical, pathologic and treatment factors. *Medicine.* **1985**, *64*, 219–227. [CrossRef]
26. Cui, Z.; Zhao, J.; Jia, X.Y.; Zhu, S.N.; Jin, Q.Z.; Cheng, X.Y.; Zhao, M.H. Anti-Glomerular Basement Membrane Disease: Outcomes of Different Therapeutic Regimens in a Large Single-Center Chinese Cohort Study. *Medicine.* **2011**, *90*, 303–311. [CrossRef]
27. Booth, A.; Harper, L.; Hammad, T.; Bacon, P.; Griffith, M.; Levy, J.; Savage, C.; Pusey, C.; Jayne, D. Prospective Study of TNFα Blockade with Infliximab in Anti-Neutrophil Cytoplasmic Antibody-Associated Systemic Vasculitis. *J. Am. Soc. Nephrol.* **2004**, *15*, 717–721. [CrossRef]
28. Van Daalen, E.E.; Jennette, J.C.; McAdoo, S.P.; Pusey, C.D.; Alba, M.A.; Poulton, C.J.; Wolterbeek, R.; Nguyen, T.Q.; Goldschmeding, R.; Alchi, B.; et al. Predicting Outcome in Patients with Anti-GBM Glomerulonephritis. *Clin. J. Am. Soc. Nephrol.* **2018**, *13*, 63–72. [CrossRef]

Permissions

All chapters in this book were first published by MDPI; hereby published with permission under the Creative Commons Attribution License or equivalent. Every chapter published in this book has been scrutinized by our experts. Their significance has been extensively debated. The topics covered herein carry significant findings which will fuel the growth of the discipline. They may even be implemented as practical applications or may be referred to as a beginning point for another development.

The contributors of this book come from diverse backgrounds, making this book a truly international effort. This book will bring forth new frontiers with its revolutionizing research information and detailed analysis of the nascent developments around the world.

We would like to thank all the contributing authors for lending their expertise to make the book truly unique. They have played a crucial role in the development of this book. Without their invaluable contributions this book wouldn't have been possible. They have made vital efforts to compile up to date information on the varied aspects of this subject to make this book a valuable addition to the collection of many professionals and students.

This book was conceptualized with the vision of imparting up-to-date information and advanced data in this field. To ensure the same, a matchless editorial board was set up. Every individual on the board went through rigorous rounds of assessment to prove their worth. After which they invested a large part of their time researching and compiling the most relevant data for our readers.

The editorial board has been involved in producing this book since its inception. They have spent rigorous hours researching and exploring the diverse topics which have resulted in the successful publishing of this book. They have passed on their knowledge of decades through this book. To expedite this challenging task, the publisher supported the team at every step. A small team of assistant editors was also appointed to further simplify the editing procedure and attain best results for the readers.

Apart from the editorial board, the designing team has also invested a significant amount of their time in understanding the subject and creating the most relevant covers. They scrutinized every image to scout for the most suitable representation of the subject and create an appropriate cover for the book.

The publishing team has been an ardent support to the editorial, designing and production team. Their endless efforts to recruit the best for this project, has resulted in the accomplishment of this book. They are a veteran in the field of academics and their pool of knowledge is as vast as their experience in printing. Their expertise and guidance has proved useful at every step. Their uncompromising quality standards have made this book an exceptional effort. Their encouragement from time to time has been an inspiration for everyone.

The publisher and the editorial board hope that this book will prove to be a valuable piece of knowledge for researchers, students, practitioners and scholars across the globe.

List of Contributors

Philipp Gauckler, Gert Mayer and Andreas Kronbichler
Department of Internal Medicine IV (Nephrology and Hypertension), Medical University Innsbruck, 6020 Innsbruck, Austria

Jae Il Shin
Department of Pediatrics, Yonsei University College of Medicine, Seoul 03722, Korea
Department of Pediatric Nephrology, Severance Children's Hospital, Seoul 03722, Korea
Institute of Kidney Disease Research, Yonsei University College of Medicine, Seoul 03722, Korea
Division of Cardiology, Emory University School of Medicine, Atlanta, GA 30322, USA

Shadi Katou, M. Haluk Morgul, Thomas Vogel, Benjamin Struecker, Jens G. Brockmann, Andreas Pascher and Volker Schmitz
Department of General, Visceral and Transplantation Surgery, Universitätsklinikum Münster, 48189 Münter, Germany

Brigitta Globke, Anja Reutzel-Selke and Marion Marksteiner
Charité – Universitätsmedizin Berlin, corporate member of Freie Universität Berlin, Humboldt-Universität zu Berlin, and Berlin Institute of Health, Department of Surgery CCM | CVK, 10117 Berlin, Germany

Natalie Maureen Otto
Department of Nephrology and Internal Intensive Care Medicine, Charité Universitätsmedizin Berlin, Campus Virchow Klinikum, 10117 Berlin, Germany

Charat Thongprayoon and Api Chewcharat
Division of Nephrology and Hypertension, Mayo Clinic, Rochester, MN 55905, USA

Javier A. Neyra
Division of Nephrology, Bone and Mineral Metabolism, Department of Internal Medicine, University of Kentucky, Lexington, KY 40506, USA
Charles and Jane Pak Center for Mineral Metabolism and Clinical Research, Dallas, TX 75390, USA
Division of Nephrology, Department of Internal Medicine, University of Texas Southwestern Medical Center, Dallas, TX 75390, USA

Juan Medaura, Paul W. Davis, Sohail Abdul Salim and Wisit Cheungpasitporn
Division of Nephrology, Department of Medicine, University of Mississippi Medical Center, Jackson, MS 39216, USA

Napat Leeaphorn
Renal Transplant Program, University of Missouri-Kansas City School of Medicine/Saint Luke's Health System, Kansas City, MO 64110, USA

Wisit Kaewput
Department of Military and Community Medicine, Phramongkutklao College of Medicine, Bangkok 10400, Thailand

Narothama Reddy Aeddula
Division of Nephrology, Department of Medicine, Deaconess Health System, Evansville, IN 47710, USA

Saraschandra Vallabhajosyula
Department of Cardiovascular Medicine, Mayo Clinic, Rochester, MN 55905, USA

Michael A. Mao
Division of Nephrology and Hypertension, Mayo Clinic, Jacksonville, FL 32224, USA

Rianne M. Douwes, António W. Gomes-Neto, Joëlle C. Schutten, Else van den Berg, Martin H. de Borst, Stefan P. Berger, Gerjan Navis, Stephan J. L. Bakker, Tim J. Knobbe, Daan Kremer, Michele F. Eisenga and Marco van Londen
Department of Internal Medicine, Division of Nephrology, University Medical Center Groningen, University of Groningen, 9700 RB Groningen, The Netherlands

Daan J. Touw
Department of Clinical Pharmacy and Pharmacology, University Medical Center Groningen, University of Groningen, 9700 RB Groningen, The Netherlands

Eelko Hak
Unit PharmacoTherapy, -Epidemiology and -Economics, Groningen Research Institute of Pharmacy, University of Groningen, 9713 AV Groningen, The Netherlands

Hans Blokzijl
Department of Gastroenterology and Hepatology, University Medical Center Groningen, University of Groningen, 9700 RB Groningen, The Netherlands

Gerold Thölking
Department of Internal Medicine and Nephrology, University Hospital of Münster Marienhospital Steinfurt, 48565 Steinfurt, Germany
Department of Medicine D, Division of General Internal Medicine, Nephrology and Rheumatology, University Hospital of Münster, 48149 Münster, Germany

Nils Hendrik Gillhaus, Katharina Schütte-Nütgen, Hermann Pavenstädt, Barbara Suwelack and Stefan Reuter
Department of Medicine D, Division of General Internal Medicine, Nephrology and Rheumatology, University Hospital of Münster, 48149 Münster, Germany

Raphael Koch
Institute of Biostatistics and Clinical Research, University of Münster, 48149 Münster, Germany

Gertrude J Nieuwenhuijs-Moeke
Department of Anesthesiology, University of Groningen, University Medical Centre Groningen, Hanzeplein 1, 9713 GZ, Groningen, The Netherlands

Tobias M Huijink, Robert A Pol and Mostafa El Moumni
Department of Surgery, University of Groningen, University Medical Centre Groningen, Hanzeplein 1, 9713 GZ, Groningen, The Netherlands

Johannes GM Burgerhof
Department of Epidemiology, University of Groningen, University Medical Centre Groningen, Hanzeplein 1, 9713 GZ, Groningen, The Netherlands

Michel MRF Struys
Department of Anesthesiology, University of Groningen, University Medical Centre Groningen, Hanzeplein 1, 9713 GZ, Groningen, The Netherlands
Department of Anesthesiology and Peri-operative Medicine, Ghent University, Corneel Heymanslaan 10, 9000 Gent, Belgium

Stefan P Berger
Department of Nephrology, University of Groningen, University Medical Centre Groningen, Groningen, The Netherlands

Panupong Hansrivijit
Department of Internal Medicine, University of Pittsburgh Medical Center Pinnacle, Harrisburg, PA 17105, USA

Camilo G. Sotomayor, Charlotte A. te Velde-Keyzer, Martin H. de Borst, Gerjan J. Navis and Stephan J.L. Bakker
Department of Internal Medicine, University Medical Center Groningen, University of Groningen, 9700 RB Groningen, The Netherlands

Kinga Musiał, Monika Augustynowicz and Danuta Zwolińska
Department of Pediatric Nephrology, Wrocław Medical University, 50-556 Wrocław, Poland

Izabella Miśkiewicz-Migoń, Krzysztof Kałwak and Marek Ussowicz
Department of Bone Marrow Transplantation, Oncology and Pediatric Hematology, Wrocław Medical University, 50-556 Wrocław, Poland

Pippa K. Bailey and Fergus J. Caskey
Population Health Sciences, Bristol Medical School, University of Bristol, Bristol BS8 2PS, UK
Southmead Hospital, North Bristol NHS Trust, Bristol BS10 5NB, UK

Stephanie MacNeill and Yoav Ben-Shlomo
Population Health Sciences, Bristol Medical School, University of Bristol, Bristol BS8 2PS, UK

Charles Tomson
The Newcastle upon Tyne Hospitals NHS Foundation Trust, Newcastle upon Tyne NE7 7DN, UK

Frank J. M. F. Dor
Imperial College Healthcare NHS Trust, London W12 0HS, UK

Tara K. Sigdel, Andrew W. Schroeder, Joshua Y. C. Yang, Reuben D. Sarwal, Juliane M. Liberto and Minnie M. Sarwal
Division of Transplant Surgery, Department of Surgery, University of California San Francisco, San Francisco, CA 94143, USA

Wisit Cheungpasitporn, Pradeep K Vaitla and Sohail Abdul Salim
Division of Nephrology, Department of Medicine, University of Mississippi Medical Center, Jackson, MS 39216, USA

Felicitas L. Koller
Department of Transplant and Hepatobiliary Surgery, University of Mississippi Medical Center, Jackson, MS 39216, USA

Michael A Mao
Division of Nephrology, Division of Nephrology and Hypertension, Mayo Clinic, Jacksonville, FL 32224, USA

Tarun Bathini
Department of Internal Medicine, University of Arizona, Tucson, AZ 85721, USA

Sreelatha Katari, Lee S Cummings, Eddie Island, Jameson Forster and Napat Leeaphorn
Renal Transplant Program, School of Medicine/Saint Luke's Health System, University of Missouri-Kansas City, Kansas City, MO 64110, USA

J. Casper Swarte
Department of Internal Medicine, Division of Nephrology, University Medical Center Groningen, University of Groningen, 9700 RB Groningen, The Netherlands
Department of Gastroenterology and Hepatology, University Medical Center Groningen, University of Groningen, 9700 RB Groningen, The Netherlands

Frans T. M. Peters and Hans Blokzijl
Department of Gastroenterology and Hepatology, University Medical Center Groningen, University of Groningen, 9700 RB Groningen, The Netherlands

Ilja M. Nolte
Department of Epidemiology, University Medical Center Groningen, University of Groningen, 9700 RB Groningen, The Netherlands

Wouter H. Hendriks
Department of Animal Sciences, Wageningen University & Research centre, 6708 PB Wageningen, The Netherlands

Hermie J. M. Harmsen
Department of Medical Microbiology, University Medical Center Groningen, University of Groningen, 9700RB Groningen, The Netherlands

Danwen Yang and Francesca Cardarelli
Division of Nephrology, Beth Israel Deaconess Medical Center and Harvard Medical School, Boston, MA 02215, USA

Natanong Thamcharoen
Section of Palliative Care, Division of General Medicine and Division of Nephrology, Beth Israel Deaconess Medical Center and Harvard Medical School, Boston, MA 02215, USA

Aureliusz Kolonko, Joanna Musialik, Magdalena Bartmańska, Natalia Słabiak- Błaż, Agata Kujawa-Szewieczek, Piotr Kuczera, Katarzyna Kwiecień-Furmańczuk and Andrzej Więcek
Department of Nephrology, Transplantation and Internal Medicine, Medical University of Silesia, Francuska 20/24, 40-027 Katowice, Poland

Jerzy Chudek
Department of Internal Medicine and Oncological Chemotherapy, Medical University of Silesia, Reymonta 8, 40-035 Katowice, Poland

Maria Irene Bellini, Aisling E Courtney and Jennifer A McCaughan
Regional Nephrology and Transplant Unit, Belfast City Hospital, 51 Lisburn Road, Belfast BT9 7AB, UK

Wisit Kaewput
Department of Military and Community Medicine, Phramongkutklao College of Medicine, Bangkok 10400, Thailand

Boonphiphop Boonpheng
Department of Medicine, David Geffen School of Medicine, University of California, Los Angeles, Los Angeles, CA 90095, USA

Patompong Ungprasert
Clinical Epidemiology Unit, Department of Research and Development, Faculty of Medicine, Siriraj Hospital, Mahidol University, Bangkok, 10700, Thailand

Narat Srivali
Department of Internal Medicine, St. Agnes Hospital, Baltimore, MD 21229, USA

Wisit Cheungpasitporn
Division of Nephrology, Department of Medicine, University of Mississippi Medical Center, Jackson, MS 39216, USA

Index

www.ingramcontent.com/pod-product-compliance
Lightning Source LLC
LaVergne TN
LVHW060542210926
848485LV00005B/1241
9781639277094